Advances in the Diagnosis of Oral and Maxillofacial Disease

Advances in the Diagnosis of Oral and Maxillofacial Disease

Guest Editor

Luis Eduardo Almeida

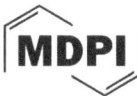

Basel • Beijing • Wuhan • Barcelona • Belgrade • Novi Sad • Cluj • Manchester

Guest Editor
Luis Eduardo Almeida
Surgical Sciences - Oral
and Maxillofacial Surgery
Marquette University
Milwaukee
United States

Editorial Office
MDPI AG
Grosspeteranlage 5
4052 Basel, Switzerland

This is a reprint of the Special Issue, published open access by the journal *Diagnostics* (ISSN 2075-4418), freely accessible at: www.mdpi.com/journal/diagnostics/special_issues/YY8NX9FH5F.

For citation purposes, cite each article independently as indicated on the article page online and using the guide below:

Lastname, A.A.; Lastname, B.B. Article Title. *Journal Name* **Year**, *Volume Number*, Page Range.

ISBN 978-3-7258-3080-0 (Hbk)
ISBN 978-3-7258-3079-4 (PDF)
https://doi.org/10.3390/books978-3-7258-3079-4

Cover image courtesy of Luis Eduardo Almeida

© 2025 by the authors. Articles in this book are Open Access and distributed under the Creative Commons Attribution (CC BY) license. The book as a whole is distributed by MDPI under the terms and conditions of the Creative Commons Attribution-NonCommercial-NoDerivs (CC BY-NC-ND) license (https://creativecommons.org/licenses/by-nc-nd/4.0/).

Contents

About the Editor vii

Preface ix

Luis Eduardo Almeida, David Lloyd, Daniel Boettcher, Olivia Kraft and Samuel Zammuto
Immunohistochemical Analysis of Dentigerous Cysts and Odontogenic Keratocysts Associated with Impacted Third Molars—A Systematic Review
Reprinted from: *Diagnostics* **2024**, *14*, 1246, https://doi.org/10.3390/diagnostics14121246 1

Ciprian Roi, Mircea Riviș, Alexandra Roi, Marius Raica, Raluca Amalia Ceaușu and Alexandru Cătălin Motofelea et al.
CD34 and Ki-67 Immunoexpression in Periapical Granulomas: Implications for Angiogenesis and Cellular Proliferation
Reprinted from: *Diagnostics* **2024**, *14*, 2446, https://doi.org/10.3390/diagnostics14212446 78

Ban A. Salih and Bashar H. Abdullah
Comparative Immunohistochemical Analysis of Craniopharyngioma and Ameloblastoma: Insights into Odontogenic Differentiation
Reprinted from: *Diagnostics* **2024**, *14*, 2315, https://doi.org/10.3390/diagnostics14202315 91

Asma Almazyad, Mohammed Alamro, Nasser Almadan, Marzouq Almutairi and Turki S. AlQuwayz
Frequency and Demographic Analysis of Odontogenic Tumors in Three Tertiary Institutions: An 11-Year Retrospective Study
Reprinted from: *Diagnostics* **2024**, *14*, 910, https://doi.org/10.3390/diagnostics14090910 100

Andrea Migliorelli, Andrea Ciorba, Marianna Manuelli, Francesco Stomeo, Stefano Pelucchi and Chiara Bianchini
Circulating HPV Tumor DNA and Molecular Residual Disease in HPV-Positive Oropharyngeal Cancers: A Scoping Review
Reprinted from: *Diagnostics* **2024**, *14*, 2662, https://doi.org/10.3390/diagnostics14232662 115

Nur Rahman Ahmad Seno Aji, Tülay Yucel-Lindberg, Ismo T. Räisänen, Heidi Kuula, Mikko T. Nieminen and Maelíosa T. C. Mc Crudden et al.
In Vivo Regulation of Active Matrix Metalloproteinase-8 (aMMP-8) in Periodontitis: From Transcriptomics to Real-Time Online Diagnostics and Treatment Monitoring
Reprinted from: *Diagnostics* **2024**, *14*, 1011, https://doi.org/10.3390/diagnostics14101011 124

Shuaa S. Alharbi and Haifa F. Alhasson
Exploring the Applications of Artificial Intelligence in Dental Image Detection: A Systematic Review
Reprinted from: *Diagnostics* **2024**, *14*, 2442, https://doi.org/10.3390/diagnostics14212442 138

Sanjeev B. Khanagar, Farraj Albalawi, Aram Alshehri, Mohammed Awawdeh, Kiran Iyer and Barrak Alsomaie et al.
Performance of Artificial Intelligence Models Designed for Automated Estimation of Age Using Dento-Maxillofacial Radiographs—A Systematic Review
Reprinted from: *Diagnostics* **2024**, *14*, 1079, https://doi.org/10.3390/diagnostics14111079 152

Milica Vasiljevic, Dragica Selakovic, Gvozden Rosic, Momir Stevanovic, Jovana Milanovic and Aleksandra Arnaut et al.
Anatomical Factors of the Anterior and Posterior Maxilla Affecting Immediate Implant Placement Based on Cone Beam Computed Tomography Analysis: A Narrative Review
Reprinted from: *Diagnostics* **2024**, *14*, 1697, https://doi.org/10.3390/diagnostics14151697 . . . . **174**

Mateusz Rogulski, Małgorzata Pałac, Tomasz Wolny and Paweł Linek
Assessment of Reliability, Agreement, and Accuracy of Masseter Muscle Ultrasound Thickness Measurement Using a New Standardized Protocol
Reprinted from: *Diagnostics* **2024**, *14*, 1771, https://doi.org/10.3390/diagnostics14161771 . . . . **192**

Ji-Song Jung, Ho-Kyung Lim, You-Sun Lee and Seok-Ki Jung
The Occurrence and Risk Factors of Black Triangles Between Central Incisors After Orthodontic Treatment
Reprinted from: *Diagnostics* **2024**, *14*, 2747, https://doi.org/10.3390/diagnostics14232747 . . . . **203**

Sandra López-Verdín, Judith A. Solorzano-López, Ronell Bologna-Molina, Nelly Molina-Frechero, Omar Tremillo-Maldonado and Victor H. Toral-Rizo et al.
The Frequency of Risk Factors for Cleft Lip and Palate in Mexico: A Systematic Review
Reprinted from: *Diagnostics* **2024**, *14*, 1753, https://doi.org/10.3390/diagnostics14161753 . . . . **216**

Lujain AlSahman, Hamad AlBagieh and Roba AlSahman
Oral Health-Related Quality of Life in Temporomandibular Disorder Patients and Healthy Subjects—A Systematic Review and Meta-Analysis
Reprinted from: *Diagnostics* **2024**, *14*, 2183, https://doi.org/10.3390/diagnostics14192183 . . . . **228**

Lujain AlSahman, Hamad AlBagieh and Roba AlSahman
Is There a Relationship between Salivary Cortisol and Temporomandibular Disorder: A Systematic Review
Reprinted from: *Diagnostics* **2024**, *14*, 1435, https://doi.org/10.3390/diagnostics14131435 . . . . **247**

About the Editor

Luis Eduardo Almeida

Dr. Luis Eduardo Almeida is a dynamic professional with an illustrious academic journey. He embarked on his pursuit of knowledge by earning a Doctorate in Dental Surgery (DDS) degree (1989–1993) from the prestigious Federal University of Parana State, UFPR, Brazil. His relentless dedication led him to achieve a Certificate in Oral and Maxillofacial Surgery (1995–1998) from the same institution.

Continuing his academic endeavors with fervor, he secured a Fellowship in Oral and Maxillofacial Surgery (1998–1999) at Northwestern University, Chicago, USA, followed by completing an official Residency Program in the same field (2001–2003) at the same esteemed institution.

He further honed his expertise by attaining a Master of Science in Health Sciences (2004–2006) and a Ph.D. in Health Sciences (2008–2013) from Pontificia Universidade Catolica do Parana, PUC-PR, Brazil.

Presently, Dr. Luis Eduardo Almeida exudes enthusiasm as a guiding force at Marquette University, School of Dentistry. Serving as a Clinical Associate Professor in Surgical Sciences, Oral and Maxillofacial Surgery. His dynamic leadership as Director of the Predoctoral Program in Oral and Maxillofacial and Oral Surgery (since 2018) ignites a fervor for excellence in his students.

Certified by the Brazilian Dental Board and the Wisconsin Dental Board and Board eligible for the American Board of Oral and Maxillofacial Surgery, Dr. Luis Eduardo Almeida stands out as a pioneer in his field. His enthusiasm extends beyond academia, as evidenced by his enriching experience as an Oral and Maxillofacial Surgeon in private practice (2003–2013).

In all his endeavors, Dr. Luis Eduardo Almeida embodies a spirit of enthusiasm, innovation, and excellence, leaving an indelible mark on the landscape of dentistry.

Preface

The complexities of oral and maxillofacial diseases demand a multidisciplinary approach, reflected in the topics covered. Advanced radiological techniques, such as cone-beam computed tomography (CBCT) and magnetic resonance imaging (MRI), are explored for their ability to provide detailed anatomical insights critical for disease localization and treatment planning. Additionally, the potential of optical imaging and non-invasive diagnostic tools is discussed, offering pathways for early disease detection and treatment response evaluation.

Pathology and biopsy techniques feature prominently, with an emphasis on the role of histopathological analysis in achieving definitive diagnoses. Innovations in biopsy methods that enhance tissue sampling accuracy are highlighted, alongside discussions on the integration of molecular diagnostics. Genetic and molecular markers are shown to be transformative in early-stage disease identification and personalized therapeutic strategies, exemplifying the shift toward precision medicine.

Another key theme is prognostic assessment, focusing on biomarkers that indicate disease progression and treatment efficacy. Understanding these markers enables clinicians to predict disease trajectories and optimize treatment strategies, ultimately leading to improved patient outcomes.

This Special Issue synthesizes cutting-edge research findings and clinical applications, aiming to bridge the gap between innovative diagnostic technologies and routine clinical practice. It serves as an essential resource for clinicians, researchers, and healthcare professionals in the oral and maxillofacial field, inspiring further research and collaboration to advance diagnostic tools and methodologies.

The overarching objective of this Special Issue is to enhance the quality of care for patients with oral and maxillofacial diseases. By integrating emerging diagnostic technologies and methodologies, it seeks to improve diagnostic precision and patient outcomes, while also fostering timely and effective interventions. As the field of diagnostics evolves, the insights shared in this edition will guide future innovations and practices, contributing to a more precise and patient-centered approach to healthcare.

Luis Eduardo Almeida
Guest Editor

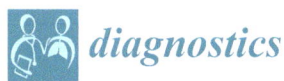

Systematic Review

Immunohistochemical Analysis of Dentigerous Cysts and Odontogenic Keratocysts Associated with Impacted Third Molars—A Systematic Review

Luis Eduardo Almeida *, David Lloyd, Daniel Boettcher, Olivia Kraft and Samuel Zammuto

Surgical Sciences Department, School of Dentistry, Marquette University, Milwaukee, WI 53233, USA
* Correspondence: luiseduardo.almeida@marquette.edu; Tel.: +1-414-288-6022

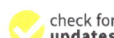

Citation: Almeida, L.E.; Lloyd, D.; Boettcher, D.; Kraft, O.; Zammuto, S. Immunohistochemical Analysis of Dentigerous Cysts and Odontogenic Keratocysts Associated with Impacted Third Molars—A Systematic Review. *Diagnostics* **2024**, *14*, 1246. https://doi.org/10.3390/diagnostics14121246

Academic Editor: Gianna Dipalma

Received: 19 April 2024
Revised: 10 May 2024
Accepted: 11 June 2024
Published: 13 June 2024

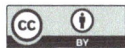

Copyright: © 2024 by the authors. Licensee MDPI, Basel, Switzerland. This article is an open access article distributed under the terms and conditions of the Creative Commons Attribution (CC BY) license (https://creativecommons.org/licenses/by/4.0/).

Abstract: Objective: This systematic review investigates the diagnostic, prognostic, and therapeutic implications of immunohistochemical markers in dentigerous cysts (DCs) and odontogenic keratocysts (OKCs) associated with impacted third molars. Materials and Methods: A comprehensive search strategy was employed across major databases including MEDLINE/PubMed, EMBASE, and Web of Science, from the inception of the databases to March 2024. Keywords and Medical Subject Heading (MeSH) terms such as "dentigerous cysts", "odontogenic keratocysts", "immunohistochemistry", "Ki-67", and "p53" were used. The PRISMA 2020 guidelines were followed to ensure methodological rigor. Inclusion criteria encompassed studies on humans and animals providing definitive diagnoses or specific signs and symptoms related to DCs and OKCs, with results on protein expression derived from immunohistochemistry, immune antibody, proteomics, or protein expression methods. Results: Of the 159 studies initially identified, 138 met the inclusion criteria. Our analysis highlighted significantly higher expressions of Ki-67 (22.1% ± 4.7 vs. 10.5% ± 3.2, $p < 0.001$), p53 (15.3% ± 3.6 vs. 5.2% ± 1.9, $p < 0.001$), and Bcl-2 (18.4% ± 3.2 vs. 8.7% ± 2.4, $p < 0.001$) in OKCs compared to DCs, indicating a higher proliferative index, increased cellular stress, and enhanced anti-apoptotic mechanisms in OKCs. Additionally, PCNA levels were higher in OKCs (25.6% ± 4.5 vs. 12.3% ± 3.1, $p < 0.001$). Genetic mutations, particularly in the PTCH1 gene, were frequently observed in OKCs, underscoring their aggressive behavior and potential malignancy. Conclusions: The findings emphasize the significant role of immunohistochemical markers in distinguishing between DCs and OKCs, with elevated levels of Ki-67, p53, Bcl-2, and PCNA in OKCs suggesting a higher potential for growth and recurrence. Genetic insights, including PTCH1 mutations, further support the need for personalized treatment approaches. These markers enhance diagnostic accuracy and inform targeted therapeutic strategies, potentially transforming patient management in oral and maxillofacial surgery.

Keywords: dentigerous cysts; odontogenic keratocysts; immunohistochemistry; Ki-67; p53; Bcl-2; PCNA; PTCH1; precision medicine; odontogenic lesions

1. Introduction

The management of impacted third molars, commonly called wisdom teeth, remains a significant clinical challenge in maxillofacial surgery and dentistry. Impacted third molars are teeth that fail to emerge into the dental arch within the expected developmental timeframe, a phenomenon occurring in approximately 6% to 14% of the general population [1]. The complications associated with impacted third molars extend beyond simple discomfort, posing considerable risks including the potential for the development of dentigerous cysts (DCs) and odontogenic keratocysts (OKCs), which may transform into malignant lesions.

Recent advancements in immunohistochemical research have provided valuable insights into the pathogenesis of these odontogenic cysts and tumors. Immunohistochemical markers, including Ki-67, p53, Bcl-2, and PCNA, have been pivotal in elucidating the cellular activities underlying the aggressive behavior of OKCs compared to DCs [2,3]. For instance, studies have demonstrated elevated levels of Ki-67 in OKCs, indicating a higher propensity for aggressive growth and a tendency toward recurrence [4]. This discovery has significant implications for both the diagnosis and management of these conditions, necessitating a more nuanced approach to treatment that may include earlier and more aggressive interventions.

Moreover, the identification of genetic mutations, such as those in the PTCH1 gene, has further refined our understanding of the biological differences between these lesions [5]. Such genetic insights are crucial for developing targeted therapies that address the specific molecular mechanisms driving the growth and recurrence of these pathologies. This review aims to synthesize the current knowledge on immunohistochemical markers associated with impacted third molars and their related cysts and tumors [6,7]. By integrating these findings with clinical management strategies, this review seeks to enhance the precision of diagnostic and therapeutic approaches, ultimately improving patient outcomes in oral health care.

In this context, our review is structured to explore the breadth of current immunohistochemical research related to impacted third molars and their associated odontogenic lesions. Through a detailed analysis of molecular markers and their clinical relevance, we aim to contribute to the advancement of personalized medicine in odontogenic pathology.

2. Materials and Methods

2.1. Search Protocol

The search protocol for this systematic review focused on the immunohistochemical analysis of dentigerous cysts (DCs) and odontogenic keratocysts (OKCs) associated with impacted third molars. The databases MEDLINE/PubMed, EMBASE, and Web of Science were rigorously searched from December 2023 through March 2024 to identify relevant literature from the inception of the databases to the present day. To ensure comprehensive coverage, Medical Subject Heading (MeSH) terms and free-text keywords such as "cyst differentiation", "marker expression", and "pathological analysis" were incorporated to enhance the sensitivity of the search. Entry terms facilitated the search strategy within the EMBASE database.

Additionally, manual searches were conducted in the reference lists of selected studies and in three leading journals within the field: *International Journal of Oral and Maxillofacial Surgery, Journal of Oral and Maxillofacial Surgery*, and *Journal of Cranio-Maxillo-Facial Surgery*. These searches provided further valuable citations.

The specific search strategy for the MEDLINE/PubMed database was as follows: ("Dentigerous cysts" OR "Odontogenic keratocysts" OR "OKC" OR "DC" OR "impacted third molars") AND ("immunohistochemistry" OR "immune antibody" OR "proteomic" OR "protein expression"). Throughout this review, the PRISMA 2020 statement served as the guideline for reporting, ensuring rigor and clarity in the synthesis of findings (Page MJ, McKenzie JE, Bossuyt PM, Boutron I, Hoffmann TC, Mulrow CD, et al. The PRISMA 2020 statement: an updated guideline for reporting systematic reviews. *Systematic Reviews* 2021; 10:89).

Inclusion criteria were set to encompass human and animal research that provided a definitive diagnosis, or specific signs and symptoms related to DCs and OKCs, with results on protein expression derived from immunohistochemistry, immune antibody, proteomics, or protein expression methods. Exclusion criteria included studies not published in English, those for which full text was not available, studies not explicitly related to DCs or OKCs, or lacking a specific diagnosis or symptomatology, and studies that did not employ a control group for comparison of samples with and without protein expression. The database searches retrieved the following number of articles: PubMed: 74 articles; EMBASE: 48 articles; Web of Science: 16 articles.

Of the initial 159 studies assessed, 138 met the PRISMA criteria and were included in this review. The excluded studies were those that either lacked a clear diagnosis related to DCs or OKCs, had inadequate methodology, were unavailable in full text, or were not written in English (Figure 1).

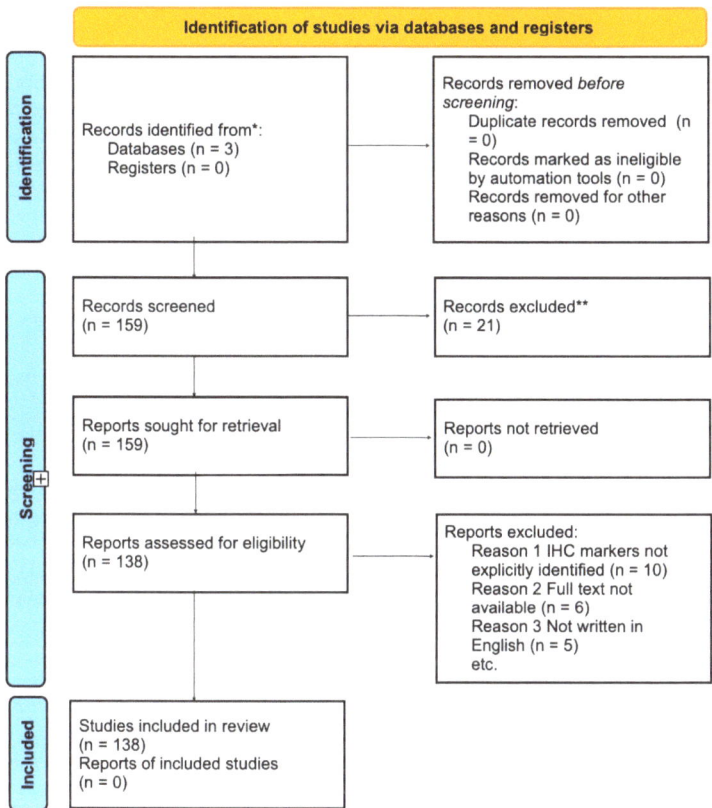

Figure 1. PRISMA 2020 flow Diagram. * MEDLINE, Web of Science, and Cochrane; ** EMBASE.

2.2. Data Analysis

The search protocol deployed for this literature review was deliberately broad to capture a comprehensive array of potential immunohistochemical markers implicated in the pathogenesis of dentigerous cysts (DCs) and odontogenic keratocysts (OKCs) associated with impacted third molars. Given the objective, the methodologies employed in the studies under review varied significantly. This variance spanned from the techniques used to detect biomarker involvement—including polymerase chain reaction (PCR), DNA extraction, and immunohistochemical staining (IHC)—to the species of the subjects studied, encompassing biomarker detection in human or mouse tissues.

Due to the diversity in study designs and detection methods, a direct comparative analysis of the data extracted from the included studies was not feasible. Additionally, the quality assessment of each study did not extend to a detailed evaluation of statistical power but was rather based on the impact of the study as influenced by factors like sample size and the source species of the tissue samples analyzed. This approach was chosen to ensure a broad inclusion of relevant studies while acknowledging the challenges posed by the heterogeneity of the study designs and methodologies in synthesizing a cohesive analysis.

Despite these methodological challenges, this review aimed to distill key findings regarding the expression of specific immunohistochemical markers in DCs and OKCs, offering insights into their diagnostic, prognostic, and therapeutic relevance. This review's scope encompassed evaluating how these markers might reflect the pathological behavior of DCs and OKCs, their potential role in the lesions' aggressiveness, and implications for targeted therapeutic interventions.

3. Results

Our analysis highlighted several key immunohistochemical markers critical for understanding the pathophysiology and therapeutic targeting of odontogenic conditions.

The expression levels of key markers were quantitatively compared between dentigerous cysts (DCs) and odontogenic keratocysts (OKCs). Ki-67 expression was significantly higher in OKCs, with a mean of 22.1% (SD $\pm$ 4.7) compared to 10.5% (SD $\pm$ 3.2) in DCs (t = 4.25, $p < 0.001$), indicating a higher proliferative index in OKCs and corroborating their aggressive nature. Similarly, p53 showed elevated levels in OKCs, with a mean of 15.3% (SD $\pm$ 3.6) versus 5.2% (SD $\pm$ 1.9) in DCs (t = 5.67, $p < 0.001$), suggesting increased cellular stress and mutation accumulation in OKCs [8].

Bcl-2 expression was also higher in OKCs, with mean levels of 18.4% (SD $\pm$ 3.2) compared to 8.7% (SD $\pm$ 2.4) in DCs, showing a significant difference (t = 4.98, $p < 0.001$). This higher expression indicates enhanced anti-apoptotic mechanisms in OKCs [9]. Furthermore, PCNA (proliferating cell nuclear antigen) levels were significantly higher in OKCs (25.6%, SD $\pm$ 4.5) compared to DCs (12.3%, SD $\pm$ 3.1) (t = 5.82, $p < 0.001$), indicating a higher proliferative rate in OKCs [10].

Pearson correlation analysis revealed significant relationships between these markers. Ki-67 and p53 showed a strong positive correlation (r = 0.68, $p < 0.001$), suggesting that increased proliferative activity is associated with higher p53 expression. Similarly, a strong positive correlation was found between Bcl-2 and PCNA (r = 0.72, $p < 0.001$), indicating linked proliferative and anti-apoptotic activities. Although the correlation between p53 and Bax was negative (r = -0.100), it was not statistically significant, indicating complex interactions between pro-apoptotic and anti-apoptotic factors [11].

Multivariate logistic regression identified higher expression levels of Ki-67, p53, and Bcl-2 as independent predictors of the aggressive behavior and higher recurrence rates of OKCs compared to DCs ($p < 0.05$ for all markers). This underscores the distinct biological profile of OKCs, characterized by heightened proliferative and anti-apoptotic activity [12].

Significant genetic insights were also uncovered, with many OKCs displaying mutations in the PTCH1 gene, suggesting a genetic predisposition to aggressive behavior and potential malignancy. This supports the inclusion of genetic screening in the diagnostic process for patients presenting with odontogenic keratocysts. Additionally, alterations in the SHH (Sonic Hedgehog) pathway were commonly associated with OKCs, implicating it in their pathogenesis and suggesting potential therapeutic targets [13].

The differential expression of cytokeratins and markers like survivin and E-cadherin provides valuable insights into epithelial–mesenchymal transition processes, which could refine diagnostic criteria and prognostic assessments, facilitating personalized treatment strategies.

An analysis of current treatment strategies revealed varying degrees of success, with approaches like enucleation combined with adjunct therapies showing promise in reducing recurrence rates. The integration of immunohistochemical data is influencing treatment protocols, suggesting more aggressive or targeted approaches based on specific marker expression.

In conclusion, the findings underscore the significance of immunohistochemical markers in understanding the biological behavior of DCs and OKCs. These insights enhance diagnostic accuracy and facilitate the development of effective, personalized therapeutic strategies, potentially transforming patient management in oral and maxillofacial surgery.

4. Discussion
4.1. Pathophysiology and Molecular Basis

The reclassification of odontogenic keratocysts (OKCs) to keratocystic odontogenic tumors (KCOTs) by the World Health Organization marks a significant advancement in our understanding of these lesions. This change highlights their invasive characteristics, unique histological features, and genetic bases [14]. Central to this reclassification is the identification of mutations in the PTCH1 gene, a critical component of the Sonic Hedgehog (SHH) signaling pathway, which plays a vital role in cell development and differentiation [14].

The SHH pathway's importance in craniofacial development is well established, with its dysregulation linked to conditions such as nevoid basal cell carcinoma syndrome (NBCCS) [15]. Anomalies in this pathway can lead to altered palatogenesis and tooth formation, emphasizing its essential role in normal facial and dental growth. Advances in genetic research have shed light on missense mutations in the PTCH1 gene across various odontogenic conditions, highlighting a direct connection to the aggressive and recurrent nature of KCOTs [15,16]. These insights have opened avenues for targeted therapeutic approaches, such as the use of inhibitors like vismodegib, which has been shown to significantly reduce the size and recurrence rates of these aggressive tumors [16].

The study by Madras and Lapointe (2008) provides an essential review of KCOTs, particularly focusing on their aggressive nature and the implications of their reclassification from cysts to tumors [14]. Their findings on the recurrence rates associated with various treatment modalities are particularly revealing:

- Enucleation and Curettage showed a recurrence rate of 30%.
- Enucleation with Carnoy's solution and marsupialization followed by enucleation/cystectomy demonstrated substantially lower recurrence rates, around 9–10% and 9–14%, respectively.
- Resection, the most definitive treatment, showed a recurrence rate of 0%.

These findings highlight the necessity for aggressive treatment strategies and are in harmony with molecular insights suggesting that targeting the SHH pathway could provide less invasive and more effective treatment options in the future. Understanding the intricate relationship between genetic mutations in the PTCH1 gene and their impact on lesion development and behavior is crucial for advancing diagnosis, management, and the development of targeted treatments. This knowledge plays a pivotal role in the evolution of precision medicine strategies that tailor treatments based on specific genetic profiles, potentially enhancing patient outcomes.

In summary, exploring the genetic and molecular framework of odontogenic lesions, with a focus on the SHH pathway and PTCH1 mutations, offers a comprehensive understanding of these conditions. It paves the way for the development of effective, targeted treatment options, ushering in a new era of personalized care characterized by enhanced treatments and outcomes. The continuous integration of these insights into clinical practice is vital to transforming the treatment landscape for odontogenic lesions, ensuring that therapeutic discoveries are swiftly translated into clinical benefits (Table 1).

Table 1. Pathophysiology and molecular basis (PTCH1, Sonic Hedgehog, NBCCS).

Authors	Objective	Study Details	Marker Identification Method	Cyst/Tumor Diagnosis Method	Results	Statistical Estimates	Conclusion
Madras et al. (2008) [14]	Review features and behavior of OKCs (now KCOTs), analyze KCOT cases, discuss reclassification and treatment implications.	Study Type: Case series and literature review. Sample Size: 21 patients, 27 KCOTs. Age Range: 1912–1986. Country/Region: Canada.	CK1, CK10, Ki-67, PTCH, bcl-2, BAX.	Radiographic and histological examination.	Recurrence rate: 29%. Lesion size: Most 0–15 cm², avg. 14 cm². Treatment: Enucleation and curettage (22), resection (2), marsupialization (3); all recurrences within 2 years—PTCH gene and SHH pathway involvement in KCOT pathophysiology indicates potential for molecular-based treatments.	Enucleation: 30%. Enucleation and Carnoy's solution: 9%. Enucleation and peripheral ostectomy: 18%. Enucleation and cryotherapy: 38%. Marsupialization: 33%. Marsupialization and cystectomy: 13%. Resection: 0%.	Aggressive treatment (enucleation with Carnoy's solution, marsupialization followed by enucleation) is effective. Long-term follow-up is essential. Molecular therapies targeting SHH pathway may offer future alternatives.
Cobourne et al. (2009) [15]	Assess the association between histopathological diagnoses of dentigerous cysts and pericoronal follicles with the positions of impacted third molars.	Study Type: Observational study. Sample Size: 151 cases. Age Range: 63.6% were 20 years or older. Gender and Ethnicity: 70.9% female; 90.1% white.	PTCH1, SHH pathway involvement.	Histopathological examination.	Pericoronal follicles: 64.9% (98 cases). Dentigerous cysts: 35.1% (53 cases). Teeth with dentigerous cysts: 84.9% in mandible, 49.1% mesioangular position, 66.0% in 20–29 years age group—SHH pathway involvement indicating potential molecular targets for treatment.	Predominance of impacted teeth and dentigerous cysts in the mandible. Increase in dentigerous cysts with age, particularly in mandibular teeth in mesioangular positions.	Mandibles are the most frequent location for impacted teeth and dentigerous cysts. Dentigerous cysts tend to increase with age, especially in mandibular teeth in mesioangular positions. Potential for molecular-based treatments targeting SHH pathway.
Shimura et al. (2020) [16]	Analyze genetic mutations in SMO, BRAF, PTCH1, and GNAS using NGS in patients with odontogenic diseases and evaluate the usefulness of genetic analysis for differential diagnosis.	Study Type: Observational study. Sample Size: 18 patients; 6 ABs; 7 OKCs; 1 odontoma. Country/Region: Japan (Department of Oral and Maxillofacial Surgery, Dokkyo Medical University School of Medicine)	SMO, BRAF, PTCH1, GNAS.	Clinical course, imaging (X-ray), histopathological, and next-generation sequencing (NGS) analysis.	Ameloblastoma (AB): BRAF mutation (T440P) in 2 patients, PTCH1 mutation (V582G) in 1 patient. Odontogenic keratocyst (OKC): PTCH1 mutation in 4 patients, BRAF mutations (T263P, K51N, Y647D) in 2 patients, SMO mutation (N396T) in 1 patient. Odontoma (1 patient): Mutations in SMO (Y394S), BRAF	Not specified.	Genetic mutations in SMO, BRAF, PTCH1, and GNAS can be identified using NGS, aiding in the differential diagnosis of odontogenic diseases. Specific mutations in these genes are associated with different types of odontogenic tumors.

4.2. Genetic and Molecular Alterations

Our review delved deeply into the genetic foundations and molecular dynamics influencing the pathogenesis of odontogenic lesions, such as ameloblastomas (ABs), adenomatoid odontogenic tumors (AOTs), and odontogenic keratocysts (OKCs). A significant focus was on the genetic mutations impacting the Sonic Hedgehog (SHH) pathway and the PTCH1 gene, which are crucially linked to the development, aggressive behavior, and response to treatment of these lesions [17,18].

The SHH pathway, critical for tissue regulation and development, has been shown to be disrupted in the invasive nature of ABs and OKCs, highlighting the potential for targeting this pathway as an effective therapeutic strategy [17,18]. Inactivating mutations in the PTCH1 gene, prevalent in keratocystic odontogenic tumors (KCOTs), directly relate to the lesions' aggressiveness and offer promising targets for novel treatments [19,20].

Identification of these genetic alterations has significantly advanced diagnostic and prognostic techniques, facilitating the development of personalized treatment plans. Biomarkers such as PTCH1 now guide clinical decision-making, demonstrating how genetic discoveries are directly applied to enhance patient care. For instance, the detection of PTCH1 mutations in patients can lead to the adoption of SHH pathway inhibitors as part of the treatment regimen, enhancing the efficacy of treatments tailored to specific genetic profiles [21].

Advances in techniques such as whole exome sequencing have enabled the differentiation of odontogenic diseases and the customization of treatment based on the genetic characteristics of each lesion, marking a significant progression towards precision medicine. This shift is promoting more effective, targeted, and patient-centered management.

Supporting evidence from Rodrigues et al. (2022) highlights the significance of SHH pathway components in epithelial odontogenic lesions, showing differential expression of SHH, SMO, and GLI-1 proteins across various odontogenic tumors, reinforcing the therapeutic potential of these pathways [17]. Similarly, Stojanov et al. (2020) identified biallelic PTCH1 inactivation as a dominant genomic change in sporadic keratocystic odontogenic tumors, supporting the classification of KCOTs as neoplasms with cystic growth and underscoring the importance of SHH pathway inhibitors in their treatment [18].

Further studies, like those by Grachtchouk et al. (2006) and Zhai et al. (2019), have demonstrated that odontogenic keratocysts in both mice and humans are associated with deregulated Hedgehog signaling due to PTCH1 mutations, suggesting that targeting the Hh signaling pathway could be a potential therapeutic approach for treating OKCs. Specifically, Zhai et al. showed that the SHH pathway inhibitor GDC-0449 effectively inhibits SHH signaling and cell proliferation in an in vitro isogenic cellular model simulating odontogenic keratocysts with a PTCH1 mutation, highlighting the therapeutic potential of SHH pathway inhibitors [19,22].

In conclusion, a deeper understanding of genetic mutations and molecular alterations within the SHH pathway and PTCH1 gene enriches our comprehension of the pathophysiology of odontogenic lesions. This knowledge not only opens the door to targeted therapies but also heralds a new era of personalized care for patients, characterized by improved treatments and outcomes. The ongoing integration of these insights into clinical practice continues to transform the landscape of treatment for odontogenic lesions, ensuring that new therapeutic discoveries are translated into clinical benefits (Table 2).

Table 2. Genetic and molecular changes (Sonic Hedgehog, PTCH1).

Authors	Objective	Study Details	Marker Identification Method	Cyst/Tumor Diagnosis Method	Results	Statistical Estimates	Conclusion
Rodrigues et al. (2022) [17]	Analyze the expression of proteins involved in the Sonic Hedgehog signaling pathway (SHH, SMO, GLI-1) in benign epithelial odontogenic lesions to identify their role in pathogenesis.	Study Type: Observational study. Sample Size: 50 samples. 20 OKCs 20 ABs 10 AOTs.	SHH, SMO, GLI-1.	Histopathology, immunohistochemistry.	SHH: Higher in AB vs. AOT ($p = 0.022$) and OKC ($p = 0.02$). No differences in SMO-GLI-1. Nuclear: Higher in AB and OKC vs. AOT ($p < 0.0001$). Positive correlations: GLI-1 in AB ($r = 0.482$, $p = 0.031$) and OKC ($r = 0.865$, $p < 0.0001$); SMO and GLI-1 in AOT ($r = 0.667$, $p = 0.035$) and OKC ($r = 0.535$, $p = 0.015$).	Kruskal–Wallis, Mann–Whitney U, Spearman's (r); $p < 0.05$.	SHH pathway involvement in pathogenesis. SHH overexpression in AB and GLI-1 in AB and OKC indicate more aggressive behavior compared to AOT.
Stojanov et al. (2020) [18]	Identify recurrent genomic aberrations in sporadic KCOTs using next-generation sequencing.	Study Type: Observational. Sample Size: 44 sporadic KCOTs; 23 females, 21 males. Age Range: Median age: 50 (range 10–82). Sites: 33 mandible, 11 maxilla.	PTCH1, SMO, SUFU, GLI1, GLI2.	Next-generation sequencing, genomic analysis.	PTCH1 mutations: 93% (41/44 cases). Biallelic PTCH1 inactivation: 80% (35 cases). 9q copy neutral loss of heterozygosity: 34% (15 cases). No aberrations in other SHH pathway members.	Not specified.	SHH pathway alterations, specifically PTCH1 inactivation, are common in sporadic KCOTs. The high frequency of PTCH1 loss suggests potential for SHH pathway inhibitors as a therapeutic target.
Zhai et al. (2019) [19]	Investigate the role of PTCH1 inactivation in OKCs and evaluate the efficacy of SHH pathway inhibitor GDC-0449 using an isogenic cellular model.	Study Type: Observational. Isogenic PTCH1R135X/+ cellular model using CRISPR/Cas9; induction of epithelial differentiation.	PTCH1, SHH pathway.	CRISPR/Cas9, in vitro cellular model, epithelial differentiation.	PTCH1R135X/+ mutation causes ligand-independent activation of SHH signaling. SHH pathway activation downregulated by GDC-0449 in a dose-dependent manner. Enhanced proliferation of induced cells suppressed by GDC-0449.	Not specified.	PTCH1 inactivation leads to SHH pathway activation in OKCs. GDC-0449 effectively inhibits SHH pathway activation and reduces cell proliferation, suggesting its potential as a therapeutic inhibitor for OKC treatment.
Ren et al. (2012) [20]	Investigate the role of SHH and NOTCH pathways in KCOTs and the effect of SMO inhibitor cyclopamine.	Study Type: Observational study. Age Range: KCOT-1 cell line established from a 53-year-old male patient.	SHH, PTCH1, SMO, GLI1, GLI2, NOTCH1, NOTCH2, NOTCH3, JAG2, DLL1, EMPs (AMELX, ENAM, AMBN, AMTN, MMP-20, KLK-4, ODAM, CK14).	Immunohistochemistry, qRT-PCR, Western blot, cell viability assays.	Cyclopamine reduced KCOT cell viability. SHH and NOTCH pathways are active in KCOT. Cyclopamine downregulated SHH and NOTCH pathway components. Cyclopamine inhibits KCOT growth dose-dependently.	Not specified.	Cyclopamine significantly inhibits SHH signaling and cell growth in KCOT, suggesting it as a potential therapeutic agent.

Table 2. Cont.

Authors	Objective	Study Details	Marker Identification Method	Cyst/Tumor Diagnosis Method	Results	Statistical Estimates	Conclusion
Yagyuu et al. (2008) [21]	Examine factors responsible for the recurrence of KCOT.	Study Type: Retrospective study. Sample Size: 74 patients. 75 sporadic KCOTs. 23 KCOTs.	SHH, PTCH1, SMO.	Immunohistochemistry.	Recurrence more frequent in multilocular lesions (64%) than unilocular (7%) ($p = 0.0350$). Recurrent lesions larger (62.8 ± 6.5 mm) than nonrecurrent (43.0 ± 4.0 mm) ($p = 0.0363$). Higher SMO expression in recurrent KCOTs ($p = 0.0475$). Inverse correlation between SHH and SMO expression in all KCOTs ($p = 0.0318$).	Not specified.	The recurrence of KCOT is associated with multilocular large lesions and high SMO expression.
Hasegawa et al. (2017) [23]	Investigate the pathophysiology of Gorlin syndrome-associated tumorigenesis and skeletal abnormalities.	Study Type: Observational study. Sample Size: 4 Gorlin syndrome patients with PTCH1 mutations.	SHH, PTCH1, SMO, GLI1, GLI2, Wnt proteins, BMP4, BMP6.	Immunohistochemistry, qRT-PCR, Western blot.	GLI1 expression is higher in fibroblasts and patient-derived iPSCs than in control cells. Patient-derived iPSCs showed lower basal levels of Hh, Wnt, BMP genes. Osteogenic activation enhanced in patient-derived iPSCs.	ANOVA, Bonferroni testing; $p < 0.05$.	Patient-derived iPSCs are hypersensitive to osteogenic induction, suggesting enhanced Hh signaling. Gorlin syndrome iPSCs could be useful for studying pathogenesis and developing new treatments.
Kesireddy et al. (2019) [24]	Assess the response and resistance mechanisms of Gorlin–Goltz Syndrome to vismodegib therapy.	Study Type: Observational case study. Sample Size: 1 patient. Age Range: 38-year-old female. Country/Region: USA.	SHH, SMO, PTCH1.	Genetic testing, clinical diagnosis, radiographic and histopathological examination.	Initial positive response to vismodegib for BCC lesions. Tumor regrowth and new lesions after 1 year. No effect on odontogenic keratocysts.	Not specified.	Vismodegib was initially effective, but resistance developed, leading to the progression of Gorlin syndrome. Optimal treatment regimens and durations need further study.
Grachtchouk et al. (2006) [22]	Investigate the role of Hh signaling in the development of odontogenic keratocysts (OKCs) using a Gli2 transgenic mouse model and human samples.	Study Type: Experimental study. Sample Size: Gli2 transgenic mice and human OKC samples.	SHH, PTCH1, GLI1, GLI2, Cyclin D1, Cyclin D2.	Immunohistochemistry, in situ hybridization.	Hh signaling is activated in both mouse and human OKCs-Gli2 overexpression in mice leads to keratocyst formation from rests of Malassez–Human OKCs show elevated expression of Hh target genes.	Not specified.	Constitutive Hh signaling, particularly through GLI2, plays a critical role in the pathogenesis of OKCs. Targeting GLI function may provide therapeutic benefits for OKCs and related disorders.

Table 2. Cont.

Authors	Objective	Study Details	Marker Identification Method	Cyst/Tumor Diagnosis Method	Results	Statistical Estimates	Conclusion
Wang et al. (2022) [25]	Report clinicopathologic profiles of OOCs and investigate PTCH1 mutations.	Study Type: Observational study. Sample Size: 167 OOCs from 159 patients.	PTCH1, SHH, Ki-67.	Immunohistochemistry and genetic analysis.	OOCs in 3rd/4th decade (60.4%), male predilection (66.7%). Mandible location predominant (posterior mandible, ramus). No PTCH1 mutations found except 3 known SNPs.	Not specified.	OOCs show lower proliferative activity than OKCs and do not harbor PTCH1 mutations, justifying their separation from OKCs.
Pan et al. (2009) [26]	Clarify the role of PTCH in NBCCS-related and non-syndromic KCOTs.	Study Type: Mutation analysis. Sample Size: 8 sporadic, 4 NBCCS-associated KCOTs. Country/Region: Peking University School and Hospital of Stomatology, Beijing, China.	PTCH.	Genetic analysis, PCR, DHPLC, sequencing.	Four novel and two known mutations in 2 sporadic and 3 syndromic cases. Germline mutations: c.2179delT, c.2824delC. Somatic mutations: c.3162dupG, c.1362–1374dup, c.1012 C > T, c.403C > T.	Not specified.	PTCH defects are associated with the pathogenesis of both syndromic and a subset of non-syndromic KCOTs.
Hellani et al. (2009) [27]	Differentiate between basaloid follicular hamartoma and nevoid basal cell carcinoma in a patient with NBCCS using genetic analysis.	Study Type: Case report. Sample Size: 1 patient. Age Range: 15-year-old boy.	PTCH1.	Histopathology, genetic analysis.	Novel PTCH1 germline mutation (c.1291delC). Clinical features: broad confluent eyebrows, frontal bossing, palmoplantar pits, multiple jaw cysts. Radiological features: calcification of falx cerebri, spina bifida, bifid ribs.	Not specified.	PTCH1 mutation confirmed NBCCS diagnosis, distinguishing it from basaloid follicular hamartoma. Genetic analysis is crucial for accurate diagnosis and management.
Asevedo Campos de Resende et al. (2018) [28]	Determine if deletion at 13q14 is a mechanism leading to miR-15a/16-1 aberrant expression in OKC.	Study Type: Observational study. Sample Size: 15 OKC cases. Country/Region: Universidade Federal de Minas Gerais, Brazil.	PTCH1, miR-15a, miR-16-1, Bcl-2.	Genetic analysis, PCR, capillary electrophoresis DNA-fragment analysis.	No LOH at D13S272 in 12 informative cases. 22% LOH at D13S273 marker in 2 out of 9 informative cases.	Not specified.	LOH at MIR15A/MIR16-1 locus is uncommon in OKC. The regulatory mechanism of miR-15a and miR-16-1 expression in OKC remains unclear.

Table 2. Cont.

Authors	Objective	Study Details	Marker Identification Method	Cyst/Tumor Diagnosis Method	Results	Statistical Estimates	Conclusion
Hong et al. (2014) [29]	Clarify the role of fibroblasts in the aggressiveness of syndromic and non-syndromic KCOTs.	Study Type: Observational study. Sample Size: 16 KCOT cases (8 syndromic, 8 non-syndromic). Country/Region: Peking University School and Hospital of Stomatology, Beijing, China.	PTCH1, vimentin, CK, Runx2, COL1A1, OCN, OPN, RANKL, OPG, COX-2, IL-1α.	Immunohistochemistry, qRT-PCR.	S-KCOT fibroblasts had higher proliferation and osteoclastogenic potential than NS-KCOT fibroblasts. NS-KCOT fibroblasts had higher osteogenic potential.	Student's t test, one-way ANOVA; $p < 0.05$.	S-KCOT fibroblasts exhibit greater aggressiveness due to higher osteoclastogenic potential, while NS-KCOT fibroblasts show higher osteogenic differentiation potential.
Shimada et al. (2013) [30]	Investigate genetic variations and clinicopathological features in KCOTs.	Study Type: Mutation analysis. Sample Size: 36 KCOT patients. Age Range: 10–81 years (median: 32 years). Country/Region: Japan.	PTCH1, PTCH2, SUFU, GLI2, CCND1, BCL2.	Histological classification, immunohistochemistry.	PTCH1 mutations were found in 9 hereditary KCOT patients. No pathogenic mutations in PTCH2 or SUFU. LOH at PTCH1 and SUFU loci correlated with epithelial budding. Nuclear GLI2 localization in germline mutation KCOTs.	PTCH1 mutations in 25% of cases. LOH at PTCH1 and SUFU loci correlate with epithelial budding.	PTCH1 and SUFU play significant roles in KCOT pathogenesis. Genotype-oriented subgroups exhibit different levels of aggressiveness.
Pastorino et al. (2012) [31]	To assess whether a combined clinical and bio-molecular approach could detect NBCCS among patients with KCOTs.	Study Type: Mutation analysis. Sample size: 70 KCOT patients. Age Range: 14–86 years. Country/Region: Italy.	PTCH1, SHH, SMO.	Histological classification, immunohistochemistry, genetic analysis.	8 of the 70 patients met the clinical criteria for NBCCS. Nine germline mutations in PTCH1, five of which were novel. Clinical evaluation of KCOTs can be used as screening for NBCCS.	PTCH1 mutations were found in 9 patients. 25.7% of patients had NBCCS.	Combined clinical and molecular screening is effective for recognizing NBCCS in patients with KCOTs.
Kaibuchi-Ando et al. (2021) [32]	To analyze the role of PTCH1 mutations in BCNS and the significance of odontogenic keratocysts in diagnosing BCNS.	Study Type: Case report. Sample Size: 2 BCNS patients. Country/Region: Japan.	PTCH1.	Whole-exome sequencing, Sanger sequencing.	Patient 1: PTCH1 mutation c.2798delC (p.Ala933fs*29). Patient 2: PTCH1 mutation c.1195T>C (p.Trp399Arg). Patient 2 had multiple BCCs and odontogenic keratocysts. Both patients had lamellar calcification of the falx cerebri.	Not specified.	Odontogenic keratocysts are a significant clue for diagnosing BCNS. Early detection of PTCH1 mutations is crucial for monitoring and early treatment of BCCs in BCNS patients.

4.3. Cell Adhesion, Proliferation, and Apoptosis Markers

Cell adhesion, proliferation, and apoptosis markers such as Bcl-2, PCNA, p53, and Ki-67 play pivotal roles in the pathogenesis of odontogenic lesions, including dentigerous cysts (DCs), radicular cysts (RCs), and odontogenic keratocysts (OKCs) [33–36]. The expression of these markers provides critical insights into the biological behaviors of these lesions and their implications for diagnosis, prognosis, and therapy.

Elevated expressions of Bcl-2 and Ki-67 are associated with the aggressiveness and likelihood of recurrence in these lesions [33,34]. Similarly, increased p53 expression is linked to greater cell proliferation and aggressiveness [35,36]. The variation in the expression of these biomarkers across different odontogenic lesions offers essential diagnostic and prognostic information, aiding in their differentiation and management.

For instance, increased levels of Ki-67 in OKCs often lead clinicians to opt for more aggressive surgical interventions and closer follow-up schedules, integrating marker profiles into personalized treatment plans. Furthermore, the presence of Bcl-2 in recurrent lesions has prompted research into adjuvant therapies that could inhibit this protein to reduce recurrence rates, directly impacting treatment protocols [33]. This demonstrates how the practical application of these biomarker insights is integrated into therapeutic strategies, enhancing the efficacy of treatments tailored to specific genetic profiles [33,34].

Additionally, changes in cell adhesion markers, such as the downregulation of E-cadherin and upregulation of N-cadherin, suggest epithelial–mesenchymal transition (EMT) in KCOTs, presenting potential therapeutic targets to control lesion progression and recurrence [34]. These changes in cellular behavior not only inform on the potential aggressiveness of the lesions but also guide the development of targeted interventions aimed at mitigating invasive growth and improving surgical outcomes.

In essence, the analysis of cell adhesion, proliferation, and apoptosis markers not only enriches our understanding of the pathogenesis of these conditions but also identifies key diagnostic and therapeutic targets. These insights are invaluable for the development of tailored treatment strategies and underscore the importance of ongoing research to find innovative management approaches for odontogenic lesions, with the goal of improving patient outcomes by addressing the molecular basis of these conditions [33–36] (Table 3).

Table 3. Cell adhesion, proliferation, and apoptosis markers (Bcl-2, PCNA, p53, Ki-67).

Authors	Objective	Study Details	Marker Identification Method	Cyst/Tumor Diagnosis Method	Results	Statistical Estimates	Conclusion
Friedlander et al. (2015) [33]	To determine the presence and distribution of VEGF and VEGFR2 in dentigerous cysts compared with normal dental follicles and to evaluate endothelial cells and proliferating cells as indicators of angiogenic activity in these tissues.	Study Type: Observational study. Sample Size: 20 dentigerous cysts, 20 dental follicles. Age Range: Mean age: 23 years; More common in males.	VEGF, VEGFR2, CD34, CD146, PCNA.	Immunohistochemistry (IHC).	VEGF and VEGFR2 are expressed in all dentigerous cysts and dental follicles. Higher positive staining in dentigerous cysts compared to dental follicles. Significant difference in VEGF and VEGFR2 expression (odds ratio = 31.24, $p < 0.001$).	CD34(+), CD146(+), and PCNA(+) cells significantly more in dentigerous cysts ($p < 0.001$). High intra- and inter-examiner agreement (kappa 0.77 and 0.75).	VEGF and VEGFR2 contribute to local bone resorption and the development and progression of dentigerous cysts.
Ruiz et al. (2010) [37]	To assess and compare the immunoexpression of VEGF and MMP-9 in radicular cysts (RCs) and residual radicular cysts (RRCs) and relate them to the angiogenic index and intensity of the inflammatory infiltrate.	Study Type: Observational study. Sample Size: 20 RCs, 10 RRCs. Country/Region: Brazil.	VEGF, MMP-9, von Willebrand factor (vWF).	Immunohistochemistry (IHC).	Higher VEGF and MMP-9 expression in RCs than in RRCs. Strong epithelial VEGF expression in RCs and RRCs. Lesions with strong MMP-9 expression had more VEGF+ cells and higher MVC. Positive correlation between VEGF+ cells, MVC, and inflammatory infiltrate intensity.	70% of RCs had inflammatory infiltrate grade III. VEGF+ cells in RCs: mean 565.05, RRCs: mean 443.90. MVC in RCs: mean 250.85, RRCs: mean 217.00. MMP-9 expression higher in RCs.	VEGF and MMP-9 are important for angiogenesis in RCs and RRCs. Expression of these molecules and MVC are closely related to the intensity of the inflammatory infiltrate.
Zhong et al. (2015) [34]	To clarify whether epithelial-mesenchymal transition (EMT) is involved in the pathogenesis and development of keratocystic odontogenic tumor (KCOT).	Study Type: Case report. Sample Size: 40 KCOT samples, 20 radicular cyst (RC) samples, 10 normal oral mucosa (OM) samples. Country/Region: China.	E-cadherin, N-cadherin, TGF-β, Slug, Pan-cytokeratin (P-CK), MMP-9.	Real-time quantitative PCR, Immunohistochemistry, Double-labeling immunofluorescence.	E-cadherin and Pan-cytokeratin downregulated, N-cadherin upregulated in KCOT compared to RC and OM. TGF-β and Slug highly expressed in KCOT. Correlation between Slug and MMP-9 demonstrated by double-labeling immunofluorescence.	Significant differences in marker expression between KCOT and RC/OM ($p < 0.0001$). Significant correlation between E-cadherin/P-CK, E-cadherin/Slug, and TGF-β/Slug.	EMT might be involved in the locally aggressive behavior of KCOT. Specific targeting of the EMT process may further advance the treatment of KCOT.

Table 3. Cont.

Authors	Objective	Study Details	Marker Identification Method	Cyst/Tumor Diagnosis Method	Results	Statistical Estimates	Conclusion
Pereira et al. (2023) [38]	To profile the expression of SOX2 in odontogenic keratocyst (OKC) and ameloblastoma, compare the intensity of these lesions, analyze their intrinsic features, and predict their recurrence.	Study Type: Comparative study. Sample Size: 20 cases of OKC, 20 cases of ameloblastoma. Age Range: OKC—32.10 years (mean); ameloblastoma—35.25 years (mean). Country/Region: India.	SOX2.	Immunohistochemistry (IHC).	45% of OKC cases exhibited strongly positive reactivity for SOX2, while 65% of ameloblastoma cases were negative. Significant differences in the frequency of SOX2 expression between OKC and ameloblastoma.	Highly significant difference ($p < 0.01$) in SOX2 expression between OKC and ameloblastoma.	High expression of SOX2 in OKC indicates the presence of stem cells with significant self-renewal and proliferative properties, potentially signifying neoplastic behavior. Weak or absent expression of SOX2 in ameloblastoma suggests different molecular pathways involved in its neoplastic behavior.
Mukhopadhyay et al. (2023) [39]	To evaluate and compare the expression of WT-1, syndecan (CD138), and Snail in ameloblastoma and odontogenic keratocyst (OKC) and analyze their potential role in pathogenesis.	Study Type: Retrospective study. Sample Size: 20 ameloblastoma cases, 20 OKC cases. Country/Region: India.	WT-1, Syndecan (CD138), Snail.	Immunohistochemistry (IHC).	WT-1 and Snail overexpression in both Ameloblastoma and OKC. Syndecan significantly downregulated in both lesions. Higher WT-1 and syndecan immunopositivity in Ameloblastoma-like cells and basal cells compared to stellate reticulum-like cells.	Statistically significant differences in expression levels of syndecan and Snail ($p < 0.0001$). WT-1, syndecan, and Snail showed varying immunoreactivity across cell types ($p < 0.05$).	Underexpression of syndecan and upregulation of Snail promote local invasion and poor prognosis. Overexpression of WT-1 results in tumorigenesis, proliferation, and localized aggressiveness. Further investigation on OKC behavior is recommended.
Escobar et al. (2023) [35]	To assess the immunohistochemical expression of p53, Bcl-2, and Bax in conventional ameloblastoma (CA), unicystic ameloblastoma (UA), and odontogenic keratocysts (OKCs) both sporadic (OKC-NS/S) and syndromic (OKC-NBSCC).	Study Type: Research. Sample Size: 66 cases: 18 CA, 15 UA, 18 OKC-NS/S, 15 OKC-NBSCC. Age Range: Mean age: 31.61 years (range 8–75 years). Country/Region: Chile and Spain.	p53, Bcl-2, Bax.	Immunohistochemistry (IHC), Shapiro–Wilk test, ANOVA with Tukey's multiple comparisons, Kruskal–Wallis with Dunn's multiple comparisons.	Higher expression of p53, Bcl-2, and Bax in CA and MUA compared to OKC-NS/S and OKC-NBSCC. Significant differences in Bcl-2 expression between OKC-NS/S vs MUA, OKC-NS/S vs I/LUA, OKC-NS/S vs CA, OKC-NBSCC vs MUA, OKC-NBSCC vs I/LUA, and I/LUA vs CA. No statistical differences in p53 expression among groups.	Statistically significant differences in Bcl-2 expression ($p < 0.05$). No significant differences in p53 and Bax expression among groups. Spearman's test showed non-statistical correlation between p53 and Bax.	Increased expression of p53 and Bcl-2 in solid tumors (CA) and focal areas of mural ameloblastomatous proliferation for UA compared to lesions with cystic morphology (OKC and LUA) could be associated with aggressive behavior. Further investigation is required to elucidate the interactions between these proteins and their role in the pathogenesis of odontogenic lesions.

Table 3. Cont.

Authors	Objective	Study Details	Marker Identification Method	Cyst/Tumor Diagnosis Method	Results	Statistical Estimates	Conclusion
Silva et al. (2020) [40]	To compare the immunohistochemical expression of SOX2 and BCL-2 in odontogenic keratocyst (OKC) and ameloblastoma (AB) specimens, and to identify a possible correlation in their expression.	Study Type: Experimental study. Sample Size: 20 OKC samples, 20 AB samples. Country/Region: Brazil.	SOX2, BCL-2.	Immunohistochemistry (IHC), quantitative and qualitative scoring system.	SOX2 and BCL-2 expression observed in all OKC specimens. SOX2 immunostaining higher in OKC compared to AB ($p < 0.05$). BCL-2 immunostaining not significantly different between OKC and AB. No significant correlation between SOX2 and BCL-2 in OKC and AB specimens.	SOX2 immunostaining higher in OKC compared to AB ($p < 0.05$). No significant difference in BCL-2 immunostaining between OKC and AB.	SOX2 and BCL-2 expressions in OKC may suggest their relationship with the biological behavior of this lesion, and the higher expression of SOX2 might be an upstream influence on the Hh signaling pathway.
Soluk Tekkeşın et al. (2012) [41]	To determine the apoptotic features and proliferation potential of odontogenic keratocysts compared with ameloblastomas and radicular cysts by analyzing the role of bax, bcl-2, and Ki-67.	Study Type: Experimental study. Sample Size: 20 OKC samples, 20 RC samples, 23 AB samples. Age Range: 7–69 years. Country/Region: Turkey.	Bax, Bcl-2, Ki-67.	Immunohistochemistry (IHC).	Ameloblastoma showed stronger bcl-2 expression than OKCs and RCs. Bcl-2 expression in the whole thickness of epithelium and connective tissue of OKC was significantly higher than RC. Bax expression in the epithelium of RC was significantly higher than OKC and AB. The lining epithelium of OKC showed stronger Ki-67 expression than AB and RC.	Significant differences in bcl-2 expression ($p < 0.001$), bax expression ($p < 0.020$), and Ki-67 expression ($p < 0.043$).	High expressions of bcl-2 and Ki-67 in OKCs accord with their aggressive clinical behavior and high recurrence rate. The proliferation potential of epithelium and the overexpression of various anti-apoptotic proteins in odontogenic epithelial tumors are significant for their clinical behavior.
Kaczmarzyk et al. (2018) [42]	To investigate the prognostic relevance of various clinicopathological features as well as immunoexpression of COX-2, bcl-2, PCNA, and p53 in sporadic odontogenic keratocysts (OKCs).	Study Type: Retrospective study. Sample Size: 41 OKC patients. Age Range Mean age: 40.24 years (range 7–65). Country/Region: Poland.	COX-2, bcl-2, PCNA, p53.	Histopathological analysis, immunohistochemistry (IHC), Fisher's exact test, Student's t-test, Mann–Whitney test, Cox proportional hazard model, Spearman correlation analysis.	Significant differences between recurrent and non-recurrent cysts in terms of multilocularity ($p = 0.029$), cortical perforation ($p = 0.001$), and lesion size ($p < 0.001$). Immunoexpression of PCNA significantly correlates with radiographic evidence of cortical perforation ($p = 0.048$). Significant positive correlation between COX-2 and bcl-2 ($p = 0.001$) and significant negative correlation between COX-2 and age ($p = 0.002$).	Recurrences in 29.27% of cases. Hazard risk for recurrence: 3.362 (95% CI 1.066–10.598) for multilocular cysts, 7.801 (95% CI 2.1–28.985) for cortical perforation, and 1.004 (1.002–1.006) for 1 mm² of lesion size on panoramic radiographs.	Larger size, multilocularity, and cortical perforation in sporadic OKC may correlate with recurrence. Immunohistochemical analyses of COX-2, bcl-2, PCNA, and p53 lack prognostic utility in sporadic OKC.

Table 3. Cont.

Authors	Objective	Study Details	Marker Identification Method	Cyst/Tumor Diagnosis Method	Results	Statistical Estimates	Conclusion
Kisielowski et al. (2023) [43]	To compare the prognostic relevance of clinicopathological factors in sporadic and syndromic odontogenic keratocysts (OKCs).	Sample Size: 43 OKC cases: 31 sporadic OKCs, 12 syndromic OKCs. Country/Region: Poland.	COX-2, Bcl-2, PCNA, p53, Ki-67, OPG, RANK, RANKL, RANKL/OPG balance.	Histological classification, immunohistochemistry.	NBCCS-associated OKCs are more prone to recur than sporadic ones. Larger size, multilocularity, cortical perforation in sporadic OKCs indicate higher recurrence risk. COX-2 upregulated in recurrent sporadic OKCs. Syndromic OKCs exhibit higher RANKL > OPG ratio.	NBCCS-associated OKCs had 83.33% recurrence rate vs. 35.48% in sporadic OKCs ($p = 0.013$). HR for recurrence in NBCCS-associated OKCs: 9.091 (95% CI: 1.682–49.123; $p = 0.01$).	Syndromic OKCs have higher recurrence risk. COX-2 upregulation in recurrent sporadic OKCs and RANKL/OPG imbalance in recurrent syndromic OKCs, though findings have no prognostic relevance.
Naz et al. (2015) [9]	To determine the biological behavior of common odontogenic cystic lesions by analyzing and comparing bcl-2 expression amongst them.	Sample Size: 90 formalin-fixed paraffin-embedded tissue samples; 26 primary cases each of radicular cysts (RCs), dentigerous cysts (DCs), and odontogenic keratocysts (OKCs), 12 recurrent OKCs. Country/Region: Pakistan.	Bcl-2.	Immunohistochemistry (IHC).	Recurrent OKCs showed strong positivity for bcl-2, absent in primary cases ($p < 0.05$). Variation in bcl-2 expression between RC and DC is not significant, but significant when compared with primary OKCs.	All 12 recurrent OKCs showed strong bcl-2 expression ($p < 0.05$).	Recurrent OKC showed more aggressive behavior than primary counterparts and RC/DC. Bcl-2 is valuable in determining aggressive biological behavior of odontogenic lesions.
Rahman et al. (2013) [10]	To evaluate and compare the proliferative index in the epithelium surrounding the impacted third molar teeth, dentigerous cysts, and gingiva.	Study Type: Case control study. Sample Size: 40 pericoronal tissues from asymptomatic impacted third molars, 20 dentigerous cysts, 20 normal gingiva samples. Country/Region: India.	Ki-67, Bcl-2.	Immunohistochemistry (IHC) using DigiPro™ version 4.0 Image analysis software.	Bcl-2 overexpressed in pericoronal tissues with squamous metaplasia and dentigerous cysts. Ki-67 labeling index (Li) is higher in pericoronal tissues with squamous metaplasia compared to reduced enamel epithelium. Ki-67 Li in pericoronal tissues with inflammation is significantly higher than in those with no-to-mild inflammation.	Ki-67 Li: pericoronal tissue with squamous metaplasia (19.87 ± 1.45), dentigerous cyst (23.81 ± 2.64), normal gingiva (3.006 ± 0.76).	Pericoronal tissues of asymptomatic impacted third molars show high proliferative activity and may develop into odontogenic cysts or tumors. Overexpression of Ki-67 and Bcl-2 indicates potential pathological changes.

Table 3. Cont.

Authors	Objective	Study Details	Marker Identification Method	Cyst/Tumor Diagnosis Method	Results	Statistical Estimates	Conclusion
Byun et al. (2013) [44]	To report on two cases of expansile keratocystic odontogenic tumors (KCOTs) in the maxilla and evaluate the immunohistochemical characteristics.	Study Type: Case report. Sample Size: 2 KCOT patients. Follow-up period: more than 2 years. Country/Region: Korea.	BCL2, BAX, Ki-67, p53, p63.	Histological classification, immunohistochemistry (IHC).	Both cases involved large KCOT occupying the entire maxilla and maxillary sinus. Strong expression of p53 and p63 in the lining epithelium. Moderate expression of BCL2 and Ki-67. BAX was almost negatively detected. These findings indicate increased anti-apoptotic activity and cell proliferation rate but decreased apoptosis in KCOT.	Not specified.	Expansile KCOT possesses increased anti-apoptotic activity and cell proliferation rate but decreased apoptosis, contributing to tumor enlargement, aggressive behavior, and high recurrence rate.
Edamatsu et al. (2005) [45]	To examine the role of apoptosis-related factors in dental follicles (DFs) and dentigerous cysts (DCs) associated with impacted third molars.	Study Type: Comparative study. Sample Size: 80 DFs, 27 DCs. Country/Region: Japan.	Fas, bcl-2, ssDNA, Ki-67.	Immunohistochemistry (IHC).	Fas and ssDNA were detected in superficial epithelial cells; bcl-2 and Ki-67 in epithelial cells near the basement membrane. bcl-2 lower in DFs than DCs. ssDNA higher in DFs; Ki-67 higher in DCs.	Significant differences in bcl-2 expression ($p < 0.05$).	Differences in apoptosis-related factors and proliferative markers suggest roles in DC pathogenesis and modulation by epithelial characteristics and inflammation in DFs.
Razavi et al. (2015) [46]	To evaluate and compare the expression of Bcl-2 and EGFR proteins in keratocystic odontogenic tumor (KCOT), dentigerous cyst (DC), and ameloblastoma (AB).	Study Type: Cross-sectional study. Sample Size: 16 KCOT, 16 DC, 16 AB. Country/Region: Iran.	Bcl-2, EGFR.	Immunohistochemistry (IHC).	All AB and KCOT cases positively stained for Bcl-2, but not DC. Bcl-2 is higher in peripheral layer of AB and basal layer of KCOT. EGFR is expressed in all AB and DC, but not KCOT. EGFR is higher in peripheral layer of AB and basal layer of DC.	Significant difference in Bcl-2 expression between KCOT and DC ($p = 0.02$). No EGFR expression in KCOT, significant EGFR expression in AB and DC ($p < 0.01$).	KCOT shows different biological activity and growth mechanisms compared to DC and AB. KCOT has high Bcl-2 expression but no EGFR, indicating less aggressive potential than AB.
Sreedhar et al. (2014) [47]	To analyze the effect of inflammation on the biological behavior of odontogenic keratocyst (OKC) and dentigerous cyst (DC) using PCNA and Bcl-2 markers.	Study Type: Retrospective study. Sample Size: 10 classical OKC, 10 inflamed OKC, 10 classical DC, 10 inflamed DC. Country/Region: India.	PCNA, Bcl-2.	Immunohistochemistry (IHC).	Inflamed OKC and DC showed significant increase in PCNA expression and decrease in Bcl-2 expression compared to non-inflamed cysts. The correlation between inflammation and proliferative and anti-apoptotic activity was statistically non-significant.	PCNA and Bcl-2 expression in inflamed OKC and DC were significantly different from non-inflamed cysts ($p < 0.05$).	Inflammation changes the behavior of neoplastic epithelium in OKC, indicating increased proliferation and survival of epithelial cells. In DC, inflammation leads to changes in the epithelial lining.

Table 3. Cont.

Authors	Objective	Study Details	Marker Identification Method	Cyst/Tumor Diagnosis Method	Results	Statistical Estimates	Conclusion
Villalba et al. (2012) [48]	To associate radiographic and histopathological features of pericoronal follicles (PFs) of asymptomatic impacted teeth and evaluate cell proliferation and apoptosis in epithelium.	Sample Size: 140 PFs. Age Range: Mean age: 20.01 years (range 9–50). Country/Region: Argentina.	Ki-67, Bcl-2.	Radiographic analysis, histopathology, immunohistochemistry (IHC).	27 normal PFs (NPFs) and 13 hyperplastic PFs (HPFs). 87.8% of PFs exhibited epithelium on the surface. Reduced enamel epithelium observed in 61.4% NPFs and 46.2% HPFs. Squamous metaplasia in 13.4% NPFs and 30.8% HPFs. Cystic epithelium in 11.8% NPFs and 23% HPFs. Ki-67 PI: NPF (1.97 ± 1.41%), DC (7.97 ± 2.05%). Bcl-2: 64.3% NPFs, 70% DCs.	p-values: Ki-67 PI ($p < 0.05$), Bcl-2 ($p > 0.05$).	Scant epithelial proliferation in PFs suggests low risk for development of odontogenic pathologies without additional stimulus.
Nimmanagoti et al. (2019) [49]	Evaluate and compare immunohistochemically, the biological behavior of KCOT with normal oral mucosa.	Sample Size: 30 KCOT cases; Control group: 30 normal oral mucosa. Country/Region: Telangana, India.	p53, Bcl-2, COX-2, CD105.	Immunohistochemistry.	73% p53 positive, 77% Bcl-2 positive, 60% COX-2 positive in KCOT samples. Mean vascular density: KCOT (13.8) vs. normal oral mucosa (4.1).	Results were statistically significant ($p < 0.05$).	Angiogenesis, cell proliferation, and anti-apoptosis contribute to the unique biological behavior of KCOT.
Phull et al. (2017) [50]	To evaluate bcl-2 expression and its distribution in the epithelial lining as well as connective tissue cells of ameloblastoma, KCOT, and radicular cyst.	Sample Size: 120 formalin-fixed paraffin-embedded tissues: 40 ameloblastoma, 40 KCOT, and 40 radicular cyst samples. Country/Region: Udaipur, Rajasthan, India.	Bcl-2.	Immunohistochemical evaluation.	Positive bcl-2 expression: all KCOTs, 38/40 ameloblastomas, 10/40 radicular cysts. Higher bcl-2 staining in KCOT vs. ameloblastoma and radicular cyst. Solid ameloblastomas showed higher expression than unicystic.	Significant differences in bcl-2 staining between ameloblastoma, KCOT, and radicular cyst (ANOVA, $p = 0.00$). Significant differences between KCOT and ameloblastoma, and between ameloblastoma and radicular cyst. There is no significant difference between radicular cyst and KCOT in connective tissue.	High bcl-2 expression in KCOT suggests neoplastic characteristics. Connective tissue cells are important in the biological behavior of odontogenic keratocyst. Further genetic studies are needed for understanding KCOT pathogenesis.

Table 3. Cont.

Authors	Objective	Study Details	Marker Identification Method	Cyst/Tumor Diagnosis Method	Results	Statistical Estimates	Conclusion
Sindura et al. (2013) [51]	To study the expression of Bcl-2 protein in ameloblastoma and keratocystic odontogenic tumor (KCOT) to determine their apoptotic behaviors and biological nature.	Study Type: Histochemical study. Sample Size: 20 ameloblastoma, 20 KCOT. Age Range: Mean age: ameloblastoma—31.6 years; KCOT—37.8 years. Country/Region: Bangalore, Karnataka, India.	Bcl-2.	Immunohistochemical evaluation.	Positive Bcl-2 expression: 85% (17/20) ameloblastoma, 85% (17/20) KCOT, 100% (3/3) lymphomas. Ameloblastoma showed expression in peripheral and intermediate cells, KCOT in basal layer.	Significant differences in Bcl-2 staining area and intensity between ameloblastoma, KCOT, and radicular cyst. Ameloblastoma showed higher expression than unicystic variants.	Bcl-2 expression indicates KCOT's neoplastic characteristics. The expression in connective tissue cells suggests a role in the biological behavior of KCOT. Further genetic studies are needed.
Cserni et al. (2020) [52]	To analyze jaw cysts for the expression of CK17 and bcl2, assessing their diagnostic value.	Study Type: Histochemical study. Sample Size: 85 cysts from 72 patients. Age Range: Median age: 44 years (range: 11–76). Country/Region: Szeged, Hungary.	CK17, Bcl-2.	Immunohistochemical evaluation.	21 OKCs with typical CK17 and bcl2 expression, non-OKCs showed varied CK17 and bcl2 positivity but weaker than OKCs. Inflammation altered IHC phenotype in OKCs.	Not specified.	CK17 and bcl2 IHC can aid in diagnosing OKCs but must be interpreted with caution. The IHC patterns are adjuncts, not definitive diagnostic tools.

Table 3. *Cont.*

Authors	Objective	Study Details	Marker Identification Method	Cyst/Tumor Diagnosis Method	Results	Statistical Estimates	Conclusion
Shetty et al. (2010) [53]	To evaluate the expression of p53 in odontogenic keratocyst (OKC) and ameloblastoma to correlate with the aggressiveness of these lesions.	Study Type: Retrospective study. Sample Size: 36 cases (18 OKC and 18 Ameloblastoma). Country/Region: Ghaziabad, Uttar Pradesh, India.	p53.	Immunohistochemical evaluation.	p53 positivity in all OKC and ameloblastoma cases. p53 positive cells predominantly in the suprabasal cell layer of OKC and peripheral pre-ameloblast-like cells in ameloblastoma. Higher total p53 count in ameloblastoma compared to OKC. There is no statistically significant difference in the intensely stained p53 cell count between the two lesions.	Significant difference in total p53 count between ameloblastoma and OKC. There is no significant difference in the intensely stained p53 cell count.	High p53 expression in OKC suggests its aggressive nature, warranting more aggressive treatment modalities.
González-Moles et al. (2006) [54]	To investigate the association between p53 alterations and HPV infection in odontogenic keratocysts (OKCs), and to study proliferation and epithelial maturation patterns by topographic analysis of Ki-67 expression.	Study Type: Immunohistochemical and molecular study. Sample Size: 83 OKC samples (29 NBCCS-associated, 29 solitary non-recurrent, 20 solitary recurrent, 5 chondroid keratocysts). Age Range: Mean age: 26 ± 14.1 years. Country/Region: Mexico.	p53 (PAb 244) and Ki-67 (MIB-1); PCR for HPV DNA.	Histopathological analysis using hematoxylin–eosin staining.	p53 protein expressed in 14.6% of cases; no HPV DNA detected; 11% had mild epithelial dysplasia. Suprabasal Ki-67 expression significantly more frequent than basal ($p < 0.001$). Significant association between p53 expression and epithelial dysplasia ($p = 0.023$). No association between Ki-67 expression and OKC type, dysplasia, or p53 expression.	$p = 0.023$ for p53 and dysplasia association, $p < 0.001$ for suprabasal vs. basal Ki-67 expression.	HPVs do not participate in OKC etiology; p53 mutations are unlikely to play a major role; OKCs show neoplasm-like behavior with local destructive capacity.

Table 3. Cont.

Authors	Objective	Study Details	Marker Identification Method	Cyst/Tumor Diagnosis Method	Results	Statistical Estimates	Conclusion
Gadbail et al. (2009) [36]	To evaluate the biological aggressiveness of odontogenic keratocyst/keratocystic odontogenic tumor (KCOT), radicular cyst (RC), and dentigerous cyst (DC) by observing the actual proliferative activity of epithelium, and p53 protein expression.	Study Type: Observational study.	Ki-67, AgNOR count, p53.	Histopathological analysis using Ki-67 Labelling Index, AgNOR count, and p53 protein expression.	Ki-67 positive cells are higher in suprabasal cell layers of KCOT, uniform distribution, fewer in basal cell layer of RC and DC. AgNOR counts significantly higher in suprabasal cell layers of KCOT. Higher actual proliferative activity in suprabasal cell layers of KCOT. Dense, scattered p53 immunolabelling in basal and suprabasal cell layers of KCOT. Weakly stained p53 positive cells diffusely distributed in KCOT, mainly in basal cell layer of RC and DC.	Not specified.	Quantitative and qualitative differences in proliferative activity and p53 protein expression in sporadic KCOT may be associated with intrinsic growth potential, explaining its locally aggressive biological behavior. AgNOR count and p53 protein detection in odontogenic lesions can predict biological behavior and prognosis.
de Oliveira et al. (2008) [55]	To analyze p53 and proliferating cell nuclear antigen (PCNA) expression in radicular and dentigerous cysts, odontogenic keratocysts, and calcifying odontogenic cysts (Gorlin cysts).	Study Type: Immunohistochemical study. Sample Size: 11 radicular cysts, 12 odontogenic keratocysts, 15 dentigerous cysts, 10 calcifying odontogenic cysts. Country/Region: Brazil.	p53, PCNA.	Histopathological analysis using hematoxylin–eosin staining.	PCNA expression was significantly greater in the basal layer of radicular cysts and in the suprabasal layer of odontogenic keratocysts. The percentage of p53 positive cells was significantly greater in the suprabasal layer of odontogenic keratocysts. p53 and PCNA expression patterns in dentigerous and radicular cysts were similar. Different patterns observed in odontogenic keratocysts and Gorlin cysts, indicating different tumor growth patterns.	Significant differences between layers in keratocysts for both p53 ($p = 0.01$) and PCNA ($p = 0.01$). Significant correlation between p53 and PCNA in basal and suprabasal layers of dentigerous and Gorlin cysts ($p < 0.05$).	PCNA and p53 expressions in radicular and dentigerous cysts show similar characteristics despite different origins. Different expression patterns in odontogenic keratocysts and Gorlin cysts suggest different growth patterns. Further studies are needed to investigate the role of inflammation in these lesions.

Table 3. Cont.

Authors	Objective	Study Details	Marker Identification Method	Cyst/Tumor Diagnosis Method	Results	Statistical Estimates	Conclusion
Gaballah et al. (2010) [56]	To investigate the immunohistochemical expression of P53 protein in odontogenic cysts.	Study Type: Immunohistochemical study. Sample Size: 16 radicular cysts (RCs), 11 odontogenic keratocysts (OKCs), 3 dentigerous cysts (DCs). Age Range: Mean age: 35.2 ± 16.5 years. Country/Region: Egypt.	Monoclonal mouse antibody to p53.	Histopathological analysis using hematoxylin–eosin staining.	P53 positive cases: 81.8% OKC, 33.3% DC, 0% RC. P53 expression seen in basal and parabasal cells of epithelial lining.	Data were analyzed using SPSS 10 software. No specific statistical values were provided.	High P53 expression in OKC suggests greater proliferative activity, supporting reclassification as keratocystic odontogenic tumor (KCOT). Low or no P53 expression in RC and DC indicates lower proliferative activity.
Chandrangsu et al. (2016) [57]	To characterize the expression of p53, p63, and p73 in KCOTs and the relationship between their expression and KCOT angiogenesis and recurrence.	Study Type: Immunohistochemical study. Sample Size: 39 KCOTs. Age Range: Mean age: 37.1 ± 21.8 years. Country/Region: Thailand.	Monoclonal antibodies specific to human p53, p63, p73, and CD105.	Histopathological analysis using hematoxylin and eosin staining.	p53 expression: 59% of cases. p63 expression: 82% of cases. p73 expression: 66.7% of cases. Mean MVD: 26.7 ± 15.8 per HPF. Significant positive relationships noted for p53, p63, and p73 expression and MVD ($p < 0.001$). Increased expression of p53, p63, and p73 significantly associated with local recurrence ($p = 0.001, 0.012,$ and 0.017, respectively).	Fisher's exact test, Mann–Whitney U test, Spearman's correlation coefficients, $p < 0.05$ considered statistically significant.	p53, p63, and p73 expression and increased angiogenesis contribute to the locally aggressive and invasive behaviors of KCOTs, supporting their classification as tumors.

Table 3. *Cont.*

Authors	Objective	Study Details	Marker Identification Method	Cyst/Tumor Diagnosis Method	Results	Statistical Estimates	Conclusion
Khan et al. (2019) [58]	To evaluate the management and follow-up of an extensive odontogenic keratocyst (OKC) over a 10-year period.	Study Type: Clinical case report. Sample Size: One case of extensive pan-mandibular OKC. Age Range: 35-year-old female. Country/Region: Saudi Arabia.	Ki-67, bcl-2.	Radiographic examination and histopathological analysis.	Initial treatment: marsupialization led to reduced Ki-67 and bcl-2 expression. Persistent area required curettage, extraction, and Carnoy's solution application. 10-year follow-up showed complete resolution with no recurrence.	Not applicable.	Marsupialization is effective as an initial treatment for extensive OKC, but additional aggressive treatment may be necessary for complete resolution. Ki-67 and bcl-2 are site-specific markers related to OKC recurrence.
Kadashetti et al. (2020) [59]	To understand the behavior of epithelial cells in pathogenesis and biological aspects of odontogenic keratocyst (OKC) in diagnosis by analyzing the expression of p53, p63, and proliferating cell nuclear antigen (PCNA).	Study Type: Immunohistochemical study. Sample Size: 21 cases of OKCs. Country/Region: India (Maharashtra).	p53, p63, PCNA.	Histopathological analysis using hematoxylin and eosin staining.	p53-positive cells mainly in suprabasal layers. p63- and PCNA-positive cells found throughout the lining epithelium, including basal and suprabasal layers. p63 and PCNA showed higher staining intensity compared to p53.	Significant difference ($p < 0.01$) between basal and suprabasal cells in OKC.	The biological behavior of OKCs may be related to the suprabasal proliferative compartment. High levels of p53, p63, and PCNA suggest that these proteins contribute to the biological profile and possibly the tumorigenesis of OKCs.
Slusarenko da Silva et al. (2021) [8]	To assess the expression of the p53 protein in odontogenic keratocysts (OKCs) compared to dentigerous cysts (DCs) and ameloblastomas (AMBs) and determine whether OKCs behave more like tumors than cysts.	Study Type: Systematic review and meta-analysis. Sample Size: 13 studies included. Country/Region: Brazil, Netherlands.	p53.	Histopathological criteria defined by WHO in 1992, 2005, and 2017.	126 records identified; 13 studies included. OKCs have a 23% higher probability of expressing p53 compared to DCs ($p < 0.003$). OKCs have a 4% higher probability of expressing p53 compared to AMBs ($p = 0.28$). p53 expressed mainly in the suprabasal layer in OKCs.	Risk Difference (RD) for OKCs vs. DCs: 0.23 [−0.39, −0.08], $p < 0.003$. RD for OKCs vs. AMBs: 0.04 [−0.11, 0.03], $p = 0.28$. Significant heterogeneity among studies ($I^2 = 78\%$ for OKCs vs. DCs, $I^2 = 27\%$ for OKCs vs. AMBs).	OKCs are more likely to express p53, indicating a behavior more like tumors rather than cysts. The classification of OKCs as keratocystic odontogenic tumors (KCOTs) should be reconsidered.

Table 3. Cont.

Authors	Objective	Study Details	Marker Identification Method	Cyst/Tumor Diagnosis Method	Results	Statistical Estimates	Conclusion
Yanatatsaneejit et al. (2015) [60]	To clarify the association between the p53 polymorphism at codon 72 and susceptibility to the sporadic keratocystic odontogenic tumor (KCOT).	Study Type: Case–control study. Sample Size: 100 KCOT samples and 160 healthy controls. Age Range: Average age of KCOT patients: 32.23 years; Average age of healthy controls: 32.51 years. Country/Region: Thailand.	Polymerase chain reaction–restriction fragment length polymorphism (PCR-RFLP), confirmed by direct sequencing.	Histopathological confirmation of KCOT.	Genotype frequencies in controls: Pro/Pro (23.8%), Arg/Pro (49.4%), Arg/Arg (26.9%). Genotype frequencies in KCOT cohort: Pro/Pro (43.0%), Arg/Pro (39.0%), Arg/Arg (18.0%). p53 Pro allele associated with increased KCOT risk (OR = 1.77, 95% CI = 1.22–2.59, $p = 0.0024$). Sex-adjusted OR = 1.71 (95% CI = 1.17–2.50, $p = 0.0046$). p53 Pro homozygous associated with twofold KCOT risk (adjusted OR = 2.17, 95% CI = 1.23–3.84, $p = 0.0062$).	OR = 1.77 (95% CI = 1.22–2.59, $p = 0.0024$); sex-adjusted OR = 1.71 (95% CI = 1.17–2.50, $p = 0.0046$); adjusted OR = 2.17 (95% CI = 1.23–3.84, $p = 0.0062$).	The C/C genotype of the p53 gene codon 72 increases the risk of developing sporadic KCOT and may be a useful tool for screening and diagnostic purposes.
Varsha et al. (2014) [61]	To investigate the expression of p63 protein in odontogenic keratocyst (OKC), solid ameloblastoma, unicystic ameloblastoma, and follicular tissue, and compare their proliferative activity and biological behavior.	Study Type: Immunohistochemical study. Sample Size: 12 OKCs, 12 solid ameloblastomas, 14 unicystic ameloblastomas, 10 follicular tissues. Country/Region: India (Bangalore, Karnataka).	Anti-p63 polyclonal antibody and super sensitive polymer HRP detection system.	Histopathological analysis using hematoxylin and eosin staining.	p63 expression in suprabasal compartment of OKC equivalent to central neoplastic cells of solid ameloblastoma and unicystic ameloblastoma type 3. Significant difference in p63 expression between OKC and unicystic ameloblastoma type 1, and between solid ameloblastoma and unicystic ameloblastoma type 1. Higher expression of p63 in OKC correlates with aggressive behavior.	Significant difference ($p < 0.05$) in p63 expression between OKC vs unicystic ameloblastoma type 1, and solid ameloblastoma vs unicystic ameloblastoma type 1.	Higher p63 expression in OKC suggests aggressive behavior, supporting the classification as keratocystic odontogenic tumor. Different expression patterns among the lesions can guide treatment modalities and prognosis.

Table 3. Cont.

Authors	Objective	Study Details	Marker Identification Method	Cyst/Tumor Diagnosis Method	Results	Statistical Estimates	Conclusion
Sajeevan et al. (2014) [62]	To assess and compare the expression of p53 and PCNA in the lining epithelium of odontogenic keratocyst (OKC) and periapical cyst (PA).	Study Type: Retrospective, immunohistochemical study. Sample Size: 10 OKCs and 10 PAs.	p53, PCNA.	Histopathological examination using hematoxylin and eosin staining.	OKC showed 100% PCNA expression; PA showed 60% PCNA expression. OKC showed 60% p53 expression; PA showed 10% p53 expression. PCNA staining intensity was more significant than p53 in both OKC and PA. Suprabasal cells in OKC showed more intense staining than basal cells with both antibodies	Chi-square test showed significant differences in staining intensity ($p = 0.013$ for PCNA vs. p53 in OKC).	OKC shows significant proliferative activity compared to PA using PCNA and p53. PCNA staining is more intense than p53 in both OKC and PA, indicating higher proliferative potential in OKC.
Razavi et al. (2014) [63]	To analyze the clinicopathological and immunohistochemical features of primary and recurrent keratocystic odontogenic tumors (KCOTs), focusing on p53 expression to identify markers predictive of recurrence.	Study Type: Descriptive analytic study. Sample Size: 78 KCOT specimens: 52 primary KCOTs and 26 recurrent KCOTs. Age Range: Mean age: Primary KCOTs: 32.15 ± 16.10 years; Recurrent KCOTs: 27.23 ± 13.04 years. Country/Region: Isfahan, Iran.	Anti-p53 monoclonal antibody.	Histopathological examination using hematoxylin and eosin staining.	No significant differences in age, gender, or anatomical location between primary and recurrent KCOTs. Histopathological features like epithelial budding ($p = 0.001$), daughter cysts ($p = 0.013$), and odontogenic rests ($p = 0.036$) were more common in recurrent KCOTs. p53 expression was significantly higher in recurrent KCOTs ($p = 0.041$).	T-test, Chi-square, and Fisher's exact tests showed significant differences in histopathological features and p53 expression between primary and recurrent KCOTs.	Predictive factors for KCOT recurrence include epithelial budding, daughter cysts, and odontogenic rests. p53 expression at diagnosis can help predict recurrence.

Table 3. *Cont.*

Authors	Objective	Study Details	Marker Identification Method	Cyst/Tumor Diagnosis Method	Results	Statistical Estimates	Conclusion
Chandrashekar et al. (2020) [64]	To investigate the clinical behavior of odontogenic keratocyst (OKC) by evaluating p53, MDM2 expression, and AgNOR staining, and to ascertain if these markers correlate with clinical outcomes and recurrence tendency.	Study Type: Retrospective, immunohistochemical study. Sample Size: 21 histologically confirmed cases of recurrent and non-recurrent OKCs. Country/Region: India (Manipal, Karnataka).	p53 and MDM2, AgNOR staining.	Histopathological examination using hematoxylin and eosin staining.	Recurrent OKCs showed higher expression of MDM2 and AgNOR compared to non-recurrent cases. Recurrent cases displayed histopathological features such as epithelial budding, daughter cysts, and odontogenic rests. Significant difference in MDM2 and AgNOR staining between recurrent and non-recurrent groups ($p = 0.001$). There is no significant difference in p53 scores between recurrent and non-recurrent groups.	Mann–Whitney U-test showed significant differences in MDM2 and AgNOR staining ($p = 0.001$), and significant correlation between p53 and MDM2, and AgNOR and MDM2.	Higher expression of MDM2 and AgNOR in recurrent lesions indicates their potential use in predicting recurrence and guiding additional surgical interventions to improve prognosis.
Deyhimi et al. (2012) [65]	To evaluate the quantity and intensity of the expression of p53 protein and transforming growth factor alpha (TGF-alpha) in odontogenic keratocyst (OKC) and orthokeratinized odontogenic cyst (OOC) to compare their biological behavior.	Study Type: Cross-sectional, descriptive analytic study. Sample Size: 15 OKC and 15 OOC. Country/Region: Iran.	Monoclonal anti-p53 and anti-TGF-alpha antibodies.	Histopathological examination using hematoxylin and eosin staining.	p53: No significant difference in the basal layer ($p = 0.076$), significant in the parabasal layer ($p = 0.003$). TGF-alpha: No significant difference in the basal layer ($p = 0.284$), significant in the parabasal layer ($p = 0.015$). Higher expression of p53 and TGF-alpha in OKC compared to OOC, suggesting higher carcinomatous potential in OKC.	Mann–Whitney and Wilcoxon tests; significant differences noted with $p < 0.05$.	OKC shows higher expression of p53 and TGF-alpha than OOC, indicating a higher theoretical potential for carcinomatous changes in OKC.

Table 3. Cont.

Authors	Objective	Study Details	Marker Identification Method	Cyst/Tumor Diagnosis Method	Results	Statistical Estimates	Conclusion
Ogden et al. (1992) [66]	To assess p53 protein expression in a range of odontogenic cysts, including developmental and inflammatory origins.	Study Type: Immunohistochemical study. Sample Size: 12 radicular cysts, 12 dentigerous cysts, 12 odontogenic keratocysts (OKC). Country/Region: Scotland.	Polyclonal antibody CM-1 and standard immunoperoxidase technique.	Histopathological examination using hematoxylin and eosin staining.	p53 expression detected in 5 of 12 OKCs, but not in radicular or dentigerous cysts. p53-positive cells actively dividing, similar regions positive for PCNA. No significant difference in clinical characteristics or recurrence between p53-positive and p53-negative OKCs. p53-positive OKCs lacked features like cholesterol clefts, hyaline bodies, or satellite cysts.	Not provided.	Increased p53 expression in some OKCs suggests higher epithelial activity and potential association with Gorlin Goltz syndrome. p53 expression may be indicative of malignant potential within OKC linings.
Aldahash (2023) [67]	To systematically review and perform a meta-analysis on the expression of p53 in odontogenic lesions, including odontogenic keratocyst (OKC), dentigerous cyst (DC), and ameloblastoma (AMB).	Study Type: Systematic review and meta-analysis. Sample Size: 18 studies included in the meta-analysis. Country/Region: Saudi Arabia.	p53.	Histopathological criteria defined by WHO in 1992, 2005, and 2017.	OKCs have a 23% higher probability of expressing p53 compared to DCs ($p = 0.003$). OKCs have a 4% lower probability of expressing p53 compared to AMBs ($p = 0.028$). p53 expression suggests that OKCs act more like tumors than cysts.	Risk difference (RD) for p53 expression between OKCs and DCs: 0.23 [0.39, 0.08], $p = 0.003$. RD between OKCs and AMBs: −0.04 [−0.11, 0.03], $p = 0.028$.	OKCs exhibit higher p53 expression compared to DCs, indicating a more tumor-like behavior. This supports reclassifying OKCs as keratocystic odontogenic tumors (KCOTs).

Table 3. Cont.

Authors	Objective	Study Details	Marker Identification Method	Cyst/Tumor Diagnosis Method	Results	Statistical Estimates	Conclusion
Gupta et al. (2019) [68]	To compare the expression pattern of p63 in the epithelium of tooth germ, dentigerous cyst (DC), and ameloblastoma (AB).	Study Type: Descriptive observational study. Sample Size: 30 tooth germs, 30 DCs, 30 ABs. Country/Region: India (Chhattisgarh, Maharashtra).	p63 antibody and Streptavidin–Biotin Detection System HRP-DAB.	Histopathological examination using hematoxylin and eosin staining.	p63 expression in 100% of tooth germs, 100% of DCs, 100% of ABs. Highest p63 labeling index (LI) in ABs, followed by tooth germs, and then DCs. Dense p63 immunolabeling in the basal and parabasal layers of DCs; peripheral cells of ameloblastic follicle in ABs; almost complete epithelium in tooth germs.	Non-significant difference in p63 LI among ABs, DCs, and tooth germs ($p > 0.05$).	p63 plays a role in the differentiation and proliferation of odontogenic epithelial cells. p63 can be used as a prognostic marker for aggressive and invasive odontogenic lesions. Different p63 isoforms may have distinct functions in developing and lesional odontogenic tissues.
Akshatha et al. (2017) [69]	To qualitatively and quantitatively analyze the expression of inducible nitric oxide synthase (iNOS) in the epithelial lining of radicular cysts (RCs), dentigerous cysts (DCs), and odontogenic keratocysts (OKCs) to determine the role of iNOS in their pathogenesis.	Study Type: Qualitative and quantitative immunohistochemical study. Sample Size: 20 RCs, 20 DCs, and 20 OKCs. Country/Region: India (Bengaluru, Karnataka).	Immunohisto-chemistry using anti-iNOS antibody.	Histopathological examination using hematoxylin and eosin staining.	iNOS-positive cells: OKCs (57.1%), RCs (28.6%), DCs (14.3%). Significant iNOS expression in OKCs ($p > 0.000$) and RCs ($p > 0.001$), but not in DCs. iNOS staining in OKCs: 47.4% showed severe intensity, mainly in basal and parabasal layers; 31.6% of RCs and 21.1% of DCs showed severe intensity. There was no significant difference in staining intensity among the three cyst types.	Mann–Whitney test and contingency coefficient showed statistically significant iNOS expression in OKCs ($p > 0.000$), RCs ($p > 0.001$), no significant values for DCs.	Increased iNOS expression in OKCs may contribute to their aggressive behavior and malignant potential, suggesting a role in bone resorption and accumulation of wild-type p53 protein.

Table 3. *Cont.*

Authors	Objective	Study Details	Marker Identification Method	Cyst/Tumor Diagnosis Method	Results	Statistical Estimates	Conclusion
Fatemeh et al. (2017) [70]	To assess and compare the expression of the tumor suppressor gene p53 in inflamed and non-inflamed types of odontogenic keratocyst (OKC) and dentigerous cyst (DC).	Study Type: Immunohistochemical study. Sample Size: 34 OKCs (18 inflamed, 16 non-inflamed), 31 DCs (16 inflamed, 15 non-inflamed), 14 dental follicles. Country/Region: Iran.	Monoclonal mouse antihuman p53 antibody.	Histopathological examination using hematoxylin and eosin staining.	Mean percentage of p53-positive cells: dental follicles (0.7%), non-inflamed OKCs (5.4%), inflamed OKCs (17.3%), non-inflamed DCs (1.2%), and inflamed DCs (2.2%). Significant differences between all groups ($p < 0.05$) except between inflamed and non-inflamed DCs, and between dental follicles and non-inflamed DCs.	Kruskal-Wallis H and Mann-Whitney U tests showed significant differences ($p < 0.05$) between the groups for p53 expression.	p53 expression is higher in OKCs than in DCs, suggesting different growth mechanisms. Inflammation increases p53 expression in OKCs, indicating a potential role in their aggressive behavior.
Seyedmajidi et al. (2013) [12]	To evaluate the expression of p53 and PCNA in keratocystic odontogenic tumors (KCOTs) compared with radicular cysts (RCs), dentigerous cysts (DCs), and calcifying cystic odontogenic tumors (CCOTs).	Study Type: Immunohistochemical study. Sample Size: 25 RCs, 23 DCs, 23 KCOTs, and 23 CCOTs. Country/Region: Iran.	p53, PCNA.	Histopathological examination using hematoxylin and eosin staining.	Highest p53 expression in the basal layer of RC and suprabasal layer of KCOT. Highest PCNA expression in the suprabasal layer of KCOT. Significant differences in p53 expression in basal and suprabasal layers, and PCNA expression in the suprabasal layer between cysts. No significant difference in PCNA expression in the basal layer among the cysts.	Kruskal-Wallis test ($p = 0.008$ for p53 in basal; $p = 0.031$ for p53 in suprabasal; $p = 0.009$ for PCNA in suprabasal). Wilcoxon signed rank test ($p = 0.007$ for p53 in basal layer RC; $p = 0.024$ for p53 in basal layer DC; $p = 0.025$ for p53 in basal layer KCOT).	The high expression of PCNA in the suprabasal layer of KCOT supports its neoplastic nature and tendency for recurrence. p53 expression in the basal layer of RC indicates an inflammatory response.

4.4. Matrix Metalloproteinases (MMPs) and Their Role

Matrix metalloproteinases (MMPs), particularly MMP-2 and MMP-9, play crucial roles in the development and progression of odontogenic lesions such as dentigerous cysts (DCs) and odontogenic keratocysts (OKCs) [71–73]. These enzymes are instrumental in the breakdown of extracellular matrix components, contributing to the rapid growth and potential recurrence of these cysts and tumors by enhancing their invasiveness. Genetic studies have linked specific gene variations of MMPs to the aggressive nature of lesions such as ameloblastomas and keratocystic odontogenic tumors (KCOTs), suggesting the potential for therapies targeting these genetic traits [72]. Additionally, the presence of MMP-7 and MMP-9 has been associated with more aggressive behavior in keratocysts related to nevoid basal cell carcinoma syndrome (NBCCS), indicating these enzymes as potential markers for distinguishing between syndromic and non-syndromic lesions [73].

The examination of MMPs in lesions like DCs and OKCs not only deepens our understanding of these conditions but also reveals how these enzymes contribute to their pathology, leading to the development of targeted treatments based on the lesions' molecular and genetic characteristics. For instance, studies have specifically linked MMP-9 to the aggressive behavior of odontogenic keratocysts, suggesting that MMP inhibitors could serve as effective therapeutic agents. Clinical case reports have demonstrated that the local application of MMP inhibitors can significantly reduce the invasiveness of these lesions, supporting their use as adjunct therapies alongside conventional surgical methods [74,75]. This practical application highlights how understanding MMP activity can lead to more targeted and effective treatment approaches, demonstrating the direct impact of molecular insights on improving clinical outcomes.

Recent studies have provided significant insights into the role of MMPs in odontogenic lesions. Ortiz-García et al. analyzed the expression levels and proteolytic activities of MMP-2 and MMP-9 in various odontogenic lesions, finding that both enzymes showed higher proteolytic activity in cystic and tumor lesions compared to dental follicles, highlighting their role in the growth and development of these lesions [71]. Aloka et al. conducted a pilot study on the gene polymorphisms of MMP-2 and MMP-9 in aggressive and nonaggressive odontogenic lesions. They found significant associations between specific polymorphisms and the aggressiveness of lesions such as ameloblastomas and KCOTs, indicating that these genetic traits could guide the development of targeted therapies [72]. Furthermore, Loreto et al. examined the expression of MMP-7 and MMP-9 in NBCCS-related, recurrent, and sporadic keratocysts. Their findings suggested that higher expressions of these MMPs in NBCCS-OKCs correlate with the more aggressive and recurrent nature of these lesions, emphasizing the potential of MMPs as therapeutic targets [73].

The practical applications of these findings are significant. The use of MMP inhibitors as adjunct therapies has been shown to reduce the invasiveness of odontogenic lesions, offering a less invasive alternative to conventional surgical methods. This integration of molecular insights into clinical practice can enhance the efficacy of treatments tailored to specific genetic profiles, ultimately improving patient outcomes [74,75].

In summary, MMPs offer key insights into the biological processes underlying odontogenic lesions. This knowledge not only aids in diagnosis but also informs the development of targeted therapeutic interventions, promising new, more effective ways to manage these conditions and improve patient outcomes [71–75] (Table 4).

Table 4. Matrix metalloproteinases (MMP-2, MMP-7, and MMP-9).

Authors	Objective	Study Details	Marker Identification Method	Cyst/Tumor Diagnosis Method	Results	Statistical Estimates	Conclusion
Ortiz-Garcia et al. (2022) [71]	To compare the expression level and proteolytic activities of MMP-2 and MMP-9 in dental follicles (DFs), dentigerous cysts (DCs), odontogenic keratocysts (OKCs), and unicystic ameloblastomas (UAs).	Study Type: Immunohistochemical and proteolytic activity study. Sample Size: 7 DFs, 8 DCs, 8 OKCs, and 8 UAs. Country/Region: Mexico.	Antibodies for MMP-2 and MMP-9, Western blot analysis.	Histopathological examination using hematoxylin and eosin staining.	MMP-2: Similar expression in all tissues, but higher activity in cystic and tumor lesions compared to DF. MMP-9: Higher expression and activity in DC, OKC, and UA compared to DF. No significant differences in MMP-2 or MMP-9 expression and activity between cystic and tumor lesions.	not specified.	MMP-2 and MMP-9 play a role in the development of DC, OKC, and UA. Their increased activity suggests involvement in lesion growth, but they do not differentiate between cystic and tumor lesions.
Aloka et al. (2019) [72]	To investigate the association of matrix metalloproteinase 2 (MMP2) and matrix metalloproteinase 9 (MMP9) gene polymorphisms with the aggressiveness of ameloblastomas, keratocystic odontogenic tumors (KCOTs), and dentigerous cysts (DCs).	Study Type: Pilot case-control study. Sample Size: 15 ameloblastomas, 11 KCOTs, 13 DCs, and 106 controls. Country/Region: India (Kerala).	PCR-restriction fragment length polymorphism (PCR-RFLP) and sequencing for MMP2 and MMP9 gene polymorphisms.	Histopathological confirmation using WHO (2005) criteria.	Ameloblastomas showed a higher frequency of the MMP9 rs3918242 T allele ($p = 0.05$). Significant differences in MMP2 rs243865 genotype ($p = 0.046$) and allele frequency ($p = 0.03$; OR = 2.06) between cases and controls. KCOT samples showed significant differences in genotype ($p = 0.01$) and allele ($p = 0.01$; OR = 3.42) frequencies compared to controls.	Chi-square analysis revealed significant associations between MMP2 rs243865 and MMP9 rs3918242 polymorphisms and odontogenic lesions ($p < 0.05$).	MMP2 rs243865 polymorphism is associated with increased aggressiveness in ameloblastomas and KCOTs. MMP9 rs3918242 polymorphism may contribute to the aggressive behavior of ameloblastomas.
Loreto et al. (2022) [73]	To analyze the immunohistochemical expression of MMP-7, MMP-9, α-SMA, desmin, and caldesmon in odontogenic keratocysts (OKCs) associated with NBCCS compared to recurrent and sporadic keratocysts.	Study Type: Immunohistochemical study. Sample Size: 40 patients (23 males, 17 females) with OKCs: 19 sporadic OKCs, 9 recurrent OKCs, and 12 NBCCS-associated OKCs. Age Range: Mean age: 32 ± 8.7 years. Country/Region: Italy.	antibodies for MMP-7, MMP-9, α-SMA, desmin, and caldesmon.	Histopathological examination using hematoxylin and eosin staining.	Significantly increased expression of α-SMA, caldesmon, MMP-7, and MMP-9 in NBCCS-OKCs compared to non-syndromic OKCs ($p < 0.001$). Desmin showed a non-significant increase in expression in non-syndromic OKCs compared to NBCCS-OKCs. NBCCS-OKCs showed greater distribution of myofibroblasts (MFs) compared to other OKC subtypes.	Statistical significance with p-values < 0.05 for α-SMA, caldesmon, MMP-7, and MMP-9 expressions in NBCCS-OKCs.	Different expression patterns of MMP-7, MMP-9, α-SMA, desmin, and caldesmon suggest distinct biological behaviors of OKC subtypes. NBCCS-OKCs showed higher levels of these markers, indicating greater aggressiveness and recurrence potential. Further studies are needed to correlate these findings with clinical behavior.

Table 4. Cont.

Authors	Objective	Study Details	Marker Identification Method	Cyst/Tumor Diagnosis Method	Results	Statistical Estimates	Conclusion
Suojanen et al. (2014) [74]	To evaluate the expression of matrix metalloproteinases (MMPs) 8, 9, 25, and 26, and tissue inhibitor of metalloproteinases-1 (TIMP-1) in dentigerous cysts (DCs) and healthy dental follicles (HDFs).	Study Type: Immunohistochemical study. Sample Size: 10 DCs and 10 HDFs. Age Range: Mean age: DC group: 39 years; HDF group: 22 years. Country/Region: Finland.	Immunohistochemistry using polyclonal antibodies for MMPs and TIMP-1.	Histopathological examination using hematoxylin and eosin staining.	MMP-8: Slightly more expressed in DC epithelium than in HDF epithelium, but not statistically significant ($p = 0.255$). MMP-9, MMP-25, MMP-26, and TIMP-1: No significant differences in expression between DCs and HDFs. TIMP-1: Strong positivity in both DCs and HDFs, no difference between groups ($p = 1.000$).	Fisher's non-parametric exact test: No significant differences found in MMP or TIMP-1 expressions between groups.	Differences in MMP expression cannot solely explain dentigerous cyst expansion, suggesting involvement of other osteolytic mechanisms.
Kuźniarz et al. (2021) [75]	To elucidate the role of MMP-2, MMP-9, and their endogenous inhibitors TIMP-1 and TIMP-2 in the pathogenesis of maxillofacial cystic lesions.	Study Type: Immunohistochemical and gelatin zymography study. Sample Size: 20 with radicular cysts (RC), 7 with retention cysts (RtC), and 3 with dentigerous cysts (DC). Age Range: 18–66 years (median age: 43.2). Country/Region: Poland.	Gelatin zymography for MMP-2 and MMP-9, ELISA for TIMP-1 and TIMP-2.	Clinical examination, CT, panoramic X-ray, histopathological examination.	MMP-9 activity and MMP-9/TIMP-1 ratio were higher in RC fluid compared to RtC fluid. No significant differences in MMP-2 activity in the wall of RtCs compared to DCs. TIMP-1 serum levels were lower in RC patients compared to DC and RtC patients, but not statistically significant.	Kruskal-Wallis test followed by Dunn's post-hoc test; significance considered at $p < 0.05$.	MMP-9 plays a significant role in the pathogenesis of RCs, while MMP-2 activity is less significant in RtCs. MMP-9 could serve as a biomarker for RC etiology. Further studies are needed to confirm these findings and their clinical implications.

Table 4. Cont.

Authors	Objective	Study Details	Marker Identification Method	Cyst/Tumor Diagnosis Method	Results	Statistical Estimates	Conclusion
de Andrade Santos et al. (2011) [76]	To compare the immunohistochemical expression of NF-κB, MMP-9, and CD105 in odontogenic keratocysts (OKCs), dentigerous cysts (DCs), and radicular cysts (RCs).	Study Type: Immunohistochemical study. Sample Size: 20 OKCs, 20 DCs, and 20 RCs.	Immunohistochemistry for NF-κB, MMP-9, and CD105.	Histopathological examination using hematoxylin and eosin staining.	NF-κB LI higher in OKCs than in DCs and RCs ($p < 0.001$). MMP-9 expression score 2 in epithelial component: OKCs (90%), DCs (70%), and RCs (65%; $p = 0.159$). No significant difference in NF-κB LI according to MMP-9 expression in epithelial lining ($p = 0.282$). Highest MMP-9 expression in fibrous capsule: OKCs ($p = 0.100$). MMP-9 expression in vessels: score 2 in OKCs (80%) and RCs (50%), score 1 in DCs (75%; $p = 0.002$). Mean microvessel count: RCs (16.9), DCs (12.1), OKCs (10.0; $p = 0.163$). No significant difference in microvessel count according to MMP-9 expression between groups ($p = 0.689$).	p-values: NF-κB LI ($p < 0.001$), MMP-9 expression in epithelial component ($p = 0.159$), NF-κB LI according to MMP-9 expression ($p = 0.282$), MMP-9 expression in fibrous capsule ($p = 0.100$), MMP-9 expression in vessels ($p = 0.002$), mean microvessel count ($p = 0.163$), microvessel count according to MMP-9 expression ($p = 0.689$).	The more aggressive biological behavior of OKCs is related to higher expression of MMP-9 and NF-κB. Differences in the biological behavior of the lesions studied do not seem to be associated with the angiogenic index.
Ribeiro et al. (2011) [77]	To evaluate the immunohistochemical expression of matrix metalloproteinases (MMPs) 1, 2, 7, 9, and 26 in calcifying cystic odontogenic tumor (CCOT).	Study Type: Immunohistochemical study. Sample Size: 10 cases of CCOT. Country/Region: Brazil.	Immunohistochemistry using monoclonal antibodies for MMP-1, MMP-2, MMP-7, MMP-9, and MMP-26.	Histopathological examination using hematoxylin and eosin staining.	MMP-1, MMP-7, and MMP-9: score 2 in 100% of cases. MMP-2: score 0 in 90% of cases. MMP-26: varied immunostaining. All MMPs except MMP-2 were expressed in the stroma, indicating their role in ECM degradation and tumor growth. Diffuse immunoreactivity observed for MMPs 1, 7, 9, and 26 in parenchymal cells, while MMP-2 showed a focal pattern.	Descriptive analysis of immunohistochemical expression, no specific statistical tests mentioned.	MMPs 1, 7, 9, and 26 contribute to tumor growth and expansion in CCOT. The presence of these MMPs in stromal cells highlights their involvement in ECM degradation and active tumor growth. Further studies using additional techniques are recommended to better understand the role of these MMPs in CCOT.

4.5. Cytokeratins and Other Markers

Cytokeratins (CKs) and markers such as survivin, E-cadherin, CD138, and CD38 are critical for understanding the development, behavior, and diagnosis of odontogenic lesions, including cysts and tumors. The expression patterns of these markers provide valuable information about the biological behavior of these lesions, influencing their management and prognosis [6,78–80].

The presence of these markers in specific lesions such as central adenoid basal (CAB), keratocystic odontogenic tumor (KCOT), dentigerous cyst (DC), and radicular cyst (RC) is crucial for accurate diagnosis and assessment of aggressiveness. For instance, increased survivin expression, typically associated with tumor survival and resistance to apoptosis, has been targeted in recent therapeutic trials with survivin inhibitors, showcasing a direct clinical application of these biomarkers in enhancing treatment efficacy. This emphasizes how differential expression of markers like survivin can inform treatment choices and potentially improve clinical outcomes by targeting specific molecular pathways involved in lesion survival and growth [6,78].

Research into markers like syndecan-1 (CD138) and CD56 (NCAM) has also revealed their roles in tumor development and their potential to help distinguish between cystic and tumorous odontogenic lesions. Studies have shown strong CD138 expression in KCOTs and dentigerous cysts, aiding in differentiating these from other lesions. Additionally, CD56 has been noted for its aberrant expression in KCOTs, particularly in syndromic cases, helping to differentiate these from orthokeratinized odontogenic cysts (OOCs) and other similar lesions [79,80].

Investigations into CK expression have emphasized its significance in differentiating between various odontogenic lesions, aiding in the identification of their histopathological features and suggesting different underlying causes for conditions such as OOCs and epithelial dysplasia cysts (EDCs). For example, CK10 and CK19 expression patterns have been useful in distinguishing OOCs from epidermoid cysts (EDCs) and odontogenic keratocysts (OKCs), which is crucial for accurate diagnosis and management. Furthermore, the expression of CK14 and CK18 has been explored in various lesions, revealing differences that help understand their pathogenesis and behavior [81–83].

The analysis of these markers not only enriches diagnostic capabilities but also points toward potential new treatments, enhancing the ability to predict and manage the outcomes of odontogenic cysts and tumors more effectively. Understanding these markers' roles in lesion pathophysiology aids clinicians in tailoring therapeutic approaches based on specific diagnostic and prognostic data, ultimately leading to more effective and personalized patient care [80,83].

In conclusion, the study of CKs, survivin, E-cadherin, CD138, and CD38 provides a deeper understanding of the molecular mechanisms underlying odontogenic lesions. This knowledge is instrumental in developing more accurate diagnostic tools and effective therapeutic strategies, leading to improved patient outcomes in the management of odontogenic cysts and tumors [6,78–83] (Table 5).

Table 5. Cytokeratins (CK7, CK10, CK13, CK14, CK17, CK18, CK19, survivin, E-cadherin, CD138, CD56, and CD38).

Authors	Objective	Study Details	Marker Identification Method	Cyst/Tumor Diagnosis Method	Results	Statistical Estimates	Conclusion
Özcan et al. (2015) [6]	To investigate the expressions of survivin, E-cadherin, CD138, and CD38 in cystic ameloblastoma, keratocystic odontogenic tumor (KCOT), dentigerous cyst (DC), and radicular cyst (RC), and their potential diagnostic usage.	Study Type: Immunohistochemical study. Sample Size: 5 RCs, 5 DCs, 5 KCOTs, 5 cystic ameloblastomas. Country/Region: Turkey.	Immunohistochemistry using antibodies for survivin, E-cadherin, CD138, and CD38.	Histopathological examination using hematoxylin and eosin staining.	Cystic ameloblastomas and KCOTs showed diffuse and strong nuclear survivin expression. No specific survivin immunoreactivity in DCs and RCs. E-cadherin expression stronger in DCs and RCs compared to other lesions. CD138 expression prominent in stromal cells of cystic ameloblastomas, gradually decreased in other lesions. All cases were negative for CD38.	Not provided.	Loss of E-cadherin expression in epithelial cells, strong CD138 expression in stromal cells, and strong nuclear survivin expression in cystic ameloblastomas and KCOTs are characteristic findings, suggesting a role in their aggressiveness and pathogenesis.
Etemad-Moghadam et al. (2017) [78]	To assess the immunohistochemical expression of CD138 (syndecan-1) in adenomatoid odontogenic tumor (AOT), ameloblastic fibroma (AF), and odontogenic myxoma (OM), and to compare it with ameloblastoma and keratocystic odontogenic tumor (KCOT).	Study Type: Immunohistochemical study. Sample Size: 7 AOTs, 5 OMs, 7 AFs, 29 KCOTs, and 10 ameloblastomas. Country/Region: Iran.	Immunohistochemistry using monoclonal antibody against syndecan-1 (CD138).	Histopathological examination using hematoxylin and eosin staining.	Syndecan-1 expressed in all samples except OMs. Significant differences in percentage and intensity of syndecan-1 expression among the studied OTs ($p < 0.001$). Pairwise comparisons showed significant difference only between OMs and each of the other tumors.	Kruskal–Wallis test followed by Bonferroni analysis for comparisons ($p < 0.05$).	Syndecan-1 may be involved in the pathogenesis of AOT, AF, KCOT, and ameloblastoma. However, its effect on clinical aggressiveness appears limited. Negative immunoexpression in OM requires further investigation.

Table 5. Cont.

Authors	Objective	Study Details	Marker Identification Method	Cyst/Tumor Diagnosis Method	Results	Statistical Estimates	Conclusion
Vera-Sirera et al. (2015) [79]	To investigate the immunohistochemical expression of neural cell adhesion molecule (NCAM, CD56) in keratin-producing odontogenic cysts (KPOCs) including keratocystic odontogenic tumors (KCOTs) and orthokeratinized odontogenic cysts (OOCs).	Study Type: Immunohistochemical study. Sample Size: 12 OOCs and 46 KCOTs (40 non-syndromic KCOTs, 6 syndromic KCOTs associated with nevoid basal cell carcinoma syndrome (NBCS)). Country/Region: Spain.	Immunohistochemistry using monoclonal antibody NCL-CD56-504 (clone CD564).	Histopathological examination using hematoxylin and eosin staining.	NCAM expression: 0% in OOCs, 36.95% in KCOTs. Focal and heterogeneous NCAM expression in 36.95% of KCOTs, especially at the basal cell level, basal budding areas, and basal cells of daughter cysts. Higher NCAM expression in syndromic KCOTs (66.66%) compared to non-syndromic KCOTs (30%). Significant difference in NCAM expression between OOCs and KCOTs ($p = 0.012$). No association between NCAM expression and lesion recurrence.	Firth's logistic regression test; significant difference with $p < 0.05$ for NCAM expression between OOCs and KCOTs.	Aberrant NCAM expression in KCOTs, especially in syndromic KCOTs, suggests a role in pathogenesis and potential impact on lesional recurrence. Further studies with homogeneously treated series are needed to confirm these findings.
Jaafari-Ashkavandi et al. (2014) [80]	To examine the expression of CD56 in ameloblastomas, dentigerous cysts, keratocystic odontogenic tumors (KCOTs), adenomatoid odontogenic tumors (AOTs), orthokeratinized odontogenic cysts, calcifying odontogenic cysts (COCs), and glandular odontogenic cysts (GOCs).	Study Type: Cross-sectional, analytical immunohistochemical study. Sample Size: 22 ameloblastomas (14 solid, 8 unicystic), 13 dentigerous cysts, 10 KCOTs, 4 AOTs, 3 orthokeratinized odontogenic cysts, 3 COCs, 1 GOC. Country/Region: Iran.	Immunohistochemistry using anti-CD56 antibody.	Histopathological examination using hematoxylin and eosin staining.	CD56 expression: 91% in ameloblastomas, 75% in AOTs, 40% in KCOTs, 100% in GOCs. No CD56 expression in dentigerous cysts, COCs, orthokeratinized odontogenic cysts. Significant difference in CD56 expression between ameloblastoma and dentigerous cysts, and between KCOT and orthokeratinized odontogenic cysts.	Chi-square test; significant differences with $p < 0.05$ in CD56 expression between specific groups.	CD56 expression is limited to more aggressive cysts and tumoral lesions, suggesting it can be a useful marker for distinguishing between cystic and tumoral odontogenic lesions.

Table 5. *Cont.*

Authors	Objective	Study Details	Marker Identification Method	Cyst/Tumor Diagnosis Method	Results	Statistical Estimates	Conclusion
Al-Otaibi et al. (2013) [84]	To analyze the expression profile of syndecan-1 (SD-1) immunohistochemically in ameloblastomas and common odontogenic cysts.	Study Type: Immunohistochemical study. Sample Size: 32 ameloblastomas, 26 keratocystic odontogenic tumors (KCOTs), 21 dentigerous cysts.	Immunohistochemistry using monoclonal antibody against SD-1 (CD138).	Histopathological examination using hematoxylin and eosin staining.	SD-1 expression in epithelial and stromal elements significantly associated with lesion extension and involvement of adjacent structures ($p = 0.025$). Higher SD-1 expression in stellate reticulum cells than ameloblasts ($p < 0.0001$). Significant difference in epithelial staining among ameloblastomas, KCOTs, and dentigerous cysts ($p < 0.0001$). Mean rank scores (Kruskal–Wallis test): ameloblastomas significantly lower than KCOTs and dentigerous cysts; non-significant comparison between KCOT and dentigerous cyst groups.	p-values: lesion extension and involvement ($p = 0.025$), stellate reticulum cells vs. ameloblasts ($p < 0.0001$), epithelial staining among groups ($p < 0.0001$).	SD-1 expression in stromal cells of ameloblastoma, KCOT, and dentigerous cyst is associated with poor prognosis.
Krishnan et al. (2023) [85]	To determine if specific patterns of CK14 and Bcl-2 staining can assist in diagnosing OKCs with altered epithelial features and provide insights into their aggressive nature.	Study Type: Immunohistochemical study.	Immunohistochemistry for CK14 and Bcl-2.	Histopathological examination.	CK14 expression: Restricted to basal and suprabasal layers near satellite cysts and areas with subepithelial split. Entire epithelial lining showed CK14 expression in areas of inflammation and after marsupialization. Bcl-2: Typical basal/suprabasal staining lost in areas of inflammation, and intensity decreased in OKCs after marsupialization.	Not specified.	Specific CK14 and Bcl-2 staining patterns could aid in diagnosing OKCs with altered epithelial features and provide insights into their aggressive behavior. Proper recognition and diagnosis are essential for treatment planning due to therapeutic consequences and high recurrence rates.

Table 5. *Cont.*

Authors	Objective	Study Details	Marker Identification Method	Cyst/Tumor Diagnosis Method	Results	Statistical Estimates	Conclusion
Padmapriya et al. (2020) [81]	To compare the cytokeratin expressions of CK10 and CK19 among orthokeratinized odontogenic cysts (OOCs), epidermoid cysts (EDCs), and odontogenic keratocysts (OKCs) by immunohistochemical study.	Study Type: Immunohistochemical study. Sample Size: 10 OOCs, 10 EDCs, 10 OKCs. Country/Region: India.	Immunohistochemistry using CK10 and CK19 markers.	Histopathological examination using hematoxylin and eosin staining.	CK10 expression: 100% in OOCs and EDCs, 50% in OKCs. CK19 expression: 40% in OOCs, 30% in EDCs, 80% in OKCs. Significant difference in CK10 expression between OKCs and OOCs/EDCs ($p = 0.009$). CK19 expression significant between EDCs and OKCs ($p = 0.028$), but not between OOCs and EDCs or OOCs and OKCs.	p-values: CK10 expression ($p = 0.002$), CK19 expression ($p = 0.061$).	CK10 expressions in OOCs and EDCs were nearly identical, indicating OOCs might not be distinguished from EDCs histologically. CK19 expression showed no significant differences between OOCs and EDCs or OOCs and OKCs, implying OOCs resemble both EDCs and OKCs.
Sheethal et al. (2019) [82]	To present a rare case of an odontogenic keratocyst (OKC) arising in the maxillary sinus and discuss its clinical, radiographic, and histopathological features.	Study Type: Case report. Sample Size: Single case. Age Range: 15-year-old female. Country/Region: India (Bengaluru, Karnataka).	Not applicable (case report).	Histopathological examination.	Patient presented with pain and pus discharge in the upper left back teeth region. Radiographs revealed an ill-defined radiolucent lesion associated with an impacted third molar in the maxillary sinus. Histopathological examination showed parakeratinized stratified squamous epithelium, nuclear hyperchromatism, and palisading of basal cells. The lesion was diagnosed as OKC in the maxillary sinus.	Not applicable.	OKC in the maxillary sinus is rare and can be mistaken for other lesions like sinusitis or antral polyps. Proper recognition and diagnosis are crucial due to its aggressive behavior and high recurrence rate. Long-term follow-up is necessary to monitor for recurrence.

Table 5. Cont.

Authors	Objective	Study Details	Marker Identification Method	Cyst/Tumor Diagnosis Method	Results	Statistical Estimates	Conclusion
Hoshino et al. (2015) [83]	To perform an immunohistochemical analysis of cytokeratins (CKs) and langerin to examine differences in the lining epithelium of dermoid cysts (DMCs), epidermoid cysts (EDMCs), orthokeratinized odontogenic cysts (OOCs), and keratocystic odontogenic tumors (KCOTs).	Study Type: Immunohistochemical study. Sample Size: 7 DMCs, 30 EDMCs, 11 OOCs, 28 KCOTs. Age Range: Mean ages: DMCs (42.9 years), EDMCs (40.8 years), OOCs (36.3 years), KCOTs (33.5 years). Country/Region: Japan.	Immunohistochemistry using antibodies against CK10, CK13, CK14, CK16, CK17, CK19, and langerin.	Histopathological examination using hematoxylin and eosin staining.	CK10: Positive in all layers except basal layer in DMCs, EDMCs, and OOCs; negative in KCOTs. CK13 and CK17: Positive in all layers except basal layer in OOCs; negative in DMCs/EDMCs. CK14 and CK16: Positive in all layers in DCs; CK14 positive in all except surface layer in DMCs, EDMCs, OOCs, and KCOTs. CK19: Negative in OOCs; positive in all layers except basal layer in KCOTs. Langerin: Positive in Langerhans cells in the spinous layer of DMCs, EDMCs, and OOCs; rarely positive in KCOTs; negative in DCs.	Not specified.	The immunohistochemical profiles of CKs and langerin in DMCs/EDMCs, OOCs, and KCOTs suggest that these are independent diseases with distinct biological characteristics.
Yamamoto et al. (2013) [86]	To report a case of keratocyst in the buccal mucosa with features of a keratocystic odontogenic tumor (KCOT).	Study Type: Case report. Sample Size: Single case. Age Range: 74-year-old male. Country/Region: Japan.	Immunohistochemistry using antibodies for CK17, CK10, and Ki-67.	Histopathological examination using hematoxylin and eosin staining, clinical and imaging examination.	The patient had a cystic lesion in the right buccal mucosa, initially diagnosed as an epidermoid cyst. Histopathological examination revealed parakeratinized squamous epithelium with palisading basal cells. Immunohistochemistry showed positive CK17 and high Ki-67 labeling, indicating high proliferation potential, and negative CK10. Features were consistent with KCOT.	Not applicable.	The keratocyst in the buccal mucosa showed characteristics of KCOT, suggesting an odontogenic origin. Accurate diagnosis and differentiation from other cystic lesions are crucial for appropriate treatment and management.

Table 5. Cont.

Authors	Objective	Study Details	Marker Identification Method	Cyst/Tumor Diagnosis Method	Results	Statistical Estimates	Conclusion
Kureel et al. (2019) [87]	To analyze the immunohistochemical (IHC) expression of cytokeratins (CK10, CK13, and CK19) and fibronectin in orthokeratinized odontogenic cyst (OOC), epidermoid cyst (EDC), dermoid cyst (DMC), dentigerous cyst (DC), and keratocystic odontogenic tumor (KCOT) to elucidate the pathogenesis of OOC.	Study Type: Immunohistochemical study. Sample Size: 25 cases for each study group: OOC, EDC, DMC, DC, KCOT. Country/Region: India.	Immunohistochemistry using CK10, CK13, CK19, and fibronectin antibodies.	Histopathological examination using hematoxylin and eosin staining.	CK10: Similar expression in OOC and EDC; negative in DC; positive only in the surface layer of KCOT. CK13: Mild expression in OOC and EDC; intense in KCOT and DC. CK19: Negative to mild in OOC; negative in EDC; positive in DC and KCOT. Fibronectin: Predominantly diffuse non-fibrillar (DN) pattern in EDC, followed by DC, KCOT, and OOC; focal non-fibrillar (FN) not detected in OOC.	Chi-square test and Spearman's correlation; significant differences in CK10, CK13, CK19, and fibronectin expressions among the study groups ($p \leq 0.05$).	The IHC profile of OOC is different from DC and KCOT but closer to EDC. CK10 expression in OOC suggests normal orthokeratinization. Strong CK19 expression in DC and KCOT confirms odontogenic origin. OOC likely represents the intraosseous counterpart of EDC.
Bhakhar et al. (2016) [88]	To evaluate the intensity and expression patterns of cytokeratins (CKs) 18 and 19 in odontogenic keratocysts (OKCs), dentigerous cysts (DCs), and radicular cysts (RCs).	Study Type: Immunohistochemical study. Sample Size: 20 OKCs, 20 DCs, 20 RCs. Country/Region: India.	Immunohistochemistry using monoclonal antibodies for CK18 and CK19.	Histopathological examination using hematoxylin and eosin staining.	CK18 expression: 25% in OKCs, 15% in DCs, 10% in RCs, mostly focal with mild intensity. CK19 expression: 75% in OKCs, 100% in DCs and RCs, with intense and "ALL" expression in DCs and RCs, and moderate in OKCs.	Z-test and Pearson's chi-square test showed significant differences in CK18 and CK19 expressions among the cysts ($p \leq 0.05$). CK18 expression in OKCs ($p = 0.001$), DCs ($p = 0.000$), and RCs ($p = 0.000$).	CK19 had higher intensity and expression in all cyst types compared to CK18, suggesting CK19 as a valuable diagnostic aid in differentiating between OKCs, DCs, and RCs.

Table 5. Cont.

Authors	Objective	Study Details	Marker Identification Method	Cyst/Tumor Diagnosis Method	Results	Statistical Estimates	Conclusion
Shruthi et al. (2014) [89]	To understand the expression pattern of cytokeratins (CKs) 14 and 18 in dentigerous cysts, dental follicular tissue, adenomatoid odontogenic tumors (AOTs), and unicystic ameloblastomas.	Study Type: Immunohistochemical study. Sample Size: 20 dentigerous cysts, 20 reduced enamel epithelium/dental follicles, 10 follicular-type AOTs, 10 unicystic ameloblastomas (UCAs). Country/Region: India (Karnataka, Madhya Pradesh).	Immunohistochemistry using monoclonal antibodies for CK14 and CK18.	Histopathological examination using hematoxylin and eosin staining.	CK14 expression: Highest in AOT, moderate in dentigerous cysts and UCA, least in dental follicle/reduced enamel epithelium (REE). CK18: Negative in all cases. Significant differences in CK14 expression among the lesions, with AOT showing more percentage, positivity, and intensity compared to dentigerous cysts and UCA.	One-way ANOVA for mean percentage of CK14-positive cells (highest in AOT, least in DF/REE); T-test for percentage, positivity, intensity, and Remmele score (statistically significant differences between AOT and dentigerous cyst/UCA).	CK14 expression in AOT, dentigerous cyst, UCA, and DF/REE suggests a potential histogenetic relationship. The absence of CK18 in these lesions indicates its limited role in their pathogenesis. Further studies are needed to explore the oncofetal transformation and histogenesis of follicular-type AOT.
Swetha et al. (2014) [90]	To analyze the expression of inducible nitric oxide synthase (iNOS) in the epithelial lining of odontogenic keratocysts (OKCs), dentigerous cysts (DCs), and radicular cysts (RCs) to understand its role in the neoplastic nature and local aggressiveness of these cysts.	Study Type: Immunohistochemical study. Sample Size: 10 OKCs, 10 DCs, 10 RCs. Country/Region: India.	Immunohistochemistry using rabbit polyclonal antibody against iNOS.	Histopathological examination using hematoxylin and eosin staining.	iNOS expression observed in entire thickness of epithelial linings in 10 OKCs (40% intensely stained, 20% moderately stained, 20% mildly stained, 20% no staining). In DCs, 10% of cases showed intense staining, 20% moderate, 30% mild, 40% no staining. In RCs, 40% of cases showed mild staining, 60% no staining. Significant difference in iNOS staining intensity between OKCs, DCs, and RCs ($p < 0.01$).	ANOVA and Chi-square tests showed significant differences in iNOS expression between the cyst groups ($p < 0.01$).	iNOS overexpression in OKCs compared to DCs and RCs suggests a role in the aggressive behavior of OKCs, supporting the view that OKCs are neoplastic in nature.
Sudhakara et al. (2016) [91]	To analyze the expression of cytokeratin 14 (CK14) and vimentin in adenomatoid odontogenic tumor (AOT) and dentigerous cyst (DC) to understand their origin and pathogenesis.	Study Type: Retrospective immunohistochemical study. Sample Size: 16 AOTs (10 follicular, 6 extrafollicular), 15 DCs. Country/Region: India.	Immunohistochemistry using monoclonal antibodies for CK14 and vimentin.	Histopathological examination using hematoxylin and eosin staining.	CK14: Positive in 90% of follicular AOTs (FAOTs) and 100% of extrafollicular AOTs (EAOTs), positive in all DC cases. Vimentin: Positive in 44% of AOT cases, negative in 56%; in DC, 73% negative, 20% intermediate positive, 7% weak positive. CK14 predominantly expressed in Type B cells in AOT, suggesting odontogenic epithelial origin.	Descriptive statistics and measures of central tendency used to analyze results.	CK14 expression in AOT and DC supports their odontogenic epithelial origin. Vimentin expression in AOT is variable, suggesting a minor role in pathogenesis. The study indicates a potential origin from reduced enamel epithelium and dental lamina.

Table 5. *Cont.*

Authors	Objective	Study Details	Marker Identification Method	Cyst/Tumor Diagnosis Method	Results	Statistical Estimates	Conclusion
Saluja et al. (2019) [92]	To elucidate the role of cytokeratin-7 (CK7) in the pathogenesis of odontogenic cysts by immunohistochemistry.	Study Type: Immunohistochemical study. Sample Size: 15 dentigerous cysts (DCs), 12 odontogenic keratocysts (OKCs), 12 radicular cysts (RCs), and 8 control specimens (periampullary carcinoma, nasopalatine duct cysts, and dental follicle). Country/Region: India.	Immunohistochemistry using monoclonal mouse anti-human cytokeratin-7 antibody.	Histopathological examination using hematoxylin and eosin staining.	CK7 expression was highest in DCs (66.66%), followed by RCs (41.66%), and least in OKCs (16.6%). CK7 positive in suprabasal (60%) and superficial layers (40%) in DCs; in superficial and spinous layers in RCs and OKCs. Statistically significant difference in CK7 expression between DCs and OKCs ($p = 0.009$), but not between RCs and DCs or RCs and OKCs.	Chi-square test; significant differences with $p \leq 0.05$.	CK7 expression correlates with the degree of epithelial differentiation. Well-differentiated epithelium (RC and DC) shows CK7 expression, while less well-differentiated epithelium (OKC) shows slight positivity. CK7 can be used to differentiate OKC from DC and RC.

4.6. Ki-67 and Other Proliferative Markers

Proliferative markers, particularly Ki-67, are instrumental in understanding the growth behavior, aggressiveness, and recurrence likelihood of odontogenic lesions such as odontogenic keratocysts (OKCs), dentigerous cysts (DCs), ameloblastomas (ABs), and unicystic ameloblastomas (UAs) [93,94]. Ki-67, a marker indicating cellular proliferation, shows notably higher levels in OKCs compared to DCs, suggesting a more aggressive growth pattern and a greater propensity for recurrence [56].

The interaction of Ki-67 with other markers like p63 and MCM3 provides deeper insights into the complex biology of these lesions, enabling clinicians to better predict their behavior and tailor treatment approaches accordingly. For instance, p63, which is associated with the regulation of epithelial cell proliferation and differentiation, shows higher expression in OKCs and ABs compared to DCs, correlating with their more aggressive behavior [95,96]. MCM3, another proliferation marker, also demonstrates higher expression in OKCs and ABs, further supporting their higher proliferative activity compared to DCs [97].

Elevated Ki-67 levels, particularly in OKCs and ABs, signal a higher risk of recurrence, guiding clinicians towards more aggressive management strategies, from surgical resections to closer post-operative monitoring. The incorporation of Ki-67 staining in routine diagnostic procedures has improved the stratification of recurrence risk, enabling clinicians to tailor follow-up intervals and treatment intensities based on individual patient profiles, thereby optimizing clinical outcomes [98,99]. For example, studies have shown that OKCs exhibit a significantly higher cellular proliferation index in the suprabasal layers compared to DCs, indicating their potential for more aggressive behavior and higher recurrence rates [56,94].

Additionally, research indicates that the expression of Ki-67 and MCM3 in different odontogenic lesions not only reflects their proliferative capacity but also aids in distinguishing between more and less aggressive types. For example, the mean Ki-67 labeling index in ameloblastomas is significantly higher than in DCs, highlighting the neoplastic nature of ameloblastomas compared to the more benign behavior of DCs [100]. Furthermore, the positive correlation between Ki-67 and p53 expression in OKCs and DCs underscores the role of these markers in understanding the pathogenesis and biological behavior of these lesions [101].

To modify and personalize therapy based on these markers, non-surgical approaches such as targeted therapies could be explored. For instance, lesions with high Ki-67 expression might benefit from treatments that inhibit cellular proliferation. The development of targeted inhibitors against specific pathways involved in cell proliferation, such as p63 or MCM3, could provide alternative or adjunctive treatments to traditional surgical methods. Additionally, personalized follow-up schedules based on Ki-67 levels could improve patient outcomes by ensuring timely intervention for recurrent lesions.

In summary, the evaluation of proliferative markers like Ki-67 marks a significant advancement in the field of oral health care. These markers provide crucial insights into how odontogenic lesions develop and respond to treatments, improving the prediction of outcomes and enabling more effective planning and execution of therapeutic strategies. Ongoing research into these markers is vital for refining management approaches and achieving better patient care outcomes [56,93–101] (Table 6).

Table 6. Proliferative markers (Ki-67, maspin, CD138, syndecan-1, p67, MCM-2, MCM-3, EGF, CD34, and COX-2).

Authors	Objective	Study Details	Marker Identification Method	Cyst/Tumor Diagnosis Method	Results	Statistical Estimates	Conclusion
Portes et al. (2020) [93]	To evaluate and compare the immunoexpression and immunostaining intensities of Ki-67 antigen in odontogenic keratocysts (OKCs) and dentigerous cysts (DCs) using computerized analysis.	Study Type: Immunohistochemical study. Sample Size: 15 OKCs, 6 DCs. Country/Region: Brazil.	Immunohistochemistry using monoclonal Ki-67 antibody (clone MIB-1) and computerized analysis with Aperio Technologies Inc. System.	Histopathological examination using hematoxylin and eosin staining.	There are no statistically significant differences in Ki-67 immunoexpression or staining intensities between OKCs and DCs. OKCs showed a significantly higher cellular proliferation index in suprabasal layers compared to basal layers. There are no significant differences in Ki-67 expression between OKCs from maxilla versus mandible or primary versus recurrent OKCs.	Mann-Whitney test, Student's t-test, and Signal test used for statistical analysis; significance level set at $\alpha = 0.05$.	Increased Ki-67 immunoexpression in the suprabasal layers of OKCs suggests a different biological behavior and more aggressive proliferation potential compared to DCs. Computerized evaluation provides a more reliable method for assessing immunoexpression.
Hammad et al. (2020) [94]	To investigate the expressions of maspin, syndecan-1, and Ki-67 in odontogenic keratocysts (OKCs) compared to dentigerous cysts (DCs) and ameloblastomas (ABs).	Study Type: Immunohistochemical analysis. Sample Size: 26 OKCs, 11 DCs, 10 ABs. Country/Region: Jordan.	Immunohistochemistry using antibodies against maspin, syndecan-1, and Ki-67.	Histopathological examination using hematoxylin and eosin staining.	Maspin: Lower expression in OKC and DC compared to AB, but not statistically significant. Syndecan-1: Lower expression in OKC and AB compared to DC, but not statistically significant. Ki-67: Significantly higher expression in OKC compared to DC ($p < 0.05$), like AB.	ANOVA and Student's t-test used; significant differences in Ki-67 scores between OKC and DC ($p < 0.05$).	Ki-67 expression indicates higher proliferative activity in OKC similar to AB, higher than in DC. Expressions of maspin and syndecan-1 are not significantly different among OKC, AB, and DC, suggesting further investigation into the biological behavior of OKC is needed.
Alsaegh et al. (2020) [95]	To investigate p63 immunoexpression and its relation to the proliferation of epithelial lining in dentigerous cyst (DC), odontogenic keratocyst (OKC), and ameloblastoma (AB).	Study Type: Immunohistochemical study. Sample Size: 12 DCs, 9 OKCs, 15 ABs. Age Range: Mean age: 40.11 years (±17.567). Country/Region: United Arab Emirates, China.	Immunohistochemistry using antibodies against p63 and Ki-67.	Histopathological examination using hematoxylin and eosin staining.	p63 expression: Significant difference among DCs, OKCs, and ABs ($p = 0.048$). Higher in OKCs compared to DCs ($p = 0.018$). Ki-67: Significant difference among DCs, OKCs, and ABs ($p = 0.022$). Higher in OKCs compared to DCs ($p = 0.007$). Positive correlation between p63 and Ki-67 in DCs ($\sigma = 0.757$, $p = 0.004$) and OKCs ($\sigma = 0.741$, $p = 0.022$). No correlation in AB group.	Kruskal-Wallis test, Mann-Whitney U test, Spearman's correlation analysis ($p < 0.05$).	The diverse expression and correlation of p63 with proliferation in odontogenic lesions suggest different roles and pathways of ΔNp63 in odontogenic tumors versus cysts, aiding in understanding their pathogenesis and behavior.

Table 6. Cont.

Authors	Objective	Study Details	Marker Identification Method	Cyst/Tumor Diagnosis Method	Results	Statistical Estimates	Conclusion
Jaafari-Ashkavandi et al. (2015) [96]	To investigate the diagnostic impact of P63 protein on dentigerous cysts and various types of ameloblastoma and compare its expression with the Ki-67 proliferation marker.	Study Type: Cross-sectional retrospective immunohistochemical study. Sample Size: 25 dentigerous cysts, 21 unicystic ameloblastomas, 17 conventional ameloblastomas. Age Range Mean age: 27 ± 15.2 years. Country/Region: Iran.	Immunohistochemistry using monoclonal anti-P63 antibody and Ki-67 antibody.	Histopathological examination using hematoxylin and eosin staining.	P63 expression higher in ameloblastoma compared to unicystic ameloblastoma and dentigerous cysts ($p < 0.05$). No significant difference in P63 expression between unicystic ameloblastoma and dentigerous cysts. A 90% cut-off point for basal layer gave 88% sensitivity and 78% specificity to distinguish more invasive lesions. No correlation between P63 and Ki-67 immunostaining in the three study groups.	Mann–Whitney test, T-test, correlation coefficient test, ROC curve analysis; significant differences with $p < 0.05$.	Higher P63 expression indicates more aggressive odontogenic lesions. No correlation found between P63 and Ki-67, suggesting different roles in tumor genesis and proliferation. P63 could be a useful diagnostic marker for aggressive odontogenic lesions.
Jaafari-Ashkavandi et al. (2019) [97]	To investigate the proliferative activity of dentigerous cysts (DCs), odontogenic keratocysts (OKCs), and ameloblastomas (ABs) using minichromosome maintenance 3 (MCM3) and Ki-67 proliferation markers.	Study Type: Cross-sectional immunohistochemical study. Sample Size: 11 DCs, 14 OKCs, 15 ABs (11 solid, 4 unicystic). Age Range Mean age: 28.9 ± 18.6 years. Country/Region: Iran.	Immunohistochemistry using anti-MCM3 and anti-Ki-67 antibodies.	Histopathological examination using hematoxylin and eosin staining.	MCM3 and Ki-67 are expressed in all cases. Higher MCM3 and Ki-67 expression in OKCs and ABs compared to DCs. MCM3 expression higher than Ki-67 in all groups. Expression more prominent in basal and parabasal layers of OKCs, peripheral cells of ameloblastomas, and basal layer of DCs. There is no significant difference in expression between inflamed and non-inflamed cysts.	ANOVA and Tukey tests showed significant differences in MCM3 and Ki-67 expression among all groups ($p < 0.000$). Spearman's correlation test showed weak positive correlation between MCM3 and Ki-67 ($\rho = 0.57$, $p = 0.002$).	MCM3 is a more sensitive proliferation marker than Ki-67. Higher expression of both markers in OKCs and ABs suggests higher proliferative activity and supports their aggressive behavior. MCM3 and Ki-67 are reliable markers for assessing proliferation in odontogenic lesions.

Table 6. Cont.

Authors	Objective	Study Details	Marker Identification Method	Cyst/Tumor Diagnosis Method	Results	Statistical Estimates	Conclusion
Brito-Mendoza et al. (2018) [98]	To compare the expression of Ki-67, syndecan-1 (CD138), and the molecular triad RANK, RANKL, and OPG in odontogenic keratocysts (OKCs), unicystic ameloblastomas (UAs), and dentigerous cysts (DCs).	Study Type: Immunohistochemical study. Sample Size: 22 OKCs, 19 UAs, 17 DCs. Country/Region: Mexico, Uruguay, Brazil.	Immunohistochemistry using antibodies for Ki-67, CD138, RANK, RANKL, and OPG.	Histopathological examination using hematoxylin and eosin staining.	Higher Ki-67 expression in OKC compared to UA and DC ($p < 0.0001$). Greater loss of CD138 in UA compared to OKC ($p = 0.0034$). Higher RANKL expression in UA epithelium and stroma ($p = 0.0002$, $p = 0.0004$). DC showed lower expression of all markers.	Chi-square test, Kruskal-Wallis test, Tukey-Kramer method, Spearman's Rho; significant differences with $p < 0.05$.	Increased RANKL expression and reduced CD138 expression in UA indicate higher invasive and destructive potential. The higher proliferation rate in OKC is related to its continuous intrabony growth. DC expansion does not seem to be related to these factors.
Modi et al. (2018) [99]	To compare the expression of Ki-67 in odontogenic keratocysts (OKCs), radicular cysts (RCs), and dentigerous cysts (DCs) to understand their proliferative activity and aggressive behavior.	Study Type: Immunohistochemical study. Sample Size: 15 OKCs, 15 RCs, 15 DCs. Country/Region: India (Gujarat and Uttar Pradesh).	Immunohistochemistry using Ki-67 monoclonal antibody (streptavidin-biotin detection system HRP-DAB).	Histopathological examination using hematoxylin and eosin staining.	Ki-67 positive cells were highest in OKC epithelium compared to DC and RC. Ki-67 labeling index (LI) in OKC: 12.76 ± 4.78; DC: 5.87 ± 4.24; RC: 5.08 ± 3.11. Ki-67 expression significantly higher in suprabasal layer of OKC (19.66 ± 7.89) compared to DC (3.60 ± 2.31) and RC (3.12 ± 2.19). No significant difference in Ki-67 LI in the basal layer among all groups.	Statistically significant differences in Ki-67 expression in suprabasal layers between OKC and DC ($p < 0.0001$), and between OKC and RC ($p < 0.0001$). No significant difference between DC and RC ($p = 0.558$).	Increased Ki-67 expression in the suprabasal cell layers of OKC indicates higher proliferative activity and aggressive behavior, suggesting that OKC may be neoplastic rather than a developmental cyst.
Alsaegh et al. (2017) [102]	To evaluate COX-2 expression and its correlation with the proliferation of odontogenic epithelium in dentigerous cysts (DCs) and ameloblastomas (ABs).	Study Type: Immunohistochemical study. Sample Size: 16 DCs, 17 ABs. Age Range: 12–74 years; mean age: 36.2 years. Country/Region: China, UAE, Iraq, Japan.	Immunohistochemistry using antibodies for COX-2 and Ki-67.	Histopathological examination using hematoxylin and eosin staining.	Ki-67 expression: DCs (absent: 25%; weak: 50%; mild: 12.5%; strong: 12.5%); ABs (absent: 23.52%; weak: 41.17%; mild: 17.64%; strong: 17.64%). COX-2 expression: DCs (absent: 18.75%; weak: 18.75%; mild: 43.75%; strong: 18.75%) ABs (absent: 5.89%; weak: 29.41%; mild: 52.94%; strong: 11.76%). Significant positive correlation between Ki-67 and COX-2 expression in DCs ($p = 0.018$) and ABs ($p = 0.004$).	Mann-Whitney U test and Spearman's rank correlation coefficient; significant differences with $p < 0.05$.	COX-2 and Ki-67 expression indicate higher proliferative activity in odontogenic epithelium of DCs and ABs, suggesting COX-2 as a potential target in managing these lesions.

Table 6. *Cont.*

Authors	Objective	Study Details	Marker Identification Method	Cyst/Tumor Diagnosis Method	Results	Statistical Estimates	Conclusion
Güler et al. (2012) [103]	To investigate the association between inflammation and the expression of cell cycle markers Ki-67 and MCM-2 in dental follicles (DF) and odontogenic cysts.	Study Type: Immunohistochemical study. Sample Size: 70 dental follicles (DF) and 20 odontogenic cysts (6 radicular cysts (RCs), 7 dentigerous cysts (DCs), 7 keratocystic odontogenic tumors (KCOTs)). Age Range: DFs: mean age 27 years (range 6–58 years); Cysts: mean age 39 years (range 22–57 years). Country/Region: Turkey.	Immunohistochemistry using Ki-67 and MCM-2 antibodies.	Histopathological examination using hematoxylin and eosin staining.	Ki-67 expression: DF (9.64 ± 5.99), RC (12.17 ± 4.49), DC (7.43 ± 3.99), KCOT (16 ± 13.46). MCM-2 expression: DF (6.34 ± 3.81), RC (19.17 ± 3.76), DC (7 ± 4.25), KCOT (15.43 ± 14.04). Significant correlation between inflammation and Ki-67/MCM-2 expressions in DFs and cysts ($p < 0.01$).	Kruskal–Wallis test, Mann–Whitney U test, Student's t-test; significant differences with $p < 0.05$.	Higher MCM-2 expression in RCs compared to KCOTs suggests a potential sensitivity to inflammation. Both Ki-67 and MCM-2 are useful in assessing proliferative activity and the influence of inflammation in odontogenic cysts and dental follicles.
Kim et al. (2003) [104]	To evaluate the comparative proliferative activity and apoptosis in odontogenic keratocysts (OKCs) associated with or without an impacted tooth and between unilocular and multilocular OKC varieties.	Study Type: Immunohistochemical study. Sample Size: 32 OKCs (16 with impacted tooth, 16 without impacted tooth), 10 dentigerous cysts (DCs).	Immunohistochemistry using Ki-67 for proliferation and TUNEL method for apoptosis.	Histopathological examination using hematoxylin and eosin staining.	OKCs showed greater proliferative potential and more apoptotic reactions than DCs. Proliferating cells primarily in the suprabasal layer and apoptotic cells in the superficial layer of OKCs. There is no significant difference in proliferative activity or apoptosis between OKCs associated with or without impacted teeth, or between unilocular and multilocular OKC varieties.	Statistical significance not explicitly stated.	OKCs are characterized by increased cell proliferation and apoptosis, indicating a unique proliferative and differentiation process. The aggressive behavior or recurrence in multilocular OKCs is likely due to incomplete removal or other contributing factors rather than intrinsic growth or apoptosis.

Table 6. *Cont.*

Authors	Objective	Study Details	Marker Identification Method	Cyst/Tumor Diagnosis Method	Results	Statistical Estimates	Conclusion
de Oliveira et al. (2011) [105]	To evaluate the biological profile of odontogenic epithelium by immunolabeling of epidermal growth factor receptor (EGFR), Ki-67, and survivin in keratocystic odontogenic tumors (KOTs), dentigerous cysts (DCs), and pericoronal follicles (PFs).	Study Type: Immunohistochemical study. Sample Size: 13 KOTs, 14 DCs, 9 PFs. Country/Region: Brazil.	Immunohistochemistry using antibodies for EGFR, Ki-67, and survivin.	Histopathological examination using hematoxylin and eosin staining.	KOTs showed the highest proliferation rate among the three groups, mainly in suprabasal layers. EGFR immunolabeling observed mainly in the cytoplasm in basal and suprabasal layers of KOTs, and in the suprabasal layer of DCs. Survivin immunolabeling showed a greater percentage of positive cells in the suprabasal layer of KOTs. PFs showed the highest percentage of survivin-positive cells, with immunolabeling in both the membrane and cytoplasm.	Chi-square test, Fisher's exact test, Spearman coefficient, Mann–Whitney test, Wilcoxon test; significant differences with $p < 0.01$.	Epithelial cells in KOTs demonstrate stimulus-independent proliferative characteristics, suggesting a suprabasal proliferative compartment maintained by inhibition of apoptosis. In DCs, the basal layer proliferates in response to stimuli. PFs, though showing low proliferative activity, have a high capacity to respond to stimuli, indicating potential for odontogenic lesion development.
Nadalin et al. (2011) [106]	To assess the immunohistochemical expression of syndecan-1 (CD138) and Ki-67 in radicular cysts (RCs), dentigerous cysts (DCs), and keratocystic odontogenic tumors (KOTs).	Study Type: Immunohistochemical study. Sample Size: 35 RCs, 22 DCs, 17 KOTs. Age Range: RC: Mean age 42.2 years; DC: Mean age 29 years; KOT: Mean age 45.8 years. Country/Region: Brazil.	Immunohistochemistry using antibodies for syndecan-1 (CD138) and Ki-67.	Histopathological examination using hematoxylin and eosin staining.	Syndecan-1: High expression in 85.7% RCs, 95.5% DCs, and 94.1% KOTs. Ki-67: Higher suprabasal expression in KOTs compared to RCs and DCs ($p < 0.0001$). Positive correlation between syndecan-1 and Ki-67 in RCs ($p = 0.01$) and KOTs ($p = 0.01$). Intense inflammation reduces syndecan-1 expression in RCs and KOTs.	Fisher's exact test, Spearman's correlation coefficient; significant differences with $p < 0.05$.	Syndecan-1 is not a determinant factor in the distinct histopathological features and biological behavior of the studied lesions. However, a positive correlation between syndecan-1 and Ki-67 indicates its potential role in cell proliferation in RCs and KOTs.

Table 6. *Cont.*

Authors	Objective	Study Details	Marker Identification Method	Cyst/Tumor Diagnosis Method	Results	Statistical Estimates	Conclusion
Naruse et al. (2017) [107]	To identify the most useful markers for predicting the recurrence of keratocystic odontogenic tumors (KCOTs) by evaluating the expression profiles of Ki-67, CD34, and podoplanin.	Study Type: Retrospective immunohistochemical study. Sample Size: 65 tumor samples from 63 patients. Age Range: Median age: 41 years (range 10–87 years). Country/Region: Japan.	Immunohistochemistry using antibodies for Ki-67, CD34, and podoplanin.	Histopathological examination using hematoxylin and eosin staining.	High Ki-67, CD34, and podoplanin expression levels were associated with tumor recurrence. Univariate analysis revealed a significant association between high CD34 expression and tumor recurrence ($p = 0.034$), as well as conservative surgical treatment ($p = 0.003$). Multivariate analysis identified conservative treatment as the greatest independent risk factor for tumor recurrence (odds ratio = 13.337, $p = 0.018$).	Univariate and multivariate logistic regression analyses; significant differences with $p < 0.05$.	Overexpression of CD34 may be a potent predictor of tumor recurrence. Radical treatment of teeth in contact with tumors is recommended to prevent recurrence. Conservative treatment was significantly associated with higher recurrence rates.
Selvi et al. (2012) [108]	To investigate the role of Ki-67 and argyrophilic nucleolar organizing regions (AgNORs) in differentiating recurrent and non-recurrent keratocystic odontogenic tumors (KCOTs) and to compare the correlation between these markers.	Study Type: Retrospective immunohistochemical study. Sample Size: 22 KCOT cases. Country/Region: Turkey.	Immunohistochemistry for Ki-67 and silver staining for AgNOR.	Histopathological examination using hematoxylin and eosin staining.	Recurrence in three patients (13.6%) during a mean follow-up period of 37.8 months (about 3 years). Significantly higher Ki-67 and AgNOR counts in recurrent lesions compared to non-recurrent lesions ($p = 0.045$ for Ki-67; $p = 0.049$ for AgNOR). Positive correlation between Ki-67 and AgNOR counts ($r = 0.853$, $p = 0.0001$).	Mann–Whitney U test, Fisher's exact test, and Spearman's correlation; significant differences with $p < 0.05$.	Ki-67 and AgNOR may serve as prognostic markers for KCOT recurrence. The findings support the classification of KCOT as an odontogenic tumor and suggest that enucleation with curettage or decompression followed by enucleation with curettage is effective despite a relatively high recurrence rate. Conservative treatment should be chosen carefully, avoiding cases with coronoid invasion, cortical lysis, or tissue invasion.

Table 6. Cont.

Authors	Objective	Study Details	Marker Identification Method	Cyst/Tumor Diagnosis Method	Results	Statistical Estimates	Conclusion
Ba et al. (2010) [109]	To investigate the relationship between radiographic appearance and epithelial cell proliferation in keratocystic odontogenic tumors (KCOTs).	Study Type: Retrospective radiographic and immunohistochemical study. Sample Size: 284 KCOT cases for radiographic analysis; 30 cases for Ki-67 immunohistochemical analysis. Age Range: Mean age: 32 years (range 9–87 years). Country/Region: China and Japan.	Immunohistochemistry using Ki-67 antibody.	Histopathological examination using hematoxylin and eosin staining.	Radiographic types: Unilocular (64.79%), multilocular (21.90%), multiple (9.79%), NBCCS-associated (3.52%). Ki-67 expression: Higher in NBCCS-associated KCOTs compared to solitary and multiple KCOTs ($p = 0.018, 0.002$). Significant difference in Ki-67 expression between multilocular and unilocular/NBCCS-associated KCOTs ($p = 0.000$). No significant difference between solitary and multiple KCOTs ($p = 0.220$).	ANOVA, least significant difference test; significant differences with $p < 0.05$.	A high correlation exists between the biological behavior of KCOTs and their imaging features. The solitary KCOTs seem less biologically aggressive and should be classified as cysts rather than tumors. More than half of KCOTs manifest as ordinary cysts.
Mendes et al. (2011) [110]	To investigate the association between the expression of cyclooxygenase-2 (COX-2) in keratocystic odontogenic tumors (KCOTs) and more commonly used markers, such as p53 and Ki-67.	Study Type: Immunohistochemical study. Sample Size: 20 KCOT biopsy specimens.	Immunohistochemistry using anti-COX-2, anti-Ki-67, and anti-p53 monoclonal antibodies.	Histopathological examination using hematoxylin and eosin staining.	COX-2 expression: Mild to strong in 100% of cases. p53 expression: Positive in 75% of cases. Ki-67 expression: Positive in 90% of cases. No statistically significant difference between the expressions of COX-2, Ki-67, and p53.	Statistical relevance of differences between COX-2, Ki-67, and p53 expressions not found.	COX-2 may be an important marker involved in the biological behavior of KCOTs. Despite its rare usage in assessing KCOTs, its role in tumorigenesis suggests its significance. Larger studies are required to understand the possible role of COX-2 in KCOT pathogenic mechanisms.
Nafarzadeh et al. (2013) [100]	To investigate the expression of PCNA and Ki-67 in dental follicle, dentigerous cyst, unicystic ameloblastoma, and ameloblastoma to assess their proliferative status.	Study Type: Immunohistochemical study. Sample Size: 60 samples: 15 each of dental follicle, dentigerous cyst, unicystic ameloblastoma, and ameloblastoma. Country/Region: Iran.	Immunohistochemistry using anti-Ki-67 and anti-PCNA monoclonal antibodies.	Histopathological examination using hematoxylin and eosin staining.	Ki-67: Weak in dental follicle (12), moderate in dentigerous cyst (14), intense in ameloblastoma (10). PCNA: Weak in dental follicle (12), moderate in dentigerous cyst (14), intense in ameloblastoma (13). Correlation coefficient between Ki-67 and PCNA: 0.88, statistically significant ($p < 0.001$).	Chi-square test, Pearson correlation, one-way ANOVA; significant differences with $p < 0.05$.	Significant differences in Ki-67 and PCNA expressions among dental follicle, dentigerous cyst, unicystic ameloblastoma, and ameloblastoma. Ki-67 and PCNA can be used to estimate proliferative status and aggressiveness, aiding in understanding the biological behavior and prognosis of these lesions.

Table 6. *Cont.*

Authors	Objective	Study Details	Marker Identification Method	Cyst/Tumor Diagnosis Method	Results	Statistical Estimates	Conclusion
Kuroyanagi et al. (2009) [111]	To determine prognostic factors for the recurrence of keratocystic odontogenic tumors (KCOTs) following simple enucleation by examining clinicopathologic and immunohistochemical findings.	Study Type: Retrospective study. Sample Size: 32 subjects diagnosed with KCOT. Country/Region: Japan.	Immunohistochemistry using antibodies for Ki-67 and p53.	Histopathological examination using hematoxylin and eosin staining.	Recurrence rate: 12.5% (4 out of 32 subjects). High Ki-67 expression (>10% LI) in basal layer: 75.0% in recurrent group vs. 14.3% in non-recurrent group ($p = 0.025$). p53 expression: 75.0% in recurrent group vs. 39.3% in non-recurrent group ($p = 0.295$). Hazard risk for recurrence with high Ki-67 expression: 4.02 (95% CI 1.42–18.14, $p = 0.009$).	Cox proportional hazard model, $p < 0.05$.	High Ki-67 expression in the basal layer of KCOTs is significantly associated with recurrence. Evaluating Ki-67 expression at diagnosis may help guide the use of appropriate adjunctive surgical procedures to prevent recurrence and serve as a prognostic marker.
Ono et al. (2022) [112]	To determine the clinical, pathological, and genetic characteristics of multiple orthokeratinized odontogenic cysts (OOCs).	Study Type: Clinical, pathological, and genetic study. Sample Size: 3 cases of multiple OOCs (total of 7 OOCs). Age Range: Mean age: 25.3 years (range 18–38 years). Country/Region: Japan.	Immunohistochemistry using antibodies for Ki-67 and Bcl-2; next-generation sequencing (NGS) for PTCH1 mutations.	Histopathological examination using hematoxylin and eosin staining.	Clinical findings: All OOCs were in posterior regions; 57.1% associated with impacted teeth; no recurrence observed. Histological findings: Cysts lined by orthokeratinized stratified squamous epithelium; no OKC features observed. Immunohistochemical findings: Low Ki-67 labeling index (mean 9.43%); no Bcl-2 expression. Genetic findings: No pathogenic PTCH1 mutations detected.	No specific statistical tests mentioned.	Multiple OOCs occur more often in younger patients and show mild biological behavior with no recurrence, distinguishing them from OKCs. Both multiple and solitary OOCs are considered related diseases within the entity of odontogenic cysts and are distinct from OKCs.

Table 6. *Cont.*

Authors	Objective	Study Details	Marker Identification Method	Cyst/Tumor Diagnosis Method	Results	Statistical Estimates	Conclusion
Park et al. (2020) [113]	To assess changes in histology and expression of proliferation markers in odontogenic keratocysts (OKCs) before and after decompression treatment.	Study Type: Clinical and immunohistochemical study. Sample Size: 38 OKC tissue samples from 19 patients. Age Range: Mean age: 38.8 years (range 19–81 years). Country/Region: South Korea.	Immunohistochemistry using antibodies for Bcl-2, EGFR, Ki-67, P53, PCNA, and SMO.	Histopathological examination using hematoxylin and eosin staining.	Decompression period: 4 to 12 months (mean 7.3 months). No significant change in Bcl-2, Ki-67, P53, PCNA, and SMO values before and after decompression. Significant change in EGFR values before and after decompression ($p = 0.040$). There is no correlation between clinical shrinkage and morphologic changes or expression of proliferation and growth markers. OKCs recurred in 3 patients' post-decompression.	Paired *t*-test, Wilcoxon signed ranks test; $p < 0.05$ considered significant.	Decompression does not significantly change the biological behavior or recurrence rate of OKCs. EGFR values changed significantly, but no other markers showed significant change, indicating decompression does not reduce the aggressive behavior of OKCs.
Coşarcă et al. (2016) [101]	To analyze the immunoexpression of Ki67, p53, MCM3, and PCNA in dental follicles of impacted teeth, dentigerous cysts (DCs), and keratocystic odontogenic tumors (KCOTs) to evaluate their proliferative capacity and evolutionary behavior.	Study Type: Immunohistochemical study. Sample Size: 62 dental follicles of impacted teeth, 20 DCs, 20 KCOTs. Country/Region: Romania.	Immunohistochemistry using antibodies for Ki67, p53, MCM3, and PCNA.	Histopathological examination using hematoxylin and eosin staining.	Dental follicles: Positive for PCNA (96.77%), Ki67 (90.32%), MCM3 (74.19%), and p53 (64.51%). Significant differences in Ki67, p53, and MCM3 between basal and parabasal layers in DCs and KCOTs. Positive correlation between Ki67 and MCM3 in basal and parabasal layers of KCOTs. Ki67 and MCM3 are useful in distinguishing between DCs and KCOTs.	Chi-square test, Mann-Whitney test, Spearman's correlation; significant differences with $p < 0.05$.	Ki67 and MCM3 are the most useful markers for evaluating the proliferative capacity and distinguishing between DCs and KCOTs. KCOTs show more aggressive behavior and higher proliferative capacity compared to DCs.

Table 6. Cont.

Authors	Objective	Study Details	Marker Identification Method	Cyst/Tumor Diagnosis Method	Results	Statistical Estimates	Conclusion
Jabbarzadeh et al. (2021) [114]	To assess the Ki-67 labeling index (LI) in odontogenic cysts and tumors through a systematic review and meta-analysis.	Study Type: Systematic review and meta-analysis. Sample Size: 608 lesions.	Immunohistochemistry for Ki-67.	Histopathological examination using hematoxylin and eosin staining.	Ki-67 LI in benign odontogenic tumors: <5%. Ki-67 LI in malignant odontogenic tumors: >15.3%. Highest Ki-67 LI in ameloblastoma (4.39 ± 0.47) among benign tumors. Highest Ki-67 LI in odontogenic cysts: odontogenic keratocyst (OKC) (3.58 ± 0.51). Significant difference in Ki-67 LI between malignant and benign odontogenic lesions ($p < 0.001$).	Random-effects model for pooled LI mean at 95% CI; significant heterogeneity ($Q = 743.03$, $df = 28$, $p < 0.001$, $I^2 = 96.23$).	Ki-67 LI is a reliable marker for distinguishing between benign and malignant odontogenic lesions. The high Ki-67 LI in OKCs suggests they are more like tumors, implying a need for tumor-like treatment plans.
Bhola et al. (2024) [115]	To compare the expression of MCM-3 and Ki-67 in odontogenic cysts and evaluate the sensitivity of these markers to inflammation.	Study Type: Immunohistochemical study. Sample Size: 37 dentigerous cysts, 37 odontogenic keratocysts (OKCs), 27 radicular cysts. Country/Region: Romania.	Immunohistochemistry using antibodies for Ki-67 and MCM-3.	Histopathological examination using hematoxylin and eosin staining.	Higher labeling index (LI) of MCM-3 compared to Ki-67 in all study groups. Positive correlation of Ki-67 LI with inflammation. MCM-3 proteins proved more accurate for determining proliferation potential and were not sensitive to external stimuli like inflammation, unlike Ki-67.	Statistical analysis with $p < 0.05$ considered significant.	MCM-3 is a more accurate marker for determining proliferation potential and is not influenced by inflammation, unlike Ki-67, making it more reliable for evaluating odontogenic cysts.

Table 6. *Cont.*

Authors	Objective	Study Details	Marker Identification Method	Cyst/Tumor Diagnosis Method	Results	Statistical Estimates	Conclusion
Embaló et al. (2018) [116]	To evaluate the metabolism and epithelial cell proliferation of odontogenic keratocyst (OKC), dentigerous cyst (DC), and unicystic ameloblastoma (UA) by quantifying the nucleolar organizing regions (AgNORs) and Ki-67 protein immunoexpression.	Study Type: Retrospective study. Sample Size: 16 OKCs, 16 DCs, 16 UAs.	Immunohistochemistry for Ki-67 and AgNOR.	Histopathological examination using hematoxylin and eosin staining.	Ki-67 and AgNOR counts were significantly higher in OKC compared to DC and UA ($p < 0.001$). Ki-67-positive cells were higher in suprabasal cell layers of OKC with uniform distribution, while a few were observed predominantly in basal cell layer in DC and UA. AgNOR count was significantly higher in the OKC basal cell layers and observed throughout the lining epithelium of DC and UA. OKC presented high metabolism and cellular proliferation compared to DC and UA, suggesting its aggressive clinical behavior and high recurrence rate.	Significant differences with $p < 0.001$.	Ki-67 and AgNOR reinforce the aggressive character of OKC, presenting high metabolism and cellular proliferation compared to DC and UA, possibly due to its more aggressive clinical behavior and high recurrence rate.
Kucukkolbasi et al. (2014) [117]	To assess the cell proliferation activity of dental follicles (DFs) surrounding asymptomatic impacted third molar teeth using the Ki-67 proliferation marker and to evaluate the variation of cell proliferation depending on age.	Study Type: Immunohistochemical study. Sample Size: 44 specimens of DFs. Age Range: 18 to 62 years (mean age: 32 years). Country/Region: Turkey.	Immunohistochemistry using Ki-67 monoclonal antibody.	Histopathological examination using hematoxylin and eosin staining.	Ki-67 expression: 60% in Group 1 (18–29 years), 75% in Group 2 (30+ years). Significant differences in Ki-67 expression between the two age groups in both basal and suprabasal layers. Histological examination showed higher squamous proliferation and inflammation in older patients. Squamous metaplasia was observed in all follicles, indicating a potential early sign of developing odontogenic lesions.	Statistically significant differences with $p < 0.05$.	DFs have more proliferative potential in older individuals compared to younger ones. Squamous metaplasia may be an early sign of developing odontogenic lesions, and histopathological changes could be found in DFs without clinical and radiographic alterations.

Table 6. *Cont.*

Authors	Objective	Study Details	Marker Identification Method	Cyst/Tumor Diagnosis Method	Results	Statistical Estimates	Conclusion
Cimadon et al. (2014) [118]	To evaluate the proliferative potential and cell proliferation rate of odontogenic epithelial cells using AgNOR and Ki-67, and to perform immunohistochemical staining for EGFR.	Study Type: Immunohistochemical study. Sample Size: 42 cases of pericoronal follicles of impacted third molars.	Silver impregnation technique for AgNOR, immunohistochemical staining for Ki-67 and EGFR.	Histopathological examination using hematoxylin and eosin staining.	Mean AgNORs per nucleus (mAgNOR): 1.43 (range: 1.0–2.42), with significant differences among pericoronal follicles from upper and lower teeth ($p = 0.041$). Ki-67 immunostaining was negative in all cases. EGFR immunolabeling was mainly cytoplasmic and more intense in islands and cords compared to the reduced epithelium of the enamel organ.	Significant differences with $p < 0.05$.	Odontogenic epithelial cells in some pericoronal follicles have proliferative potential, suggesting their association with the development of odontogenic lesions. Non-erupted teeth, especially of the lower jaw, should be monitored and possibly removed.
Chaturvedi et al. (2022) [119]	To distinguish aggressive from nonaggressive benign odontogenic tumors using the immunohistochemical expression of Ki-67 and Glypican-3 (GPC3).	Study Type: Immunohistochemical study. Sample Size: 20 solid ameloblastomas (8 follicular, 8 plexiform, 4 acanthomatous), 4 unicystic ameloblastomas, 28 keratocystic odontogenic tumors (KCOTs), 5 adenomatoid odontogenic tumors, and 2 calcifying cystic odontogenic tumors. Country/Region: India.	Immunohistochemistry using antibodies for Ki-67 and GPC3.	Histopathological examination using hematoxylin and eosin staining.	Ki-67: Positive correlation with aggressiveness ($p < 0.001$). GPC3: More useful than Ki-67 in distinguishing aggressiveness among aggressive tumors ($p < 0.001$). Intensity of GPC3: Maximum in plexiform ameloblastoma, followed by follicular and acanthomatous ameloblastomas, and KCOTs. GPC3 is not expressed in unicystic ameloblastomas.	Pearson correlation coefficient; $p < 0.001$ considered highly significant.	Ki-67 and GPC3 are valuable markers for differentiating aggressive from nonaggressive benign odontogenic tumors. GPC3 is more sensitive in determining the aggressiveness among aggressive odontogenic tumors.

Table 6. Cont.

Authors	Objective	Study Details	Marker Identification Method	Cyst/Tumor Diagnosis Method	Results	Statistical Estimates	Conclusion
Yamasaki et al. (2024) [120]	To describe the transformation of an odontogenic keratocyst (OKC) into a solid variant of odontogenic kerato-cyst/keratoameloblastoma (SOKC/KA) during long-term follow-up and analyze genetic mutations.	Study Type: Case report and genetic analysis. Sample Size: Single case study. Age Range: 26-year-old man at initial presentation. Country/Region: Japan.	Immunohistochemistry (IHC) for p53, Ki-67, BRAF, calretinin, β-catenin, CD56, p-S6, p-ERK1/2; Genetic panel sequencing for mutations.	Histopathological examination using hematoxylin and eosin staining; CT imaging.	Initial diagnosis: OKC. Recurrence: transformed to SOKC/KA with higher Ki-67 (~10%) and p53 positivity compared to primary lesion. Genetic mutations: APC (p.Arg876*), KRAS (p.Gly13Asp), and TP53 (p.Val31Ile). IHC: p-S6 and p-ERK1/2 positive in recurrent lesions.	Not applicable.	OKC can transform into SOKC/KA upon recurrence, indicated by increased proliferative activity and genetic mutations. The study suggests a close histogenetic relationship between OKC and SOKC/KA, and emphasizes the importance of genetic analysis in understanding tumor behavior.
Dong et al. (2010) [121]	To analyze the clinicopathologic features of 61 cases of orthokeratinized odontogenic cysts (OOCs) in a Chinese population.	Study Type: Clinicopathologic analysis and immunohistochemical study. Sample Size: 61 cases of OOC. Age Range: 13 to 75 years (average 38.93 years). Country/Region: China.	Immunohistochemical expression of Ki-67 and p63.	Clinicopathologic features and radiographic records.	90.16% of cases are mandible, 9.84% are maxilla. 87.04% unilocular radiolucencies, 12.96% multilocular. 50% associated with an impacted tooth. No recurrence in 42 patients after 76.8 months (about 6 and a half years) follow-up	Expression levels of Ki-67 and p63 were significantly lower in OOCs compared to KCOTs ($p < 0.001$).	OOC is clinicopathologically distinct from KCOT and should constitute its own clinical entity.
Mustansir-Ul-Hassnain et al. (2021) [122]	1. Analysis of histopathological findings in odontogenic cysts before and after decompression. 2. Analysis of Ki-67 expression in odontogenic jaw cysts before and after decompression.	Study Type: Original Research Article. Sample Size: 10 cases of odontogenic cysts. Age Range: Average age 26 ± 9.2 years (range not specified). Country/Region: Greater Noida, Uttar Pradesh, India.	Immunohistochemistry using Ki-67 monoclonal antibody.	Histopathologic examination of incisional and excisional biopsies before and after decompression.	Fewer Ki-67 + cells in radicular cysts, dentigerous cysts, and sialo-odontogenic cyst compared to odontogenic keratocysts (OKCs). Average scores were 2.2 before and 1 after decompression (statistically significant difference).	Two-tailed p value < 0.0001. Confidence interval 95%. Hazard ratio for recurrence not applicable.	The proliferative activity, evaluated by Ki-67 marker, was significantly greater in the epithelial lining before decompression compared to after decompression. Decompression significantly diminishes the proliferative rate of the cystic epithelial lining.

Table 6. Cont.

Authors	Objective	Study Details	Marker Identification Method	Cyst/Tumor Diagnosis Method	Results	Statistical Estimates	Conclusion
Trujillo-González et al. (2022) [123]	To evaluate the histological effects of decompression treatment on OKC, including cell proliferation and apoptosis of epithelial cyst.	Study Type: Original Study. Sample Size: 21 samples. Age Range: 9–58 years. Country/Region: Venezuela, Uruguay.	Immunohistochemistry (Ki-67, MCM4/7, Bax, Bcl2).	Surgical decompression with histological evaluation and immunohistochemical staining.	Increased inflammation ($p = 0.029$), loss of parakeratinization ($p = 0.007$), absence of palisade cell distribution ($p = 0.002$). No significant changes in expression of Ki-67 ($p = 0.323$), MCM4/7, Bax, or Bcl-2.	p values: 0.029 (inflammation), 0.007 (parakeratinization), 0.002 (palisade cell distribution), 0.323 (Ki-67), 0.079 (MCM4/7), 0.392 (Bax), Bcl-2 not specified.	Surgical decompression induces structural changes in OKC but does not significantly alter cell proliferation or apoptosis.
Zhou et al. (2022) [124]	To demonstrate the clinicopathological and radiological features of orthokeratinized odontogenic cysts (OOCs) and analyze the epithelial cell proliferative activity between OOCs and odontogenic keratocysts (OKCs).	Study Type: retrospective clinicopathological and radiological analysis. Sample Size: 48 OOC cases and 20 OKC cases. Age Range: 13 to 61 years. Country/Region: Shanghai Ninth People's Hospital.	Immunohistochemistry was performed using a DAKO AutostainerLink 48, with paraffin-embedded samples cut into 4-μm sections, deparaffinized, and rehydrated. Ki-67 and cyclin D1 antibodies were used for staining.	Histological examination and radiological imaging (panoramic radiographs and CT) were used to diagnose OOCs. The presence of orthokeratinized stratified squamous epithelial lining characterized OOCs.	Demographic Findings: 28 males and 20 females, with an average age of 33.50 years. Location: 40 cases in the mandible and 8 in the maxilla. Radiological Features: All OOCs were unilocular radiolucencies with well-defined margins, 83.33% showed buccolingual expansion. Histological Features: Thin, uniform orthokeratinized epithelium with a prominent granular cell layer. Proliferative Activity: Ki-67 and cyclin D1 expression were significantly lower in OOCs compared to OKCs ($p < 0.001$). Treatment: 40 cases treated with enucleation, 8 with decompression followed by enucleation. Follow-Up: Average follow-up of 32.50 ± 27.58 months (about 2 and a half years), with a 4.44% recurrence rate.	Ki-67 Expression: OOCs: $2.50\% \pm 0.25\%$; OKCs: $12.50\% \pm 1.42\%$, $p < 0.001$. Cyclin D1 Expression: OOCs: $9.71\% \pm 1.38\%$. OKCs: $32.50\% \pm 3.98\%$, $p < 0.001$.	OOCs predominantly affect the mandible, exhibit lower proliferative activity than OKCs, and are associated with buccolingual expansion and cortical bone destruction. Due to their lower aggressiveness and recurrence rate, minimally invasive surgical methods like enucleation or decompression followed by enucleation are recommended for treating OOCs.

Table 6. Cont.

Authors	Objective	Study Details	Marker Identification Method	Cyst/Tumor Diagnosis Method	Results	Statistical Estimates	Conclusion
Orikpete et al. (2020) [125]	To compare the proliferative capacity and antiapoptotic capacity of unicystic ameloblastoma (UA), odontogenic keratocyst (OKC), dentigerous cyst (DC), and radicular cyst (RC) by assessing the Ki-67 labeling index (LI) and Bcl-2 LI, respectively.	Study Type: Retrospective analysis. Sample Size: 23 histopathologically diagnosed UAs, 6 OKCs, 8 DCs, and 10 RCs were selected from archival specimens. Country/Region: Nigeria.	Five micrometer thick sections were made from the tissue blocks and mounted on silanized glass slides. Immunohistochemistry was performed using Ki-67 and Bcl-2 primary antibodies, followed by appropriate detection and staining procedures.	Histopathological examination was used for diagnosis, confirmed by hematoxylin and eosin staining of fresh sections from the tissue blocks.	Ki-67 Expression: UA: 26.1%. OKC: 66.7%; DC: 12.5%; RC: 10.0%. The mean Ki-67 LI was 1.3% for UA, 7.7% for OKC, 1.7% for DC, and 15.3% for RC. Bcl-2 Expression: UA: 69.6%. OKC: 83.3%. DC: 62.5%. RC: 50.0%. The mean Bcl-2 LI was 44.7% for UA, 58.8% for OKC, 5.2% for DC, and 10.3% for RC. Statistical Significance: Significant differences in Ki-67 LI between UA and OKC ($p = 0.024$). Significant differences in Bcl-2 LI between UA and DC ($p = 0.048$), and between OKC and both DC ($p = 0.026$) and RC ($p = 0.049$).	Ki-67 LI: UA: 1.3%. OKC: 7.7%. DC: 1.7%. RC: 15.3%. Significant difference between UA and OKC ($p = 0.024$). Bcl-2 LI: UA: 44.7%. OKC: 58.8%. DC: 5.2%. RC: 10.3%. Significant differences between UA and DC ($p = 0.048$), and between OKC and both DC ($p = 0.026$) and RC ($p = 0.049$).	The Ki-67 LI may help differentiate OKC from UA, and the Bcl-2 LI may be useful in differentiating UA from DC, as well as OKC from DC and RC.
Lafuente-Ibáñez de Mendoza et al. (2022) [126]	The aim of this study is to present and discuss the salient clinicopathological features, differential diagnosis, and epithelial immunohistochemical profile of three additional cases of peripheral odontogenic keratocyst (POKC) and to present a review of the literature.	Study Type: Case series and literature review. Sample Size: 3 new cases of POKC (2 women and 1 man; age range: 14–74 years).	Immunohistochemical study included CK7, CK14, CK19, and Ki-67. A systematic review of the literature was performed using PubMed, Scopus, and Web of Science databases.	Diagnosis of POKC was based on clinicopathological features and immunohistochemical profile.	All cases were in the anterior gingiva (2 in maxilla and 1 in mandible). None of the cases corresponded to Gorlin-Goltz syndrome. High expression of CK14 in all cases, CK19 and CK7 were only focally positive, and Ki-67 expression was in the basal and parabasal cells in all cases.	Not applicable.	POKC is a rare gingival lesion that seems to originate from remnants of dental lamina or from the basal cells of the gingival epithelium and presents a similar histopathology as compared to intraosseous OKC.

4.7. Therapeutic Insights and Surgical Management

Understanding the molecular and biochemical underpinnings of odontogenic lesions, particularly odontogenic keratocysts (OKCs), has significantly improved their therapeutic management and surgical outcomes. Insights into the biochemical behavior of these lesions have led to the refinement of surgical techniques and the development of treatments tailored to their specific pathophysiological features.

Marsupialization, a pre-surgical technique used for OKCs, not only reduces the size of the lesion but also induces biochemical changes within the cyst, such as increased Slug expression [127]. These changes are associated with fibrosis of the cyst wall, which facilitates easier surgical removal and reduces the likelihood of aggressive recurrence. The biochemical insights gained from studying odontogenic lesions have led to significant improvements in surgical management. Techniques like marsupialization, which have been shown to alter biochemical markers within the cyst, are now routinely used to prepare lesions for less invasive surgery, reducing the risk of recurrence. The use of pre-surgical marsupialization based on biochemical marker changes exemplifies how molecular insights are integrated into surgical planning, enhancing therapeutic outcomes by modifying the biological behavior of lesions before more definitive surgical interventions.

These therapeutic insights emphasize the importance of considering the biological behavior of lesions in surgical planning, moving beyond mere removal to positively influencing the lesion's biochemical environment. Utilizing biochemical markers like Slug in surgical planning allows for more customized and effective interventions, aiming to minimize the risk of recurrence and enhance overall treatment outcomes.

Research into the effects of marsupialization has shown that this procedure significantly increases epithelial thickness and collagen production within the cyst wall [127]. These changes are crucial for reducing the size and aggressiveness of OKCs, facilitating their surgical management. Furthermore, the study by Baris et al. highlighted that marsupialization leads to a significant reduction in the radiographic size of OKCs and an increase in fibrosis, which are key factors in preventing recurrence [127].

The potential for new therapeutic targets based on the molecular and biochemical profiles of odontogenic lesions points towards an era of targeted, specific treatments. For instance, targeting pathways involved in epithelial–mesenchymal transition (EMT) and inflammation could provide new avenues for therapy. The increased expression of Slug post-marsupialization indicates its role in EMT and fibrosis, suggesting that therapies targeting Slug could enhance the efficacy of marsupialization and other surgical interventions.

The advancements in understanding the molecular and biochemical behavior of odontogenic lesions have significant implications for personalized therapy. By integrating molecular insights into surgical planning and postoperative management, clinicians can tailor interventions to the specific characteristics of each lesion, improving patient outcomes. The use of targeted therapies alongside traditional surgical methods could further reduce recurrence rates and enhance the overall effectiveness of treatment.

In summary, the study of the molecular and biochemical aspects of odontogenic lesions, particularly OKCs, has led to significant advancements in their therapeutic management. The integration of biochemical markers into surgical planning and the development of targeted therapies promise to improve patient outcomes by aligning treatment strategies with the underlying causes of lesion behavior [127] (Table 7).

Table 7. Therapeutic and surgical management (OKCs).

Authors	Objective	Study Details	Marker Identification Method	Cyst/Tumor Diagnosis Method	Results	Statistical Estimates	Conclusion
Baris et al. (2022) [127]	To assess the effect of marsupialization on histomorphological and biochemical markers of odontogenic keratocysts (OKCs).	Study Type: Retrospective analysis. Sample Size: 48 paraffin blocks of 24 OKC cases between 2012 and 2018. Country/Region: Turkey.	Immunohistochemical staining with E-cadherin, Ki67, IL1α, TNFα, Slug, and Snail was performed on 4 μm thick sections of formalin-fixed paraffin OKC sections. The BOND Polymer Refine Detection Kit and BOND Polymer Refine Red Detection Kit were used for staining on the Leica BOND-MAX fully automated IHC and ISH staining system.	Diagnosis was based on histological and histomorphometric analysis, and radiological data including measurements on orthopantomographs.	The majority (70.8%) of OKC cases were in the mandibular posterior region. Marsupialization Period: Mean period was 8.8 ± 6.5 months (range: 3–25 months). Radiographic Findings: Mean size of OKC significantly reduced from 57.1 ± 53.5 mm to 22.6 ± 19.9 mm after marsupialization ($p = 0.002$). Histological Findings: Increased epithelial thickness ($p = 0.002$) and collagen production ($p = 0.034$) post-marsupialization. Positive correlation of inflammation score with TNFα (r: 0.69, $p < 0.001$) and IL-1α (r: 0.58, $p = 0.008$) expressions in connective tissue. Significant increase in Slug expression after marsupialization ($p = 0.019$).	Epithelial Thickness: Increased from 83.46 ± 45.05 μm to 167.39 ± 110.08 μm ($p = 0.002$). Collagen Production: Increased significantly post-marsupialization ($p = 0.034$). Inflammation Scores: Positive correlations with TNFα and IL-1α expressions ($p < 0.001$ and $p = 0.008$, respectively). Slug Expression: Significantly higher in the connective tissue post-marsupialization ($p = 0.019$).	Marsupialization can lead to significant changes in the histomorphology of OKCs, including increased epithelial thickness and collagen production. The increase in Slug expression may contribute to fibrosis, potentially aiding in subsequent surgical procedures.

4.8. Emerging Markers and Therapeutic Targets

The treatment landscape for odontogenic lesions, such as odontogenic keratocyst (OKC), adenomatoid odontogenic tumor (AOT), and ameloblastoma (AB), is evolving rapidly due to new discoveries in molecular markers and therapeutic targets like survivin, EGFR, BMP4, FOXN1, and paxillin [128–131]. These markers are shifting treatment paradigms from traditional surgical interventions to innovative, targeted therapies that address the underlying molecular and genetic drivers of these lesions.

Research into these molecular pathways and genetic mutations has unveiled new therapeutic opportunities. For instance, the roles of molecules such as survivin and EGFR suggest novel approaches for managing lesion growth. Studies have demonstrated that survivin expression is highest in ameloblastoma, followed by OKC, AOT, and reduced enamel epithelium, suggesting that survivin plays a role in inhibiting apoptosis and influencing the biological behavior of these lesions [128]. Similarly, EGFR and survivin have been shown to play crucial roles in the pathogenesis of ameloblastoma, OKC, and calcifying odontogenic cyst, highlighting the potential of targeting these markers in therapeutic approaches [129].

Differences in BMP4 and FOXN1 expression are opening new diagnostic and treatment avenues, potentially allowing for the modulation of cellular behaviors within lesions. Higher expression of BMP4 and FOXN1 in orthokeratinized odontogenic cysts (OOCs) compared to OKCs suggests a higher level of activation of pathways involved in more mature epithelial differentiation in OOCs, potentially contributing to their more benign behavior [130]. This distinction could aid in differential diagnosis and guide targeted therapeutic strategies.

The discovery of new molecular markers and therapeutic targets is transforming the treatment landscape for odontogenic lesions. The identification of EMT-related markers such as Snail and Slug in odontogenic cysts has prompted the exploration of EMT inhibitors as potential therapeutic options, aiming to prevent the invasive progression of these lesions. Significant expression of EMT markers like Snail and Slug in keratocystic odontogenic tumors (KOTs) suggests their role in EMT induction and potential as targets for therapeutic intervention [132].

The exploration of markers related to cell growth, apoptosis, and EMT is leading to therapies that directly target these cellular processes. Such targeted approaches are part of a broader shift towards precision medicine in the treatment of odontogenic lesions, aiming for more effective management with fewer adverse effects and more personalized treatment plans. Differential protein expressions in peripheral ameloblastoma and oral basal cell carcinoma have been shown to aid in accurate classification and tailored treatments [133].

Understanding the molecular and biochemical underpinnings of odontogenic lesions, particularly OKCs, has significantly improved their therapeutic management and surgical outcomes. Insights into the biochemical behavior of these lesions have led to the refinement of surgical techniques and the development of treatments tailored to their specific pathophysiological features. For example, marsupialization, a pre-surgical technique used for OKCs, not only reduces the size of the lesion but also induces biochemical changes within the cyst, such as increased Slug expression [127]. These changes are associated with fibrosis of the cyst wall, which facilitates easier surgical removal and reduces the likelihood of aggressive recurrence. Marsupialization significantly reduces the size of OKCs and increases epithelial thickness and collagenization, suggesting fibrosis and cyst wall strengthening, thus supporting its use as an effective treatment for reducing OKC size and potential recurrence [127].

The potential for new therapeutic targets based on the molecular and biochemical profiles of odontogenic lesions points towards an era of targeted, specific treatments. These advancements promise to align therapeutic strategies more closely with the underlying causes of a lesion's behavior, enhancing the effectiveness of interventions and leading to better patient outcomes [128–131].

In summary, the evaluation and incorporation of molecular and biochemical markers in the management of odontogenic lesions represents a significant advancement in the field. These markers provide crucial insights into how these lesions develop and respond to treatments, improving the prediction of outcomes and enabling more effective planning and execution of therapeutic strategies. Ongoing research into these markers is vital for refining management approaches and achieving better patient care outcomes (Table 8).

Table 8. Markers and therapeutic targets (OKC, AOT, AB, Survivin, EGFR, BMP4, FOXN1, and paxillin).

Authors	Objective	Study Details	Marker Identification Method	Cyst/Tumor Diagnosis Method	Results	Statistical Estimates	Conclusion
Latha et al. (2023) [128]	To assess the anti-apoptotic survivin expression in reduced enamel epithelium, adenomatoid odontogenic tumor, odontogenic keratocyst, and ameloblastoma.	Study Type: Quantitative analysis. Sample Size: 48 samples (12 each) of reduced enamel epithelium (REE), adenomatoid odontogenic tumor (AOT), odontogenic keratocyst (OKC), and ameloblastoma. Country/Region: India.	Immunohistochemistry was performed using survivin antibody. The sections were stained with hematoxylin and eosin for confirmatory diagnosis before immunohistochemical analysis. The slides were examined under a BX43 microscope with a ProgRes microscope camera, and the survivin expression was analyzed.	Histopathological examination using routine hematoxylin and eosin staining, followed by immunohistochemical analysis with survivin antibody.	Survivin Expression: Total Positive Cells: REE: 313.3; AOT: 1930.16; OKC: 2153.583; ameloblastoma: 2399.5823. Nuclear Expression: REE: 73.91; AOT: 270.83; OKC: 358.66; ameloblastoma: 379.663. Cytoplasmic Expression: REE: 169.833; AOT: 1029.833; OKC: 1003.58; ameloblastoma: 1180.50. Membrane Expression: REE: 20.67; AOT: 89.66; OKC: 174; ameloblastoma: 180.0833. Cytoplasm Membrane Expression: REE: 67.9167; AOT: 453.583; OKC: 617.33; ameloblastoma: 659.416. Intensity of Staining: Mild: REE: 50%; AOT: 25%; OKC: 25%; ameloblastoma: 17%. Moderate: REE: 33%; AOT: 33%; OKC: 25%; ameloblastoma: 42%. Intense: REE: 17%; AOT: 42%; OKC: 50%; ameloblastoma: 50%. Survivin expression was highest in Ameloblastoma, followed by OKC, AOT, and REE. The expression showed significant statistical differences ($p < 0.05$).	Total Positive Cells: $p = 0.00657$. Nuclear Expression: $p = 0.00219$. Cytoplasmic Expression: $p = 0.00213$. Membrane Expression: $p = 0.000542$. Cytoplasm Membrane Expression: $p = 0.00101$. Intensity of Staining: $p = 0.00005987$.	High survivin expression was observed in Ameloblastoma, followed by OKC, AOT, and REE. The expression of survivin in these odontogenic cysts and tumors suggests its role in the inhibition of apoptosis and its potential as a therapeutic target. Higher survivin expression indicates worse prognosis, and its study may aid in understanding the biological behavior of odontogenic cysts and tumors.

Table 8. Cont.

Authors	Objective	Study Details	Marker Identification Method	Cyst/Tumor Diagnosis Method	Results	Statistical Estimates	Conclusion
Baddireddy et al. (2023) [129]	To assess and compare the expression of EGFR and survivin in ameloblastoma (AB), odontogenic keratocyst (OKC), and calcifying odontogenic cyst (COC).	Study Type: Immunohistochemical study. Sample Size: 30 ABs, 15 OKCs, and 10 COCs. Country/Region: India and USA	Immunohistochemistry was performed using primary antibodies against EGFR and survivin. The staining procedure included dewaxing, rehydration, antigen retrieval, blocking, primary and secondary antibody incubation, and chromogen development. The slides were examined under an Olympus BX51 research microscope.	Diagnosis was confirmed by examining archival hematoxylin and eosin (H&E) slides.	EGFR Expression: EGFR positivity was found in all cases. Predominant cytoplasmic staining with variations in intensity. Intensity: AB ($p = 0.007$), OKC ($p = 0.005$), COC ($p = 0.006$). IRS Scores: Significant difference between lesions ($p = 0.02$). Survivin Expression: 96% positive in AB, 100% positive in OKC and COC. Predominant cytoplasmic staining with variations in intensity. Intensity: Significant difference in AB peripheral and central cells ($p = 0.03$). IRS Scores: Significant difference between study groups ($p = 0.001$).	EGFR: IRS Scores: AB ($p = 0.02$), OKC ($p = 0.005$), COC ($p = 0.006$). Intensity: AB ($p = 0.007$), OKC ($p = 0.005$), COC ($p = 0.006$). Survivin: IRS Scores: AB ($p = 0.03$), OKC ($p = 0.09$), COC ($p = 0.06$). Intensity: AB ($p = 0.03$), OKC ($p = 0.09$), COC ($p = 0.06$).	The study provides insight into the role of EGFR and survivin in the pathogenesis of AB, OKC, and COC. OKC appears to be more aggressive than AB and COC due to its higher IRS scores. The study highlights the potential for EGFR and survivin as targets for therapeutic interventions in these lesions.
Thermos et al. (2022) [130]	To compare BMP4 and FOXN1 expression in orthokeratinized odontogenic cysts (OOCs) and odontogenic keratocysts (OKCs) to investigate their role in epithelial differentiation.	Study Type: Immunohistochemical comparison. Sample Size: 20 primary sporadic OKCs and 16 OOCs.	Immunohistochemistry was used to assess the expression of BMP4 and FOXN1 in the epithelial and connective tissues of OKC and OOC samples.	The diagnosis was based on histological examination.	BMP4 Expression: Epithelial: Detected in 81.25% OOC vs. 35% OKC. Connective Tissue: Observed in 65% OKC and 75% OOC. FOXN1 Expression: Detected in 75% OOC vs. 30% OKC. BMP4 epithelial and connective tissue positivity and FOXN1 epithelial positivity: 56.25% OOC vs. 10% OKC. Greater expression of BMP4 and FOXN1 in OOC suggests greater activation of this pathway in OOC, contributing to its more mature epithelium and resemblance to an epidermal phenotype.	Not specified.	The greater expression of BMP4 and FOXN1 in OOC suggests a more mature epithelial phenotype and a greater activation of the BMP4/FOXN1 pathway in OOC compared to OKC. This indicates a role in the differing biological behavior and differentiation of these cysts.

Table 8. Cont.

Authors	Objective	Study Details	Marker Identification Method	Cyst/Tumor Diagnosis Method	Results	Statistical Estimates	Conclusion
Zhang et al. (2018) [131]	To explore the potential involvement of Fra-1, c-Jun, and c-Fos, three vital members of the AP-1 complex, in the pathogenesis of odontogenic keratocysts (OKCs).	Study Type: Immunohistochemical and RT-qPCR analysis. Sample Size: 10 normal oral mucosa (OM), 10 dentigerous cysts (DC), and 32 OKC specimens.	Immunohistochemistry and real-time-quantitative polymerase chain reaction (RT-qPCR) were used to investigate the expression levels of Fra-1, c-Jun, and c-Fos. Double-labelling immunofluorescence analysis was also used to confirm the associations.	Diagnosis was based on histological examination and immunohistochemical analysis.	Fra-1, c-Jun, and c-Fos Expression: Increased significantly in OKCs compared to OM and DC tissue samples. Positively associated with the expression levels of Ki-67, PCNA, and Bcl-2. Analysis Methods: Double-labelling immunofluorescence analysis Hierarchical analysis.	Not specified.	This study revealed for the first time that Fra-1, c-Jun, and c-Fos were overexpressed in OKCs and had a close correlation with proliferation and anti-apoptosis potential of OKCs.
Pinheiro et al. (2020) [134]	To evaluate tryptase and E-cadherin protein expression in odontogenic keratocysts (OKCs) and radicular cysts (RCs) and their relationship with lesion size.	Study Type: Immunohistochemical analysis. Sample Size: 30 OKCs and 30 RCs. Country/Region: Brazil.	Immunohistochemistry was used to assess the expression of tryptase and E-cadherin in tissue samples. Tryptase expression was quantitatively assessed by counting mast cells, and E-cadherin expression was semi-quantitatively analyzed by estimating the proportion of positive cells.	The diagnosis was based on histological examination and radiographic measurements of the cystic lesion sizes.	Tryptase Expression: Higher mast cell means were found in RCs compared to OKCs. Degranulated mast cells were predominant in both OKCs and RCs. Negative correlation between E-cadherin expression and total number of mast cells, degranulated mast cells, and lesion size. E-cadherin Expression: Negative correlation with total number of mast cells ($p = 0.011$), degranulated mast cells ($p = 0.040$), and degranulated mast cells in both superficial ($p = 0.035$) and deep connective tissues ($p = 0.009$). Lesion Size: RCs: 67% ≤ 2 cm, 27% > 2 to 4 cm, 6% > 4 cm. OKCs: 47% ≤ 2 cm, 37% > 2 to 4 cm, 16% > 4 cm. Negative correlation between lesion size and total number of mast cells in the epithelium ($p = 0.016$) and degranulated mast cells in the epithelium ($p = 0.049$).	p-values: <Total number of mast cells in epithelium: $p = 0.016$. Degranulated mast cells in epithelium: $p = 0.049$. E-cadherin expression and total number of mast cells: $p = 0.011$. E-cadherin expression and degranulated mast cells: $p = 0.040$. E-cadherin expression and degranulated mast cells in superficial connective tissue: $p = 0.035$. E-cadherin expression and degranulated mast cells in deep connective tissue: $p = 0.009$.	The higher expression of tryptase in degranulated mast cells is linked to lower expression of E-cadherin, suggesting a change in epithelial permeability and contributing to increased cystic content and lesion growth. Mast cells in RCs may initiate cystic formation, while in OKCs, they act in more advanced stages, contributing to bone resorption and lesion expansion.

Table 8. Cont.

Authors	Objective	Study Details	Marker Identification Method	Cyst/Tumor Diagnosis Method	Results	Statistical Estimates	Conclusion
Porto et al. (2016) [132]	To evaluate the epithelial–mesenchymal transition (EMT) in keratocystic odontogenic tumors (KOTs) by assessing the immunoexpression of E-cadherin, N-cadherin, Snail, and Slug and comparing them to radicular cysts and dental follicles.	Study Type: Immunohistochemical study. Sample Size: 32 KOTs, 15 radicular cysts, and 8 dental follicles.	Immunohistochemistry was used to evaluate the expression levels of E-cadherin, N-cadherin, Snail, and Slug in tissue samples.	Diagnosis was based on histological examination and immunohistochemical analysis of the collected samples.	E-cadherin: Preserved in most cases of KOT. N-cadherin: Increased in the tumor epithelium, positively correlated with heterogeneous and nuclear immunoexpression of Slug in the epithelium. Also correlated with high Snail immunoexpression. Slug: Heterogeneous and nuclear expression in the epithelium, correlated with high Snail expression. Snail: High immunoexpression in KOTs. Stroma: N-cadherin positively correlated with Slug.	Not specified.	The high immunoexpression of Snail and nuclear Slug in KOTs suggests these proteins act as transcription factors without necessarily participating in "cadherin switching". However, the understanding of their role in inducing EMT in odontogenic tumors is still limited.
Singh et al. (2023) [13]	To analyze the immunohistochemical expression of paxillin in ameloblastoma (AB) and odontogenic keratocyst (OKC) to appraise their roles in cell-matrix interactions.	Study Type: Observational study. Sample Size: 60 cases (30 AB and 30 OKC). Age Range: OKC: 10–20 years: 2 cases. 21–30 years: 16 cases. 31–40 years: 6 cases. 41–50 years: 3 cases. 50 years: 3 cases. AB: 10–20 years: 6 cases. 21–30 years: 11 cases. 31–40 years: 5 cases. 41–50 years: 5 cases. 50 years: 3 cases. Country/Region: India.	Immunohistochemistry was used to stain tissue sections with a paxillin antibody. Staining intensity and quantitative staining were evaluated and scored.	Diagnosis was confirmed using histopathological criteria and hematoxylin and eosin staining.	Staining Intensity: Score 0 (No staining): OKC 1 (3%), AB 0 (0%). Score 1 (Weak staining): OKC 13 (43%), AB 6 (20%). Score 2 (Moderate staining): OKC 10 (33%), AB 6 (20%). Score 3 (Strong staining): OKC 5 (17%), AB 8 (27%). Score 4 (Very strong staining): OKC 1 (3%), AB 10 (33%). Statistical Comparison: Significant ($p = 0.013$). Quantitative Staining: Score 0 (No staining): OKC 1 (3%), AB 0 (0%). Score 1 (<25% of cells): OKC 9 (30%), AB 5 (17%). Score 2 (25–50% of cells): OKC 5 (17%), AB 5 (17%).	p-values: Staining Intensity: $p = 0.013$. Quantitative Staining: $p = 0.432$. Final Summation Score: $p = 0.503$. Gender-wise Comparison in OKC: $p < 0.05$. Gender-wise Comparison in AB: Quantitative staining $p < 0.001$, Final summation $p = 0.027$, Staining intensity $p = 0.091$.	Paxillin expression is significant in the epithelial lining of both OKC and AB, suggesting its role in cell-matrix interactions and tumorigenesis. The expression pattern indicates its involvement in the biological behavior of these odontogenic lesions. Further studies with larger sample sizes and molecular analyses are needed to confirm paxillin's exact role and potential as a therapeutic target.

Table 8. *Cont.*

Authors	Objective	Study Details	Marker Identification Method	Cyst/Tumor Diagnosis Method	Results	Statistical Estimates	Conclusion
					Score 3 (50–75% of cells): OKC 5 (17%), AB 10 (33%).		
					Score 4 (>75% of cells): OKC 10 (33%), AB 10 (33%).		
					Statistical Comparison: Non-significant ($p = 0.432$).		
					Final Summation Score: Score 0 (No staining): OKC 1 (3%), AB 0 (0%).		
					Score 1–4 (Weak staining): OKC 16 (53%), AB 11 (37%).		
					Score 5–8 (Strong staining): OKC 13 (43%), AB 19 (63%).		
					Statistical Comparison: Non-significant ($p = 0.503$).		
					Gender-wise Comparison: OKC: Significant ($p < 0.05$). AB: Quantitative staining and final summation significant ($p < 0.001$ and $p = 0.027$), staining intensity non-significant ($p = 0.091$).		
					Age-wise Comparison: OKC: Weak staining predominant in 21–30 years (53%). AB: Strong staining predominant in 21–30 years (66%)		

Table 8. *Cont.*

Authors	Objective	Study Details	Marker Identification Method	Cyst/Tumor Diagnosis Method	Results	Statistical Estimates	Conclusion
Cesinaro et al. (2020) [135]	To assess the expression of calretinin in odontogenic keratocysts (OKCs) and basal cell carcinomas (BCCs) in sporadic and Gorlin–Goltz syndrome (GGS) cases.	Study Type: Immunohistochemical analysis. Sample Size: 28 OKCs: 16 sporadic OKCs from 15 patients, 12 GGS-related OKCs from 11 patients. 34 BCCs: 19 BCCs and 2 cutaneous keratocysts from 4 GGS patients, 15 sporadic BCCs and 3 steatocystomas. Age Range: Sporadic OKCs: 10 to 61 years (Mean: 39.6 years, SD: 14.71) GGS-OKCs: 26 to 44 years (Mean: 32.7 years, SD: 5.82) Country/Region: Italy.	Immunohistochemistry was performed on 4-μm thick sections using anti-calretinin SP65 pre-diluted monoclonal rabbit antibody. Immunostaining was evaluated as negative, focally positive (<5% of cells), or positive (>5% of cells).	Diagnosis was based on histological examination according to the WHO classification of head and neck tumors.	Calretinin Expression in OKCs: GGS-OKCs: 10 negative, 2 focally positive. Sporadic OKCs: 6 negative, 6 focally positive, 4 diffusely positive. Significant difference between sporadic and GGS-OKCs ($p = 0.02$). Calretinin Expression in BCCs: GGS-BCCs: 14 negative, 4 focally positive, 1 diffusely positive. Sporadic BCCs: 7 negative, 8 focally positive. No significant difference between GGS and sporadic BCCs. Calretinin Expression in Cutaneous Cysts: GGS–cutaneous keratocysts: 2 negatives. Sporadic Steatocystomas: 1 negative, 1 focally positive, 1 diffusely positive	*p*-values: Calretinin expression in OKCs: $p = 0.02$. Calretinin expression in BCCs: Not significant. Calretinin expression in cutaneous cysts: Not significant.	Calretinin expression is significantly lower in GGS-OKCs compared to sporadic OKCs, suggesting a potential link between SHH pathway dysfunction and calretinin expression in GGS-related tumors. However, calretinin's value in differential diagnosis between sporadic and syndromic tumors appears limited.
Galvão et al. (2013) [136]	To perform an immunohistochemical assessment of protein 53 (p53), proliferating cell nuclear antigen (PCNA), B-cell lymphoma 2 (bcl-2), and murine double minute 2 (MDM2) expression in odontogenic cysts and keratocystic odontogenic tumor (KCOT), analyzing their correlation with the biological behavior of these lesions.	Study Type: Immunohistochemical analysis. Sample Size: 11 radicular cysts, 11 dentigerous cysts, 11 KCOTs.	The streptavidin-biotin-peroxidase method was used with antibodies against p53, PCNA, bcl-2, and MDM2 proteins.	Diagnosis was based on histological examination and immunohistochemical analysis.	PCNA: Immunopositivity observed in all cases, predominantly in the suprabasal layer of KCOT epithelial lining (SD ± 19.44), but no significant differences among the groups. Bcl-2: Immunoexpression observed especially in the basal layer of KCOT. PCNA LI: Significantly higher than bcl-2 LI in KCOT. MDM2 and p53: Immunoexpression not detected in the lesions studied. KCOT: Showed different immunoexpression of proliferation and apoptosis markers compared to other odontogenic cysts.	Non-parametric Mann–Whitney U-test and Kruskal–Wallis test ($p \leq 0.05$).	The results suggest that KCOT presents distinct biological behavior compared to odontogenic cysts, in terms of proliferation, apoptosis, and differentiation. This supports the neoplastic nature of KCOT.

Table 8. Cont.

Authors	Objective	Study Details	Marker Identification Method	Cyst/Tumor Diagnosis Method	Results	Statistical Estimates	Conclusion
Tenório et al. (2018) [11]	To investigate the expression of Bcl-2, Bax, and p53 to better understand the possible role of these proteins in ameloblastomas (AMBs), odontogenic keratocysts (OKCs), and adenomatoid odontogenic tumors (AOTs).	Study Type: Immunohistochemical analysis. Sample Size: 20 AMBs, 20 OKCs, 20 AOTs.	Immunohistochemistry technique was performed for the antibodies p53, Bcl-2, and Bax. Immunoreactivity was observed in the epithelial component.	Diagnosis was based on histological examination and immunohistochemical analysis.	Expression of Proteins: All lesions exhibited staining for p53, Bcl-2, and Bax. Statistical Analysis: No statistically significant associations between the expression of proteins and the lesions. Correlations: Positive correlation between the expression of p53 and Bcl-2 ($r = 0.200$). Negative correlation between p53 and Bax expressions ($r = -0.100$). p53 and Bax were similarly expressed between AMBs and OKCs. Bcl-2 was similarly expressed in AMBs and AOTs.	Kruskal–Wallis and Spearman tests ($p < 0.05$). Correlation Coefficients: p53 and Bcl-2: $r = 0.200$. p53 and Bax: $r = -0.100$	Apoptosis regulatory proteins, as well as cell cycle proteins, are differently expressed in epithelial odontogenic lesions. Their expression is possibly related to the biological behavior of AMBs, OKCs, and AOTs.
Ghafouri-Fard et al. (2021) [137]	To summarize the current data on the expression patterns of genes in ameloblastoma (AB), dentigerous cyst (DC), and odontogenic keratocyst (OKC), and to examine the association between genetic polymorphisms and the development of these lesions.	Study Type: Review. Sample Size: Various studies and samples were mentioned within the review. Country/Region: Iran.	Gene expression profiling, immunohistochemistry, cDNA microarray, RT-qPCR, Western blotting, loss of heterozygosity (LOH), PCR-RFLP, next-generation sequencing, methylation-specific PCR, and microarray studies.	Diagnosis was based on histological examination and various genetic and molecular assays.	Ameloblastoma (AB): Dysregulation of genes such as FOS, TNFRSF1A, SHH, TRAF3, ARHGAP4, DCC, CDH12 and 13, TDGF1, TGFB1, WNT1, IGF2, P63, WT1, IL-6, PTEN, COX-2, and many others. High incidence of BRAF V600E and SMO L412F mutations. Overexpression of long non-coding RNAs (lncRNAs) such as ENST00000512916 and KIAA0125. Genetic polymorphisms in genes like MMP9, APC, XRCC1, P53, RECK, and PTCH1. Dentigerous Cysts (DCs): Differential expression of genes related to extracellular matrix formation, adhesion, invasion, metabolic pathways, cell signalling, cytokine functions, inflammation, and immune responses. Genetic polymorphisms are associated with the PTCH gene region.	Not specified.	The review highlights the significant role of dysregulated genes, genetic polymorphisms, and miRNA/lncRNA expressions in the pathogenesis of AB, DC, and OKC. These molecular markers can potentially aid in the diagnosis, prognosis, and development of therapeutic approaches for these odontogenic lesions.

Table 8. Cont.

Authors	Objective	Study Details	Marker Identification Method	Cyst/Tumor Diagnosis Method	Results	Statistical Estimates	Conclusion
					Odontogenic Keratocysts (OKCs): Overexpression of genes like PTCH, SHH, SMO, GLI1, CCND1, and BCL2. Genetic polymorphisms and mutations in PTCH1, P53, IL-1, survivin gene promoter, and MIR15A/MIR16-1. Lower expression of calretinin in syndromic OKCs compared to sporadic cases.		
Kim et al. (2014) [133]	To compare the protein expression profiles of peripheral ameloblastoma (PA) and oral basal cell carcinoma (OBCC) occurring in the same mandibular molar area to better understand their tumorigenesis.	Study Type: Case study with immunohistochemical examination. Sample Size: One case of PA in a 61-year-old male and one case of OBCC in a 33-year-old male. Country/Region: Korea.	Immunohistochemistry using 50 antisera selected for important signaling pathways. Staining was evaluated and confirmed through repeated testing.	Histological examination and immunohistochemical analysis based on tissue samples.	PA: Strong positive for ameloblastin, KL1, p63, carcinoembryonic antigen (CEA), focal adhesion kinase (FAK), and cathepsin K. Slightly positive for amelogenin, Krox-25, E-cadherin, and PTCH Exhibited odontogenic differentiation and active ectomesenchymal interaction. Higher positivity for proteins associated with odontogenic epithelium, epithelial adhesion, and bone resorption. OBCC: Strong positive for EpCam, MMP-1, α1-antitrypsin, CK-7, p53, survivin, pAKT1, TGF-β1, N-RAS, TGase-1, and TNFα. Consistently positive for β-catenin, MMP-2, cathepsin G, TGase-2, SOS-1, SHH, and β-defensins 1, 2, and 3 exhibited basaloid epidermal differentiation influenced by growth factor/cytokine-related signals. Higher positivity for proteins associated with proliferation, apoptosis, and inflammation. Common Markers: Both PA and OBCC showed positive reactions for PCNA, NFkB, MMP-9, eIF5A, BCL-2, PARP, PIM1, NF-1, HSP-70, 14-3-3, HIF, vWF, and VEGF, indicating similar tumor growth potential.	Not specified.	PA and OBCC differ in their protein expression profiles, with PA showing odontogenic differentiation and OBCC exhibiting basaloid epidermal differentiation. These differences suggest distinct tumorigenesis pathways and could aid in differential diagnosis. Further investigations are required to fully elucidate characteristic protein expressions in these tumors.

5. Conclusions

This systematic review has comprehensively explored the roles of immunohistochemical markers in dentigerous cysts (DCs) and odontogenic keratocysts (OKCs) associated with impacted third molars. By synthesizing data from 138 articles, this review highlights the diagnostic, prognostic, and therapeutic importance of markers such as Ki-67, p53, Bcl-2, and PCNA. These markers have proven instrumental in predicting aggressive behavior and guiding management strategies for OKCs, which are prone to aggressive growth and recurrence.

The findings indicate that the elevated expressions of Ki-67 and p53 in OKCs are particularly significant, suggesting that these markers can critically inform clinical decisions regarding the timing and extent of surgical interventions. Additionally, the identification of PTCH1 gene mutations and alterations in the SHH pathway presents promising targets for developing novel therapeutic approaches, potentially leading to more effective treatments tailored to the genetic profiles of individual lesions.

However, this review acknowledges several limitations, including the heterogeneity of the study designs, sample sizes, and methodologies used, which may affect the generalizability of the findings. Most studies were limited by small sample sizes and the retrospective nature of data collection, which can introduce bias and limit the applicability of the results to a broader population. Furthermore, the predominance of research from high-resource settings may not accurately represent the global burden and characteristics of these conditions.

To address these limitations, future research should focus on conducting large-scale, multicentric prospective studies that include diverse populations to enhance the external validity of the findings. There is also a pressing need for longitudinal studies to assess the long-term outcomes of different therapeutic interventions and their impact on the patient's quality of life. Exploring the molecular mechanisms driving the expression of these immunohistochemical markers could uncover additional therapeutic targets. Furthermore, the development of non-invasive diagnostic tools based on these markers could revolutionize the early detection and management of DCs and OKCs, offering substantial improvements in patient care.

In summary, while this review makes significant strides toward understanding the complex pathology of odontogenic cysts and tumors, it also underscores the crucial need for continued research and innovation in this field. Ensuring that future studies address the identified limitations will be essential for producing findings that are robust, replicable, and applicable to diverse patient populations. By integrating immunohistochemical data into clinical practice, clinicians can optimize therapeutic outcomes and reduce the recurrence rates of these potentially aggressive conditions, ultimately advancing patient care in oral and maxillofacial surgery.

Author Contributions: Conceptualization, L.E.A. and S.Z.; methodology, L.E.A. and S.Z.; software, L.E.A.; validation, L.E.A., D.L., D.B. and O.K.; formal analysis L.E.A.; investigation, L.E.A. and S.Z.; resources, L.E.A.; data curation, L.E.A.; writing—original draft preparation, L.E.A. and S.Z.; writing—review and editing, S.Z.; visualization, D.B.; supervision, L.E.A.; project administration, L.E.A. All authors have read and agreed to the published version of the manuscript.

Funding: This research received no external funding.

Institutional Review Board Statement: Not applicable.

Data Availability Statement: Data can be found on PubMed.

Acknowledgments: We would like to acknowledge the Marquette University School of Dentistry for their support with this research.

Conflicts of Interest: The authors declare no conflicts of interest.

References

1. Vigneswaran, A.T.; Shilpa, S. The incidence of cysts and tumors associated with impacted third molars. *J. Pharm. Bioallied Sci.* **2015**, *7* (Suppl. S1), S251–S254. [CrossRef] [PubMed]
2. Passi, D.; Singh, G.; Dutta, S.; Srivastava, D.; Chandra, L.; Mishra, S.; Srivastava, A.; Dubey, M. Study of pattern and prevalence of mandibular impacted third molar among Delhi-National Capital Region population with newer proposed classification of mandibular impacted third molar: A retrospective study. *Natl. J. Maxillofac. Surg.* **2019**, *10*, 59–67. [PubMed]
3. Miranda da Rosa, F.; Oliveira, M.G.; Palmeira da Silva, V.; Rados, P.V.; Sant'Ana Filho, M. Relationship between the positions of impacted third molars and the presence of dentigerous cysts. *Gen. Dent.* **2015**, *63*, 43–46. [PubMed]
4. Mehta, D.N.; Thakkar, V.C.; Mandviya, P.; Jadav, B.; Goswami, R.; Chavda, R. Dermatoglyphic Patterns in Patients Having Impacted and Erupted Third Molars—A Comparative Study. *J. Pharm. Bioallied Sci.* **2023**, *15* (Suppl. S2), S1142–S1144. [CrossRef] [PubMed]
5. Li, K.; Xu, W.; Zhou, T.; Chen, J.; He, Y. The radiological and histological investigation of the dental follicle of asymptomatic impacted mandibular third molars. *BMC Oral Health* **2022**, *22*, 642. [CrossRef]
6. Özcan, A.; Yavan, İ.; Günhan, Ö. Immunohistochemical characteristics of cystic odontogenic lesions: A comparative study. *Turk Patoloji Derg.* **2015**, *31*, 104–110. [PubMed]
7. Hunter, K.D.; Speight, P.M. The diagnostic usefulness of immunohistochemistry for odontogenic lesions. *Head Neck Pathol.* **2014**, *8*, 392–399. [CrossRef]
8. Slusarenko da Silva, Y.; Stoelinga, P.J.W.; Grillo, R.; da Graça Naclério-Homem, M. Cyst or Tumor? A systematic review and meta-analysis on the expression of p53 marker in Odontogenic Keratocysts. *J. Cranio-Maxillo-Facial Surg.* **2021**, *49*, 1101–1106. [CrossRef] [PubMed]
9. Naz, I.; Mahmood, M.K.; Nagi, A.H. Expression of Bcl-2 in Primary and Recurrent Odontogenic Keratocysts in Comparison with Other Odontogenic Lesions. *Asian Pac. J. Cancer Prev.* **2015**, *16*, 6289–6292. [CrossRef]
10. Rahman, F.; Bhargava, A.; Tippu, S.R.; Kalra, M.; Bhargava, N.; Kaur, I.; Srivastava, S. Analysis of the immunoexpression of Ki-67 and Bcl-2 in the pericoronal tissues of impacted teeth, dentigerous cysts and gingiva using software image analysis. *Dent. Res. J.* **2013**, *10*, 31–37.
11. Tenório, J.R.; Santana, T.; Queiroz, S.I.; de Oliveira, D.H.; Queiroz, L.M. Apoptosis and cell cycle aberrations in epithelial odontogenic lesions: An evidence by the expression of p53, Bcl-2 and Bax. *Med. Oral Patol. Oral Cir. Buccal* **2018**, *23*, e120–e125. [CrossRef] [PubMed]
12. Seyedmajidi, M.; Nafarzadeh, S.; Siadati, S.; Shafaee, S.; Bijani, A.; Keshmiri, N. p53 and PCNA Expression in Keratocystic Odontogenic Tumors Compared with Selected Odontogenic Cysts. *Int. J. Mol. Cell. Med.* **2013**, *2*, 185–193. [PubMed]
13. Singh, A.; Astekar, M.S.; Sapra, G.; Agarwal, A.; Murari, A. Immunohistochemical expression of paxillin in ameloblastoma and odontogenic keratocyst: An observational study. *J. Oral Maxillofac. Pathol.* **2023**, *27*, 727–734. [CrossRef] [PubMed]
14. Madras, J.; Lapointe, H. Keratocystic odontogenic tumour: Reclassification of the odontogenic keratocyst from cyst to tumour. *J. Can. Dent. Assoc.* **2008**, *74*, 165–165h. [PubMed]
15. Cobourne, M.T.; Xavier, G.M.; Depew, M.; Hagan, L.; Sealby, J.; Webster, Z.; Sharpe, P.T. Sonic hedgehog signalling inhibits palatogenesis and arrests tooth development in a mouse model of the nevoid basal cell carcinoma syndrome. *Dev. Biol.* **2009**, *331*, 38–49. [CrossRef] [PubMed]
16. Shimura, M.; Nakashiro, K.I.; Sawatani, Y.; Hasegawa, T.; Kamimura, R.; Izumi, S.; Komiyama, Y.; Fukumoto, C.; Yagisawa, S.; Yaguchi, E.; et al. Whole Exome Sequencing of SMO, BRAF, PTCH1 and GNAS in Odontogenic Diseases. *In Vivo* **2020**, *34*, 3233–3240. [CrossRef]
17. Rodrigues, K.S.; Santos, H.B.P.; Morais, E.F.; Freitas, R.A. Immunohistochemical analysis of SHH, SMO and GLI-1 proteins in epithelial odontogenic lesions. *Braz. Dent. J.* **2022**, *33*, 91–99. [CrossRef] [PubMed]
18. Stojanov, I.J.; Schaefer, I.M.; Menon, R.S.; Wasman, J.; Gokozan, H.N.; Garcia, E.P.; Baur, D.A.; Woo, S.B.; Sholl, L.M. Biallelic PTCH1 Inactivation Is a Dominant Genomic Change in Sporadic Keratocystic Odontogenic Tumors. *Am. J. Surg. Pathol.* **2020**, *44*, 553–560. [CrossRef]
19. Zhai, J.; Zhang, H.; Zhang, J.; Zhang, R.; Hong, Y.; Qu, J.; Chen, F.; Li, T. Effect of the sonic hedgehog inhibitor GDC-0449 on an in vitro isogenic cellular model simulating odontogenic keratocysts. *Int. J. Oral Sci.* **2019**, *11*, 4. [CrossRef]
20. Ren, C.; Amm, H.M.; DeVilliers, P.; Wu, Y.; Deatherage, J.R.; Liu, Z.; MacDougall, M. Targeting the sonic hedgehog pathway in keratocystic odontogenic tumor. *J. Biol. Chem.* **2012**, *287*, 27117–27125. [CrossRef]
21. Yagyuu, T.; Kirita, T.; Sasahira, T.; Moriwaka, Y.; Yamamoto, K.; Kuniyasu, H. Recurrence of keratocystic odontogenic tumor: Clinicopathological features and immunohistochemical study of the Hedgehog signaling pathway. *Pathobiol. J. Immunopathol. Mol. Cell. Biol.* **2008**, *75*, 171–176. [CrossRef] [PubMed]
22. Grachtchouk, M.; Liu, J.; Wang, A.; Wei, L.; Bichakjian, C.K.; Garlick, J.; Paulino, A.F.; Giordano, T.; Dlugosz, A.A. Odontogenic keratocysts arise from quiescent epithelial rests and are associated with deregulated hedgehog signaling in mice and humans. *Am. J. Pathol.* **2006**, *169*, 806–814. [CrossRef] [PubMed]
23. Hasegawa, D.; Ochiai-Shino, H.; Onodera, S.; Nakamura, T.; Saito, A.; Onda, T.; Watanabe, K.; Nishimura, K.; Ohtaka, M.; Nakanishi, M.; et al. Gorlin syndrome-derived induced pluripotent stem cells are hypersensitive to hedgehog-mediated osteogenic induction. *PLoS ONE* **2017**, *12*, e0186879. [CrossRef] [PubMed]
24. Kesireddy, M.; Mendiola, V.L.; Jana, B.; Patel, S. Long-term Response to Vismodegib in a Patient with Gorlin-Goltz Syndrome: A Case Report and Review of Pathological Mechanisms Involved. *Cureus* **2019**, *11*, e5383. [CrossRef] [PubMed]

25. Wang, Y.J.; Zhang, J.Y.; Dong, Q.; Li, T.J. Orthokeratinized odontogenic cysts: A clinicopathologic study of 159 cases and molecular evidence for the absence of PTCH1 mutations. *J. Oral Pathol. Med. Off. Publ. Int. Assoc. Oral Pathol. Am. Acad. Oral Pathol.* **2022**, *51*, 659–665. [CrossRef] [PubMed]
26. Pan, S.; Xu, L.L.; Sun, L.S.; Li, T.J. Identification of known and novel PTCH mutations in both syndromic and non-syndromic keratocystic odontogenic tumors. *Int. J. Oral Sci.* **2009**, *1*, 34–38. [CrossRef] [PubMed]
27. Hellani, A.; Baghdadi, H.; Dabbour, N.; Almassri, N.; Abu-Amero, K.K. A novel PTCH1 germline mutation distinguishes basal cell carcinoma from basaloid follicular hamartoma: A case report. *J. Med. Case Rep.* **2009**, *3*, 52. [CrossRef] [PubMed]
28. Asevedo Campos de Resende, T.; de Fátima Bernardes, V.; Carolina da Silva, J.; De Marco, L.A.; Santiago Gomez, R.; Cavalieri Gomes, C.; Gonçalves Diniz, M. Loss of heterozygosity of MIR15A/MIR16-1, negative regulators of the antiapoptotic gene BCL2, is not common in odontogenic keratocysts. *Oral Surg. Oral Med. Oral Pathol. Oral Radiol.* **2018**, *125*, 313–316. [CrossRef] [PubMed]
29. Hong, Y.Y.; Yu, F.Y.; Qu, J.F.; Chen, F.; Li, T.J. Fibroblasts regulate variable aggressiveness of syndromic keratocystic and non-syndromic odontogenic tumors. *J. Dent. Res.* **2014**, *93*, 904–910. [CrossRef]
30. Shimada, Y.; Katsube, K.; Kabasawa, Y.; Morita, K.; Omura, K.; Yamaguchi, A.; Sakamoto, K. Integrated genotypic analysis of hedgehog-related genes identifies subgroups of keratocystic odontogenic tumor with distinct clinicopathological features. *PLoS ONE* **2013**, *8*, e70995. [CrossRef]
31. Pastorino, L.; Pollio, A.; Pellacani, G.; Guarneri, C.; Ghiorzo, P.; Longo, C.; Bruno, W.; Giusti, F.; Bassoli, S.; Bianchi-Scarrà, G.; et al. Novel PTCH1 mutations in patients with keratocystic odontogenic tumors screened for nevoid basal cell carcinoma (NBCC) syndrome. *PLoS ONE* **2012**, *7*, e43827. [CrossRef] [PubMed]
32. Kaibuchi-Ando, K.; Takeichi, T.; Ito, Y.; Takeuchi, S.; Yamashita, Y.; Yamada, M.; Muro, Y.; Ogi, T.; Akiyama, M. Odontogenic keratocysts are an important clue for diagnosing basal cell nevus syndrome. *Nagoya J. Med. Sci.* **2021**, *83*, 393–396. [PubMed]
33. Friedlander, L.T.; Hussani, H.; Cullinan, M.P.; Seymour, G.J.; De Silva, R.K.; De Silva, H.; Cameron, C.; Rich, A.M. VEGF and VEGFR2 in dentigerous cysts associated with impacted third molars. *Pathology* **2015**, *47*, 446–451. [CrossRef] [PubMed]
34. Zhong, W.Q.; Chen, G.; Zhang, W.; Ren, J.G.; Wu, Z.X.; Zhao, Y.; Liu, B.; Zhao, Y.F. Epithelial-mesenchymal transition in keratocystic odontogenic tumor: Possible role in locally aggressive behavior. *BioMed Res. Int.* **2015**, *2015*, 168089. [CrossRef] [PubMed]
35. Escobar, E.; Gómez-Valenzuela, F.; Peñafiel, C.; Chimenos-Küstner, E.; Pérez-Tomás, R. Aberrant immunoexpression of p53 tumour-suppressor and Bcl-2 family proteins (Bcl-2 and Bax) in ameloblastomas and odontogenic keratocysts. *J. Clin. Exp. Dent.* **2023**, *15*, e125–e134. [PubMed]
36. Gadbail, A.R.; Chaudhary, M.; Patil, S.; Gawande, M. Actual Proliferating Index and p53 protein expression as prognostic marker in odontogenic cysts. *Oral Dis.* **2009**, *15*, 490–498. [CrossRef] [PubMed]
37. Ruiz, P.A.; Toledo, O.A.; Nonaka, C.F.; Pinto, L.P.; Souza, L.B. Immunohistochemical expression of vascular endothelial growth factor and matrix metalloproteinase-9 in radicular and residual radicular cysts. *J. Appl. Oral Sci. Rev. FOB* **2010**, *18*, 613–620. [CrossRef] [PubMed]
38. Pereira, T.; Shetty, S.J.; Punjabi, V.; Vidhale, R.G.; Gotmare, S.S.; Kamath, P. Immunohistochemical expression of SOX2 in OKC and ameloblastoma: A comparative study. *J. Oral Maxillofac. Pathol.* **2023**, *27*, 685–692. [CrossRef] [PubMed]
39. Mukhopadhyay, A.; Panda, A.; Mishra, P.; Chowdhary, G.; Mohanty, A.; Sahoo, P.D. Comparative immunohistochemical analysis of WT-1, Syndecan and Snail in Ameloblastoma and odontogenic keratocyst: A retrospective study. *J. Oral Maxillofac. Pathol.* **2023**, *27*, 295–301. [PubMed]
40. Silva, B.S.; Silva, L.R.; Lima, K.L.; Dos Santos, A.C.; Oliveira, A.C.; Dezzen-Gomide, A.C.; Batista, A.C.; Yamamoto-Silva, F.P. SOX2 and BCL-2 Expressions in Odontogenic Keratocyst and Ameloblastoma. *Med. Oral Patol. Oral Cir. Bucal* **2020**, *25*, e283–e290. [CrossRef]
41. Soluk Tekkeşın, M.; Mutlu, S.; Olgaç, V. Expressions of bax, bcl-2 and Ki-67 in odontogenic keratocysts (Keratocystic Odontogenic Tumor) in comparison with ameloblastomas and radicular cysts. *Turk Patoloji Derg.* **2012**, *28*, 49–55. [PubMed]
42. Kaczmarzyk, T.; Kisielowski, K.; Koszowski, R.; Rynkiewicz, M.; Gawełek, E.; Babiuch, K.; Bednarczyk, A.; Drozdzowska, B. Investigation of clinicopathological parameters and expression of COX-2, bcl-2, PCNA, and p53 in primary and recurrent sporadic odontogenic keratocysts. *Clin. Oral Investig.* **2018**, *22*, 3097–3106. [CrossRef] [PubMed]
43. Kisielowski, K.; Drozdzowska, B.; Szuta, M.; Kaczmarzyk, T. Prognostic relevance of clinicopathological factors in sporadic and syndromic odontogenic keratocysts: A comparative study. *Adv. Clin. Exp. Med.* **2023**, *32*, 245–259. [CrossRef] [PubMed]
44. Byun, J.H.; Kang, Y.H.; Choi, M.J.; Park, B.W. Expansile keratocystic odontogenic tumor in the maxilla: Immunohistochemical studies and review of literature. *J. Korean Assoc. Oral Maxillofac. Surg.* **2013**, *39*, 182–187. [CrossRef] [PubMed]
45. Edamatsu, M.; Kumamoto, H.; Ooya, K.; Echigo, S. Apoptosis-related factors in the epithelial components of dental follicles and dentigerous cysts associated with impacted third molars of the mandible. *Oral Surg. Oral Med. Oral Pathol. Oral Radiol. Endod.* **2005**, *99*, 17–23. [CrossRef]
46. Razavi, S.M.; Torabinia, N.; Mohajeri, M.R.; Shahriyary, S.; Ghalegolab, S.; Nouri, S. Expression of Bcl-2 and epithelial growth factor receptor proteins in keratocystic odontogenic tumor in comparison with dentigerous cyst and ameloblastoma. *Dent. Res. J.* **2015**, *12*, 342–347.
47. Sreedhar, G.; Raju, M.V.; Metta, K.K.; Manjunath, S.; Shetty, S.; Agarwal, R.K. Immunohistochemical analysis of factors related to apoptosis and cellular proliferation in relation to inflammation in dentigerous and odontogenic keratocyst. *J. Nat. Sci. Biol. Med.* **2014**, *5*, 112–115. [CrossRef]
48. Villalba, L.; Stolbizer, F.; Blasco, F.; Mauriño, N.R.; Piloni, M.J.; Keszler, A. Pericoronal follicles of asymptomatic impacted teeth: A radiographic, histomorphologic, and immunohistochemical study. *Int. J. Dent.* **2012**, *2012*, 935310. [CrossRef]

49. Nimmanagoti, R.; Nandan, S.; Kulkarni, P.G.; Reddy, S.P.; Keerthi, M.; Pupala, G. Protein 53, B-Cell Lymphoma-2, Cyclooxygenase-2, and CD105 Reactivity in Keratocystic Odontogenic Tumors: An Immunohistochemical Analysis. *Int. J. Appl. Basic Med. Res.* **2019**, *9*, 27–31.
50. Phull, K.; Metgud, R.; Patel, S. A study of the distribution of B-cell lymphoma/leukemia-2 in odontogenic cyst and tumors: Histochemical study. *J. Cancer Res. Ther.* **2017**, *13*, 570–575.
51. Sindura, C.; Babu, C.; Mysorekar, V.; Kumar, V. Study of immunohistochemical demonstration of Bcl-2 protein in ameloblastoma and keratocystic odontogenic tumor. *J. Oral Maxillofac. Pathol.* **2013**, *17*, 176–180. [CrossRef]
52. Cserni, D.; Zombori, T.; Vörös, A.; Stájer, A.; Rimovszki, A.; Daru, K.; Baráth, Z.; Cserni, G. A Clinicopathological Approach to Odontogenic Cysts: The Role of Cytokeratin 17 and bcl2 Immunohistochemistry in Identifying Odontogenic Keratocysts. *Pathol. Oncol. Res.* **2020**, *26*, 2613–2620. [CrossRef] [PubMed]
53. Shetty, D.C.; Urs, A.B.; Godhi, S.; Gupta, S. Classifying odontogenic keratocysts as benign cystic neoplasms: A molecular insight into its aggressiveness. *J. Maxillofac. Oral Surg.* **2010**, *9*, 30–34. [CrossRef] [PubMed]
54. González-Moles, M.A.; Mosqueda-Taylor, A.; Delgado-Rodríguez, M.; Martínez-Mata, G.; Gil-Montoya, J.A.; Díaz-Franco, M.A.; Bravo-Pérez, J.J.; M-González, N. Analysis of p53 protein by PAb240, Ki-67 expression and human papillomavirus DNA detection in different types of odontogenic keratocyst. *Anticancer Res.* **2006**, *26*, 175–181. [PubMed]
55. de Oliveira, M.G.; Lauxen, I.d.S.; Chaves, A.C.; Rados, P.V.; Sant'Ana Filho, M. Immunohistochemical analysis of the patterns of p53 and PCNA expression in odontogenic cystic lesions. *Med. Oral Patol. Oral Cir. Buccal* **2008**, *13*, E275–E280.
56. Gaballah, E.T.; Tawfik, M.A. Immunohistochemical analysis of P53 protein in odontogenic cysts. *Saudi Dent. J.* **2010**, *22*, 167–170. [CrossRef] [PubMed]
57. Chandrangsu, S.; Sappayatosok, K. p53, p63 and p73 expression and angiogenesis in keratocystic odontogenic tumors. *J. Clin. Exp. Dent.* **2016**, *8*, e505–e511. [CrossRef]
58. Khan, A.A.; Qahtani, S.A.; Dawasaz, A.A.; Saquib, S.A.; Asif, S.M.; Ishfaq, M.; Kota, M.Z.; Ibrahim, M. Management of an extensive odontogenic keratocyst: A rare case report with 10-year follow-up. *Medicine* **2019**, *98*, e17987. [CrossRef]
59. Kadashetti, V.; Patil, N.; Datkhile, K.; Kanetakar, S.; Shivakumar, K.M. Analysis of expression of p53, p63 and proliferating cell nuclear antigen proteins in odontogenic keratocyst: An immunohistochemical study. *J. Oral Maxillofac. Pathol.* **2020**, *24*, 273–278. [CrossRef]
60. Yanatatsaneejit, P.; Boonsrang, A.; Mutirangura, A.; Patel, V.; Kitkumthorn, N. P53 polymorphism at codon 72 is associated with keratocystic odontogenic tumors in the Thai population. *Asian Pac. J. Cancer Prev.* **2015**, *16*, 1997–2001. [CrossRef]
61. Varsha, B.; Gharat, A.L.; Nagamalini, B.; Jyothsna, M.; Mothkur, S.T.; Swaminathan, U. Evaluation and comparison of expression of p63 in odontogenic keratocyst, solid ameloblastoma and unicystic ameloblastoma. *J. Oral Maxillofac. Pathol.* **2014**, *18*, 223–228. [CrossRef] [PubMed]
62. Sajeevan, T.P.; Saraswathi, T.R.; Ranganathan, K.; Joshua, E.; Rao, U.D. Immunohistochemical study of p53 and proliferating cell nuclear antigen expression in odontogenic keratocyst and periapical cyst. *J. Pharm. Bioallied Sci.* **2014**, *6* (Suppl. S1), S52–S57. [CrossRef] [PubMed]
63. Razavi, S.M.; Khalesi, S.; Torabinia, N. Investigation of clinicopathological parameters alongside with p53 expression in primary and recurrent keratocysticodontogenic tumours. *Malays. J. Pathol.* **2014**, *36*, 105–113. [PubMed]
64. Chandrashekar, C.; Patel, P.; Thennavan, A.; Radhakrishnan, R. Odontogenic keratocyst: Analysis of recurrence by AgNOR, p53 and MDM2 profiling. *J. Oral Maxillofac. Pathol.* **2020**, *24*, 184–185.
65. Deyhimi, P.; Hashemzade, Z. Comparative study of TGF-alpha and P53 markers' expression in odontogenic keratocyst and orthokeratinaized odontogenic cyst. *Dent. Res. J.* **2012**, *9* (Suppl. S1), S39–S44.
66. Ogden, G.R.; Chisholm, D.M.; Kiddie, R.A.; Lane, D.P. p53 protein in odontogenic cysts: Increased expression in some odontogenic keratocysts. *J. Clin. Pathol.* **1992**, *45*, 1007–1010. [CrossRef] [PubMed]
67. Aldahash, F. Systematic review and meta-analysis of the expression of p53 in the odontogenic lesions. *J. Oral Maxillofac. Pathol. JOMFP* **2023**, *27*, 168–172. [CrossRef] [PubMed]
68. Gupta, R.; Chaudhary, M.; Patil, S.; Fating, C.; Hande, A.; Suryawanshi, H. Expression of p63 in tooth germ, dentigerous cyst and ameloblastoma. *J. Oral Maxillofac. Pathol.* **2019**, *23*, 43–48. [CrossRef]
69. Akshatha, B.K.; Karuppiah, K.; Manjunath, G.S.; Kumaraswamy, J.; Papaiah, L.; Rao, J. Immunohistochemical evaluation of inducible nitric oxide synthase in the epithelial lining of odontogenic cysts: A qualitative and quantitative analysis. *J. Oral Maxillofac. Pathol.* **2017**, *21*, 375–381.
70. Fatemeh, M.; Sepideh, A.; Sara, B.S.; Nazanin, M. P53 Protein Expression in Dental Follicle, Dentigerous Cyst, Odontogenic Keratocyst, and Inflammatory Subtypes of Cysts: An Immunohistochemical Study. *Oman Med. J.* **2017**, *32*, 227–232. [CrossRef]
71. Ortiz-García, J.Z.; Munguía-Robledo, S.; Estrada-Orozco, J.J.; Licéaga-Escalera, C.; Rodríguez, M.A. Expression level and proteolytic activity of MMP-2 and MMP-9 in dental follicles, dentigerous cysts, odontogenic keratocysts and unicystic ameloblastomas. *J. Oral Biol. Craniofacial Res.* **2022**, *12*, 339–342. [CrossRef] [PubMed]
72. Aloka, D.; Padmakumar, S.K.; Sathyan, S.; Sebastian, M.; Banerjee, M.; Beena, V.T. Association of matrix metalloproteinase 2 and matrix metalloproteinase 9 gene polymorphism in aggressive and nonaggressive odontogenic lesions: A pilot study. *J. Oral Maxillofac. Pathol.* **2019**, *23*, 158. [CrossRef] [PubMed]
73. Loreto, C.; Polizzi, A.; Filetti, V.; Pannone, G.; Dos Santos, J.N.; Venezia, P.; Leonardi, R.; Isola, G. Expression of Matrix Metalloproteinases 7 and 9, Desmin, Alpha-Smooth Muscle Actin and Caldesmon, in Odontogenic Keratocyst Associated with NBCCS, Recurrent and Sporadic Keratocysts. *Biomolecules* **2022**, *12*, 775. [CrossRef] [PubMed]

74. Suojanen, J.; Lehtonen, N.; Färkkilä, E.; Hietanen, J.; Teronen, O.; Sorsa, T.; Hagström, J. Common Matrix Metalloproteinases (MMP-8, -9, -25, and -26) Cannot Explain Dentigerous Cyst Expansion. *J. Clin. Diagn. Res.* **2014**, *8*, ZC82–ZC85. [PubMed]
75. Kuźniarz, K.; Luchowska-Kocot, D.; Tomaszewski, T.; Kurzepa, J. Role of matrix metalloproteinases and their tissue inhibitors in the pathological mechanisms underlying maxillofacial cystic lesions. *Biomed. Rep.* **2021**, *15*, 65. [CrossRef] [PubMed]
76. de Andrade Santos, P.P.; de Aquino, A.R.; Oliveira Barreto, A.; de Almeida Freitas, R.; Galvão, H.C.; de Souza, L.B. Immunohistochemical expression of nuclear factor κB, matrix metalloproteinase 9, and endoglin (CD105) in odontogenic keratocysts, dentigerous cysts, and radicular cysts. *Oral Surg. Oral Med. Oral Pathol. Oral Radiol. Endod.* **2011**, *112*, 476–483. [CrossRef] [PubMed]
77. Ribeiro, B.F.; Ferreira de Araújo, C.R.; dos Santos, B.R.; de Almeida Freitas, R. Immunohistochemical expression of matrix metalloproteinases 1, 2, 7, 9, and 26 in the calcifying cystic odontogenic tumor. *Oral Surg. Oral Med. Oral Pathol. Oral Radiol. Endod.* **2011**, *112*, 609–615. [CrossRef] [PubMed]
78. Etemad-Moghadam, S.; Alaeddini, M. A comparative study of syndecan-1 expression in different odontogenic tumors. *J. Oral Biol. Craniofacial Res.* **2017**, *7*, 23–26. [CrossRef] [PubMed]
79. Vera-Sirera, B.; Forner-Navarro, L.; Vera-Sempere, F. NCAM (CD56) expression in keratin-producing odontogenic cysts: Aberrant expression in KCOT. *Head Face Med.* **2015**, *11*, 3. [CrossRef] [PubMed]
80. Jaafari-Ashkavandi, Z.; Dehghani-Nazhvani, A.; Razmjouyi, F. CD56 Expression in Odontogenic Cysts and Tumors. *J. Dent. Res. Dent. Clin. Dent. Prospect.* **2014**, *8*, 240–245.
81. Padmapriya, V.M.; Kavitha, B.; Sivapathasundram, B.; Nagaraj, J. Comparison of cytokeratin expressions among orthokeratinized odontogenic cysts, epidermoid cysts and odontogenic keratocysts: An immunohistochemical study. *J. Oral Maxillofac. Pathol.* **2020**, *24*, 472–478. [CrossRef]
82. Sheethal, H.S.; Rao, K.; Umadevi, H.S.; Chauhan, K. Odontogenic keratocyst arising in the maxillary sinus: A rare case report. *J. Oral Maxillofac. Pathol.* **2019**, *23* (Suppl. S1), 74–77. [CrossRef]
83. Hoshino, M.; Inoue, H.; Kikuchi, K.; Miyazaki, Y.; Yoshino, A.; Hara, H.; Terui, T.; Kusama, K.; Sakashita, H. Comparative study of cytokeratin and langerin expression in keratinized cystic lesions of the oral and maxillofacial regions. *J. Oral Sci.* **2015**, *57*, 287–294. [CrossRef]
84. Al-Otaibi, O.; Khounganian, R.; Anil, S.; Rajendran, R. Syndecan-1 (CD 138) surface expression marks cell type and differentiation in ameloblastoma, keratocystic odontogenic tumor, and dentigerous cyst. *J. Oral Pathol. Med.* **2013**, *42*, 186–193. [CrossRef] [PubMed]
85. Krishnan, R.P.; Pandiar, D.; Sagar, S. Immunohistochemical Expression of CK14 and Bcl-2 in Odontogenic Keratocyst and Its Variants. *Appl. Immunohistochem. Mol. Morphol.* **2024**, *32*, 151–156. [CrossRef] [PubMed]
86. Yamamoto, K.; Matsusue, Y.; Kurihara, M.; Takahashi, Y.; Kirita, T. A keratocyst in the buccal mucosa with the features of keratocystic odontogenic tumor. *Open Dent. J.* **2013**, *7*, 152–156. [CrossRef] [PubMed]
87. Kureel, K.; Urs, A.B.; Augustine, J. Cytokeratin and fibronectin expression in orthokeratinized odontogenic cyst: A comparative immunohistochemical study. *J. Oral Maxillofac. Pathol.* **2019**, *23*, 65–72.
88. Bhakhar, V.P.; Shah, V.S.; Ghanchi, M.J.; Gosavi, S.S.; Srivastava, H.M.; Pachore, N.J. A Comparative Analysis of Cytokeratin 18 and 19 Expressions in Odontogenic Keratocyst, Dentigerous Cyst and Radicular Cyst with a Review of Literature. *J. Clin. Diagn. Res.* **2016**, *10*, ZC85–ZC89. [CrossRef]
89. Shruthi, D.K.; Shivakumar, M.C.; Tegginamani, A.S.; Karthik, B.; Chetan, B.I. Cytokeratin 14 and cytokeratin 18 expressions in reduced enamel epithelium and dentigerous cyst: Possible role in oncofetal transformation and histogenesis- of follicular type of adenomatoid odontogenic tumor. *J. Oral Maxillofac. Pathol.* **2014**, *18*, 365–371. [CrossRef]
90. Swetha, P.; Ramesh, K.; Madhavan, N.; Veeravarmal, V.; Sameera, A. Expression of inducible nitric oxide synthase in the epithelial linings of odontogenic keratocyst, dentigerous cyst and radicular cyst: A pathological insight. *Ann. Med. Health Sci. Res.* **2014**, *4*, 583–589. [CrossRef]
91. Sudhakara, M.; Rudrayya, S.P.; Vanaki, S.S.; Bhullar, R.K.; Shivakumar, M.S.; Hosur, M. Expression of CK14 and vimentin in adenomatoid odontogenic tumor and dentigerous cyst. *J. Oral Maxillofac. Pathol.* **2016**, *20*, 369–376. [CrossRef] [PubMed]
92. Saluja, P.; Arora, M.; Dave, A.; Shetty, V.P.; Khurana, C.; Madan, A.; Rai, R.; Katiyar, A. Role of Cytokeratin-7 in the pathogenesis of odontogenic cysts—An immunohistochemical study. *Med. Pharm. Rep.* **2019**, *92*, 282–287. [CrossRef] [PubMed]
93. Portes, J.; Cunha, K.S.G.; da Silva, L.E.; da Silva, A.K.F.; Conde, D.C.; Silva Junior, A. Computerized Evaluation of the Immunoexpression of Ki-67 Protein in Odontogenic Keratocyst and Dentigerous Cyst. *Head Neck Pathol.* **2020**, *14*, 598–605. [CrossRef] [PubMed]
94. Hammad, H.M.; Nagrash, O.M.; Safadi, R.A. Maspin, Syndecan-1, and Ki-67 in the Odontogenic Keratocyst: An Immunohistochemical Analysis. *Int. J. Dent.* **2020**, *2020*, 7041520. [CrossRef]
95. Alsaegh, M.A.; Altaie, A.M.; Zhu, S. p63 Expression and its Relation to Epithelial Cells Proliferation in Dentigerous Cyst, Odontogenic Keratocyst, and Ameloblastoma. *Pathol. Oncol. Res.* **2020**, *26*, 1175–1182. [CrossRef] [PubMed]
96. Jaafari-Ashkavandi, Z.; Geramizadeh, B.; Ranjbar, M.A. P63 and Ki-67 Expression in Dentigerous Cyst and Ameloblastomas. *J. Dent.* **2015**, *16*, 323–328.
97. Jaafari-Ashkavandi, Z.; Mehranmehr, F.; Roosta, E. MCM3 and Ki67 proliferation markers in odontogenic cysts and ameloblastoma. *J. Oral Biol. Craniofacial Res.* **2019**, *9*, 47–50. [CrossRef] [PubMed]
98. Brito-Mendoza, L.; Bologna-Molina, R.; Irigoyen-Camacho, M.E.; Martinez, G.; Sánchez-Romero, C.; Mosqueda-Taylor, A. A Comparison of Ki67, Syndecan-1 (CD138), and Molecular RANK, RANKL, and OPG Triad Expression in Odontogenic Keratocyts, Unicystic Ameloblastoma, and Dentigerous Cysts. *Dis. Mrk.* **2018**, *2018*, 7048531. [CrossRef]

99. Modi, T.G.; Chalishazar, M.; Kumar, M. Expression of Ki-67 in odontogenic cysts: A comparative study between odontogenic keratocysts, radicular cysts and dentigerous cysts. *J. Oral Maxillofac. Pathol.* **2018**, *22*, 146. [CrossRef]
100. Nafarzadeh, S.; Seyedmajidi, M.; Jafari, S.; Bijani, A.; Rostami-Sarokolaei, A. A comparative study of PCNA and Ki-67 expression in dental follicle, dentigerous cyst, unicystic ameloblastoma and ameloblastoma. *Int. J. Mol. Cell. Med.* **2013**, *2*, 27–33.
101. Coşarcă, A.S.; Mocan, S.L.; Păcurar, M.; Fülöp, E.; Ormenişan, A. The evaluation of Ki67, p53, MCM3 and PCNA immunoexpressions at the level of the dental follicle of impacted teeth, dentigerous cysts and keratocystic odontogenic tumors. *Rom. J. Morphol. Embryol. = Rev. Roum. Morphol. Embryol.* **2016**, *57*, 407–412.
102. Alsaegh, M.A.; Miyashita, H.; Taniguchi, T.; Zhu, S.R. Odontogenic epithelial proliferation is correlated with COX-2 expression in dentigerous cyst and ameloblastoma. *Exp. Ther. Med.* **2017**, *13*, 247–253. [CrossRef] [PubMed]
103. Güler, N.; Comunoğlu, N.; Cabbar, F. Ki-67 and MCM-2 in dental follicle and odontogenic cysts: The effects of inflammation on proliferative markers. *Sci. World J.* **2012**, *2012*, 946060. [CrossRef] [PubMed]
104. Kim, D.K.; Ahn, S.G.; Kim, J.; Yoon, J.H. Comparative Ki-67 expression and apoptosis in the odontogenic keratocyst associated with or without an impacted tooth in addition to unilocular and multilocular varieties. *Yonsei Med. J.* **2003**, *44*, 841–846. [CrossRef] [PubMed]
105. de Oliveira, M.G.; Lauxen, I.d.S.; Chaves, A.C.; Rados, P.V.; Sant'Ana Filho, M. Odontogenic epithelium: Immunolabeling of Ki-67, EGFR and survivin in pericoronal follicles, dentigerous cysts and keratocystic odontogenic tumors. *Head Neck Pathol.* **2011**, *5*, 1–7. [CrossRef] [PubMed]
106. Nadalin, M.R.; Fregnani, E.R.; Silva-Sousa, Y.T.; Perez, D.E. Syndecan-1 (CD138) and Ki-67 expression in odontogenic cystic lesions. *Braz. Dent. J.* **2011**, *22*, 223–229. [CrossRef] [PubMed]
107. Naruse, T.; Yamashita, K.; Yanamoto, S.; Rokutanda, S.; Matsushita, Y.; Sakamoto, Y.; Sakamoto, H.; Ikeda, H.; Ikeda, T.; Asahina, I.; et al. Histopathological and immunohistochemical study in keratocystic odontogenic tumors: Predictive factors of recurrence. *Oncol. Lett.* **2017**, *13*, 3487–3493. [CrossRef] [PubMed]
108. Selvi, F.; Tekkesin, M.S.; Cakarer, S.; Isler, S.C.; Keskin, C. Keratocystic odontogenic tumors: Predictive factors of recurrence by Ki-67 and AgNOR labelling. *Int. J. Med. Sci.* **2012**, *9*, 262–268. [CrossRef] [PubMed]
109. Ba, K.; Li, X.; Wang, H.; Liu, Y.; Zheng, G.; Yang, Z.; Li, M.; Shimizutani, K.; Koseki, T. Correlation between imaging features and epithelial cell proliferation in keratocystic odontogenic tumour. *Dento Maxillo Facial Radiol.* **2010**, *39*, 368–374.
110. Mendes, R.A.; Carvalho, J.F.; van der Waal, I. A comparative immunohistochemical analysis of COX-2, p53, and Ki-67 expression in keratocystic odontogenic tumors. *Oral Surg. Oral Med. Oral Pathol. Oral Radiol. Endod.* **2011**, *111*, 333–339. [CrossRef]
111. Kuroyanagi, N.; Sakuma, H.; Miyabe, S.; Machida, J.; Kaetsu, A.; Yokoi, M.; Maeda, H.; Warnakulasuriya, S.; Nagao, T.; Shimozato, K. Prognostic factors for keratocystic odontogenic tumor (odontogenic keratocyst): Analysis of clinico-pathologic and immunohistochemical findings in cysts treated by enucleation. *J. Oral Pathol. Med.* **2009**, *38*, 386–392. [CrossRef] [PubMed]
112. Ono, S.; Hirose, K.; Sukegawa, S.; Nakamura, S.; Motooka, D.; Iwamoto, Y.; Hori, Y.; Oya, K.; Fukuda, Y.; Toyosawa, S. Multiple orthokeratinized odontogenic cysts: Clinical, pathological, and genetic characteristics. *Diagn. Pathol.* **2022**, *17*, 82. [CrossRef] [PubMed]
113. Park, S.; Jung, H.S.; Jung, Y.S.; Nam, W.; Cha, J.Y.; Jung, H.D. Changes in Cellular Regulatory Factors before and after Decompression of Odontogenic Keratocysts. *J. Clin. Med.* **2020**, *10*, 30. [CrossRef] [PubMed]
114. Jabbarzadeh, M.; Hamblin, M.R.; Pournaghi-Azar, F.; Vakili Saatloo, M.; Kouhsoltani, M.; Vahed, N. Ki-67 expression as a diagnostic biomarker in odontogenic cysts and tumors: A systematic review and meta-analysis. *J. Dent. Res. Dent. Clin. Dent. Prospect.* **2021**, *15*, 66–75. [CrossRef]
115. Bhola, R.; Narwal, A.; Kamboj, M.; Devi, A. Immunohistochemical Comparison of Ki-67 and MCM-3 in Odontogenic Cysts: An Observational Study. *Appl. Immunohistochem. Mol. Morphol.* **2024**, *32*, 111–116. [CrossRef]
116. Embaló, B.; Parize, H.N.; Rivero, E.R.C. Evaluation of cell proliferation in cystic lesions associated with impacted third molars. *Microsc. Res. Tech.* **2018**, *81*, 1241–1245. [CrossRef] [PubMed]
117. Kucukkolbasi, H.; Esen, A.; Erinanc, O.H. Immunohistochemical analysis of Ki-67 in dental follicle of asymptomatic impacted third molars. *J. Oral Maxillofac. Pathol.* **2014**, *18*, 189–193. [PubMed]
118. Cimadon, N.; Lauxen, I.S.; Carrard, V.C.; Sant'Ana Filho, M.; Rados, P.V.; Oliveira, M.G. Analysis of the proliferative potential of odontogenic epithelial cells of pericoronal follicles. *J. Contemp. Dent. Pract.* **2014**, *15*, 761–765. [CrossRef] [PubMed]
119. Chaturvedi, T.P.; Gupta, K.; Agrawal, R.; Naveen Kumar, P.G., Gupta, J. Immunohistochemical expression of Ki-67 and Glypican-3 to distinguish aggressive from nonaggressive benign odontogenic tumors. *J. Cancer Res. Ther.* **2022**, *18* (Suppl. S2), S205–S209. [PubMed]
120. Yamasaki, S.; Shintani, T.; Ando, T.; Miyauchi, M.; Yanamoto, S. Transformation of an odontogenic keratocyst into a solid variant of odontogenic keratocyst/keratoameloblastoma during long-term follow-up: A case report. *Mol. Med. Rep.* **2024**, *29*, 44. [CrossRef]
121. Dong, Q.; Pan, S.; Sun, L.S.; Li, T.J. Orthokeratinized odontogenic cyst: A clinicopathologic study of 61 cases. *Arch. Pathol. Lab. Med.* **2010**, *134*, 271–275. [CrossRef] [PubMed]
122. Mustansir-Ul-Hassnain, S.; Chandavarkar, V.; Mishra, M.N.; Patil, P.M.; Bhargava, D.; Sharma, R. Histopathologic and immunohistochemical findings of odontogenic jaw cysts treated by decompression technique. *J. Oral Maxillofac. Pathol.* **2021**, *25*, 272–278. [PubMed]
123. Trujillo-González, D.; Villarroel-Dorrego, M.; Toro, R.; Vigil, G.; Pereira-Prado, V.; Bologna-Molina, R. Decompression induces inflammation but do not modify cell proliferation and apoptosis in odontogenic keratocyst. *J. Clin. Exp. Dent.* **2022**, *14*, e100–e106. [CrossRef] [PubMed]
124. Zhou, Q.; Xu, L.; Li, H.; Xia, R.H. Orthokeratinized odontogenic cyst (OOC): Clinicopathological and radiological features of a series of 48 cases. *Pathol. Res. Pract.* **2022**, *236*, 153969. [CrossRef] [PubMed]

125. Orikpete, E.V.; Omoregie, O.F.; Ojo, M.A. Proliferative and anti-apoptotic indices of unicystic ameloblastoma, odontogenic keratocyst, dentigerous cyst and radicular cyst. *J. Oral Maxillofac. Pathol.* **2020**, *24*, 399. [CrossRef] [PubMed]
126. Lafuente-Ibáñez de Mendoza, I.; Aguirre-Urizar, J.M.; Villatoro-Ugalde, V.; Magaña-Quiñones, J.J.; Lana-Ojeda, J.; Mosqueda-Taylor, A. Peripheral odontogenic keratocyst: Clinicopathological and immunohistochemical characterization. *Oral Dis.* **2022**, *28*, 1198–1206. [CrossRef] [PubMed]
127. Baris, E.; Secen, A.; Karabulut, S.; Gultekin, S.E. Investigation of the effects of marsupialization on histomorphological and immunohistochemical markers of odontogenic keratocysts. *Niger. J. Clin. Pract.* **2022**, *25*, 1548–1556. [CrossRef] [PubMed]
128. Latha, H.A.; Prakash, A.R.; Kanth, M.R.; Reddy, A.V.S.; Sreenath, G.; Vidya, K.S. Expression of anti—Apoptotic survivin in odontogenic keratocyst, adenomatoid odontogenic tumor and ameloblastoma. *J. Oral Maxillofac. Pathol.* **2023**, *27*, 601.
129. Baddireddy, S.M.; Manyam, R.; Thomas, D.C. Expression of EGFR and survivin in ameloblastoma, odontogenic keratocyst and calcifying odontogenic cyst—An immunohistochemical study. *J. Oral Maxillofac. Pathol.* **2023**, *27*, 424. [PubMed]
130. Thermos, G.; Piperi, E.; Tosios, K.I.; Nikitakis, N.G. Expression of BMP4 and FOXN1 in orthokeratinized odontogenic cyst compared to odontogenic keratocyst suggests an epidermal phenotype. *Biotech. Histochem.* **2022**, *97*, 584–592. [CrossRef]
131. Zhang, L.Z.; Man, Q.W.; Liu, J.Y.; Zhong, W.Q.; Zheng, Y.Y.; Zhao, Y.F.; Liu, B. Overexpression of Fra-1, c-Jun and c-Fos in odontogenic keratocysts: Potential correlation with proliferative and anti-apoptotic activity. *Histopathology* **2018**, *73*, 933–942. [CrossRef] [PubMed]
132. Porto, L.P.; dos Santos, J.N.; Ramalho, L.M.; Figueiredo, A.L.; Carneiro Júnior, B.; Gurgel, C.A.; Paiva, K.B.; Xavier, F.C. E-cadherin regulators are differentially expressed in the epithelium and stroma of keratocystic odontogenic tumors. *J. Oral Pathol. Med.* **2016**, *45*, 302–311. [CrossRef] [PubMed]
133. Kim, Y.S.; Lee, S.K. Different Protein Expressions between Peripheral Ameloblastoma and Oral Basal Cell Carcinoma Occurred at the Same Mandibular Molar Area. *Korean J. Pathol.* **2014**, *48*, 151–158. [CrossRef] [PubMed]
134. Pinheiro, J.C.; de Carvalho, C.H.P.; Galvão, H.C.; Pereira Pinto, L.; de Souza, L.B.; de Andrade Santos, P.P. Relationship between mast cells and E-cadherin in odontogenic keratocysts and radicular cysts. *Clin. Oral Investig.* **2020**, *24*, 181–191. [CrossRef]
135. Cesinaro, A.M.; Burtini, G.; Maiorana, A.; Rossi, G.; Migaldi, M. Expression of calretinin in odontogenic keratocysts and basal cell carcinomas: A study of sporadic and Gorlin-Goltz syndrome-related cases. *Ann. Diagn. Pathol.* **2020**, *45*, 151472. [CrossRef] [PubMed]
136. Galvão, H.C.; Gordón-Núñez, M.A.; de Amorim, R.F.; de Almeida Freitas, R.; de Souza, L.B. Immunohistochemical expression of protein 53, murine double minute 2, B-cell lymphoma 2, and proliferating cell nuclear antigen in odontogenic cysts and keratocystic odontogenic tumor. *Indian J. Dent. Res. Off. Publ. Indian Soc. Dent. Res.* **2013**, *24*, 369–374. [CrossRef]
137. Ghafouri-Fard, S.; Atarbashi-Moghadam, S.; Taheri, M. Genetic factors in the pathogenesis of ameloblastoma, dentigerous cyst and odontogenic keratocyst. *Gene* **2021**, *771*, 145369. [CrossRef]

Disclaimer/Publisher's Note: The statements, opinions and data contained in all publications are solely those of the individual author(s) and contributor(s) and not of MDPI and/or the editor(s). MDPI and/or the editor(s) disclaim responsibility for any injury to people or property resulting from any ideas, methods, instructions or products referred to in the content.

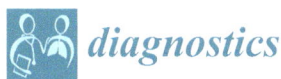

Article

CD34 and Ki-67 Immunoexpression in Periapical Granulomas: Implications for Angiogenesis and Cellular Proliferation

Ciprian Roi [1], Mircea Riviș [1], Alexandra Roi [2,*], Marius Raica [3], Raluca Amalia Ceaușu [3], Alexandru Cătălin Motofelea [4] and Pușa Nela Gaje [3]

[1] Department of Anesthesiology and Oral Surgery, Multidisciplinary Center for Research, Evaluation, Diagnosis and Therapies in Oral Medicine, "Victor Babeș" University of Medicine and Pharmacy, Eftimie Murgu Sq. no. 2, 300041 Timisoara, Romania; ciprian.roi@umft.ro (C.R.); rivis.mircea@umft.ro (M.R.)

[2] Department of Oral Pathology, Multidisciplinary Center for Research, Evaluation, Diagnosis and Therapies in Oral Medicine, "Victor Babeș" University of Medicine and Pharmacy, Eftimie Murgu Sq. no. 2, 300041 Timisoara, Romania

[3] Department of Microscopic Morphology/Histology, Angiogenesis Research Center, "Victor Babeș" University of Medicine and Pharmacy, 300041 Timisoara, Romania; marius.raica@umft.ro (M.R.); ra.ceausu@umft.ro (R.A.C.); gaje.nela@umft.ro (P.N.G.)

[4] Department of Internal Medicine, Faculty of Medicine, "Victor Babeș" University of Medicine and Pharmacy, 300041 Timisoara, Romania; alexandru.motofelea@umft.ro

* Correspondence: alexandra.moga@umft.ro

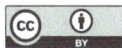

Citation: Roi, C.; Riviș, M.; Roi, A.; Raica, M.; Ceaușu, R.A.; Motofelea, A.C.; Gaje, P.N. CD34 and Ki-67 Immunoexpression in Periapical Granulomas: Implications for Angiogenesis and Cellular Proliferation. *Diagnostics* **2024**, *14*, 2446. https://doi.org/10.3390/diagnostics14212446

Academic Editors: Luis Eduardo Almeida and Siu Wai Choi

Received: 24 September 2024
Revised: 18 October 2024
Accepted: 28 October 2024
Published: 31 October 2024

Copyright: © 2024 by the authors. Licensee MDPI, Basel, Switzerland. This article is an open access article distributed under the terms and conditions of the Creative Commons Attribution (CC BY) license (https://creativecommons.org/licenses/by/4.0/).

Abstract: Background/Objectives: The main mechanism of the formation of granulation tissue is the progression of an infection from the tooth to the periapical bone. At this level, the immune system tries to localize and annihilate the microorganism's injury. Ki-67 is a protein directly associated with the cell proliferation rate, while CD34 is a biomarker involved in angiogenesis, and studies suggest that they both have a positive correlation with the intensity of the local inflammatory infiltrate. This study will determine the immunoexpression of CD34 and Ki-67 in periapical granulomas and assess their impact on the growth and development of this tissue, as well as consider their roles in the proliferative process and aggressiveness of evolution. Methods: In the present study, 35 periapical granulomas obtained after a tooth extraction were included. The specimens were analyzed via histopathology and immunohistochemistry. Results: A positive reaction for the Ki-67 antibody was observed in 32 (86.5%) of the 35 periapical granuloma cases included in our study. We identified the overexpression of Ki-67 and CD34 and further calculated the Ki-67 index to evaluate and correlate the proliferation potential and angiogenesis with regard to the presence of an inflammatory infiltrate. Conclusions: These findings suggest that the persistence of an inflammatory environment directly influences Ki-67 and CD34 expression, sustaining the proliferative capacity of cells and abnormal angiogenesis. This study is the first to evaluate the presence of the CD34+ and Ki-67+ proliferating vessels in periapical granulomas.

Keywords: CD34; Ki-67; periapical granuloma; granulation tissue; cell proliferation; angiogenesis

1. Introduction

One frequently encountered pathology affecting the alveolar bone is periapical periodontitis, a reaction caused by the invasion and proliferation of microorganisms due to untreated pulp necrosis [1]. The interaction between these microorganisms and the immune system's response to their action determines periapical periodontitis development. The persistence of the infection determines local bone resorption, followed by the replacement of bone tissue with granulation tissue [2]. It is estimated that, worldwide, 52% of adults have at least one periapical periodontitis-affected tooth [3]. Nair et al. classified periapical radiolucency into apical abscesses, acute apical periodontitis, apical cysts, and chronic apical periodontitis, identified as periapical granulomas. The World Health Organization does not include the term "periapical lesion" in their classification [4,5].

These modifications can also be explained by an alteration in the eubiosis of an oral cavity. In the past, only the concept of probiotics and their important roles were known; nowadays, novel products, such as paraprobiotics (tyndallized probiotics) and postbiotics, have been created, and they can play a protective role in the occurrence of periapical pathologies [6].

Granulation tissue, as a precursor of periapical granulomas, predominantly includes the lymphocytes, plasma cells, macrophages, and mast cells that influence the development of periapical granulomas [7]. Nevertheless, the presence of mast cells in inflammatory granulomas highlights their role in this inflammatory process [8].

A histological analysis of periapical granulomas shows a strong angiogenesis process affecting the newly formed vessels, and that significant immune cell infiltration secretes the growth factors and cytokines that affect cells' continued proliferation and migration [9].

The presence of an inflammatory infiltrate and the activation of neo-angiogenesis have direct implications for the continuous development of periapical granulomas. As the inflammatory stage continues, it triggers the release of multiple angiogenic factors that directly act upon different cells [10]. Angiogenesis in oral pathologies potentiates progression and sustains inflammation, and it is linked to an unfavorable prognosis. During its progress, it determines the formation of new blood vessels through the proliferation and migration of endothelial cells. The formation of new vessels is accompanied by the introduction, among oxygen and nutrients, of pro-inflammatory cells into pathological tissue [11].

Since different pathological mechanisms and changes are involved in periapical granulomas' occurrence, persistence, and progression, multiple markers linked to these could be targeted to evaluate this pathological lesion. Studies have focused on evaluating CD34 to assess the presence of endothelial cells and the progress of angiogenesis in pathological tissue [12,13].

CD34 is a macromolecular transmembrane sialomucin protein, and it was first discovered in human hematopoietic progenitor cells [14]. Besides the bloodstream, it is found in vascular endothelial cells, keratinocytes, fibrocytes, interstitial cells, and epithelial progenitors [15]. The presence of the CD34 marker has significant involvement in angiogenesis, and studies also suggest that it has a positive correlation with the intensity of the local inflammatory infiltrate [16].

Ki-67 is a protein directly associated with the cell proliferation rate. The presence of this protein has been reported at all evolution stages of cells [17], making it a viable marker responsible for the growth rates of cells [18]. To outline this aspect, past research identified highly expressed Ki-67 in all phases of a cell cycle, being outlined in G1, S, G2, and mitosis. One important aspect was the absence of Ki-67 expression in the resting cell stage (G0) [19].

To assess the level of Ki-67, the percentage of cells labeled with a representative antibody for Ki-67 must be quantified [20]. Through the evaluation of Ki-67 and its presence in odontogenic inflammatory lesions, important information regarding the proliferative potential of the cells and the recurrence rate can be obtained [20]. Nevertheless, several studies have identified the presence of high levels of Ki-67, showing that it is a potential biomarker for acknowledging the aggressive behavior of odontogenic cystic lesions [21]. In addition, a positive Ki-67 reaction has been identified as a predictor of proliferation as a result of a chronic inflammatory environment [22]. Several studies have discussed the effects of higher levels of Ki-67 on the aggressive behavior of these granulomas as a consequence of the continuous activation of the inflammatory cells by the existing microorganisms [23].

In the development of periapical granulomas, the inflammatory environment plays a key role, maintaining the proper conditions and cell populations required for the further progression of this pathological entity. Based on the involvement of several bacterial populations that trigger cytokine and growth factor production, the cell proliferation rate is directly influenced and sustained. The release of cytokines will determine the rate of increase in cellular stress and the increased immunoexpression of inflammatory markers, such as Ki-67 [24] and CD34 [16]. This aspect appears to directly influence the proliferation rate of pathological tissue, as well as further immunopathological interactions.

The present study aims to identify and evaluate the immunoexpression of CD34 and Ki-67 in periapical granulomas, as well as determine their influence on the development and progress of this type of tissue, considering their influence on the proliferative process and aggressiveness of evolution. By understanding this pathogenesis, cellular and molecular interactions, and the existing changes related to periapical granulomas, treatment approaches can be optimized.

2. Materials and Methods

This cross-sectional study was conducted during September 2022–March 2024 and approved by the Ethics Committee of "Victor Babeș" University of Medicine and Pharmacy Timișoara (no. 39/2022). All the patients included in the present study signed an informed consent form that followed the guidelines of the Declaration of Helsinki.

2.1. Patients

The inclusion and exclusion criteria were as follows:
The inclusion criteria:

- Age: 18–70 years;
- Both males and females;
- Teeth with an indication of exodontia due to the impossibility of restorative treatment and presence of a periapical granuloma;
- Non-vital teeth;
- Teeth without endodontic treatment.

The exclusion criteria:

- Minor patients;
- Patients with cervico-facial or/and oral cancers;
- Patients with mucositis;
- Patients with altered general conditions: acute leukemia, recent myocardial infarction, or a stroke in the last 6 months;
- Patients undergoing drug treatment for bone pathologies (e.g., bisphosphonates).

Based on the inclusion and exclusion criteria, 35 patients were included in this study, namely 17 females and 18 males, with an age range from 24 to 72 years. Regarding smoking status, 25 patients were non-smokers and 10 were smokers.

2.2. Clinical Assessment and Granuloma Harvesting

Patients with preoperative periapical radiological radio transparency specific to an odontogenic granuloma and clinically evident or suspected periapical lesions involving non-vital teeth (as determined by an electric pulp tester) were included in this study. In addition, only teeth with no clinical indications of restauration were included. All the patients underwent a standardized preoperative orthopantomogram radiography. All radiographic films were exposed and processed under similar conditions. A radiographic evaluation was performed based on the Periapical Index (PAI) scoring system [24].

After tooth exodontia, the periapical granulomas were removed via the curettage of the root socket. In our study, 29 patients had one tooth extracted, 5 patients had two teeth extracted and 1 patient had three teeth extracted. In this study, 22 teeth were maxillary teeth and 13 were mandibular teeth.

After socket curettage, the periapical granulomas were immersed in formalin, and a fixation of the specimens was carried out with 10% buffered formalin for 48–72 h.

2.3. Primary Probe Processing

We performed an observational study on the paraffin-embedded periapical tissue slices of the 35 periapical granuloma specimens processed according to a standard histology technique. The probes were cleaned, dried, clarified, and imbedded in paraffin. The Thermo Shandon standardized inclusion automat (Thermo Fisher Scientific Inc., Aren-dalsvägen 16–418 78 Gothenburg, Sweden) was utilized for the inclusion stage. The Shandom ME microtome was used to perform sectioning. Two slices, each measuring around 3 to 5 μm in thickness, were cut from each paraffin block. Hematoxylin–eosin staining of one set of sections was performed using the Leica automatic system on a regular basis to verify the clinical diagnosis.

2.4. Immunohistochemistry

For all the cases included in this study, double immunostaining was performed through a fully automated and standardized procedure for all the cases, using a Leica Bond-Max auto-stainer (Leica Biosystems, Newcastle upon Tyne, UK). Paraffin sections were treated for 20 min with a Bond Epitope Retrieval 2 solution (Leica Biosystems, Newcastle Ltd., Newcastle Upon Tyne, UK). Endogenous peroxidase was blocked with 3% hydrogen peroxide for 5 min. Then, the sections were incubated for 30 min with the CD34 primary antibody (Leica Bond, RTU, clone QBEnd/10, Leica Biosystems Nussloch GmbH, Nußloch, Germany).

For visualization, we used the Bond Polymer Refine Detection System, including the secondary antibody (8 min) and the polymer, with an 8 min incubation time. After peroxidase blocking, we applied the second Ki-67 antibody (Leica Bond, RTU, clone MM1). The Bond Polymer Refine Red detection system containing 3,3-diamino-benzidine dihydrochloride and hematoxylin was used for visualization. Stained sections were permanently mounted with Canada balsam.

2.5. Microscopic Evaluation and Image Analysis

Sections stained morphologically with hematoxylin–eosin and immunohistochemically via CD34-Ki-67 double immunostaining were analyzed using the Zeiss Axiocam 506 (Jena, Germany) and Nikon AY260 microscopes (Nikon Europe B.V., Amstelveen, The Netherlands). Both microscopes are equipped with a real-time imaging system and software for the digital analysis of microscopic images.

The assessment of microvascular density was performed according to the modified Weidner method [25]. Three microscopic fields with maximum vascular densities were chosen, and they had a ×400 magnification. The arithmetic mean represented the final result.

Ki-67 was assessed via the original semi-automated method [26] on the immunohistochemically stained sections. Each slide was initially examined with a ×100 magnification, and the areas with the highest densities of Ki-67-positive nuclei were selected. The Ki-67 proliferation index was calculated using the digital images captured with a ×400 magnification. The percentage of positive cells expressing Ki-67 was calculated, and the expression level was evaluated using a scoring system developed by the American Association for the Study of Cell Biology [27,28]. Applying this approach gave a score for the proportion of positively immunostained cells [(absent 1%), (mild 1–10%), (moderate > 10–30%) and (strong > 30%)] ranging from 0 to 3.

2.6. Statistical Analysis

The continuous variables following a normal distribution were presented as means with standard deviations (SDs), while non-normally distributed data were presented as medians with interquartile ranges (IQRs). The distribution's normality was evaluated using the Shapiro–Wilk test. The differences among the groups for the normally distributed continuous data were assessed using the Welch's t-test for two groups or the ANOVA for more than two groups. Post hoc analyses, when necessary, were performed using the Bonferroni correction to adjust for multiple comparisons. For the non-normally distributed continuous data, the Mann–Whitney U test and the Wilcoxon signed rank test were used for two-group comparisons, while the Kruskal–Wallis test was applied for comparisons involving three or more groups. The false discovery rate was applied to adjust for multiple comparisons in the Mann–Whitney U test, Wilcoxon signed rank test, and Kruskal–Wallis test. The categorical data were analyzed using the χ^2 test or Fisher's exact test, particularly when the expected cell counts were below five. The categorical data were reported as frequencies (n) and percentages (%). A prior power analysis was performed with at least 80% statistical power and a 95% confidence interval. All statistical analyses were performed using R Studio version 3.6.0, using the packages stats, dplyr, coin, multcomp, and pwr. For the logistic regression model analyzing the Ki-67 score, model fit measures included deviance, AIC, and McFadden's R^2. The deviance was 62.8, the AIC was 119, and McFadden's R^2 was 0.330.

3. Results

In the present study, 35 periapical granulomas obtained after the extraction of teeth were included. The patients were enrolled, and the details related to demographic data and potential associated risk factors were further analyzed to identify the potential correlations. The histopathological examination of the samples involved describing the existing cellular population and evaluating CD34 and Ki-67 expression.

The median age of the patients included in this study was 43 years old, with an interquartile range (IQR) of 36 to 50 years. Out of the 35 patients, 17 (49%) were female. Ten patients (27%) were smokers, and among the smokers, the median daily cigarette consumption was 20 cigarettes, with an IQR of 16.3 to 20 cigarettes per day (Table 1).

Table 1. Patient baseline characteristics.

	$N = 35$
Age	43 (36, 50)
Sex	
M	18 (51%)
F	17 (49%)
Smoking status	
Non-smoker	25 (71%)
Smoker	10 (29%)
Daily cigarette consumption	20 (16, 3–20)
Extracted tooth	
1	29 (83%)
2	5 (14%)
3	1 (3%)

For the average proliferating vessels, significant differences were observed between the Ki-67 score groups, with the highest values being found in the >30 group (mean = 8.0), followed by the 20–30 group (mean = 6.0). The statistical test had a significant effect, with $p < 0.011$.

The connective tissue vessels had a consistent median across the groups, with the highest value recorded in the >30 group (median = 15.0); however, the differences were not significant ($p = 0.821$).

The results indicate that the majority of patients across all the Ki-67 score groups had one tooth extracted, with 83.8% of patients placed in this category. Regarding sex distribution, females comprised 49% of the total sample, and they were more highly represented in the 10–20 Ki-67 group (100%). Males made up 51% of the sample, and all the patients in the >10 group were male.

Figure 1 shows a bimodal distribution, with 34.4% of the subjects having Ki-67 scores greater than 30, 31.2% having scores less than 10, and smaller proportions falling within the intermediate ranges.

In the logistic regression model for the Ki-67 score groups, significant predictors included "Proliferant vessels" for the <10 vs. 20–30 comparison (estimate = -35.637, $p < 0.001$), and "Connective tissue vessels" for the >20 vs. 20–30 comparison (estimate = -8.333, $p = 0.048$). The other predictors did not show significant effects.

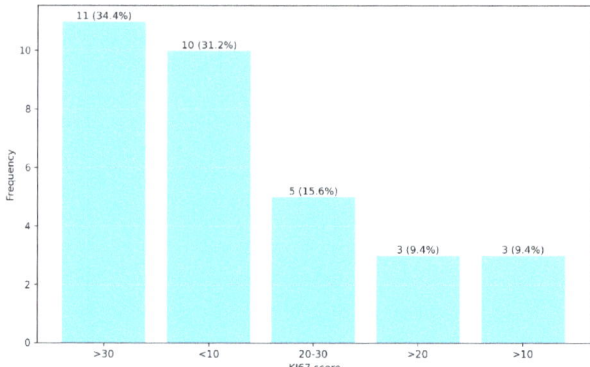

Figure 1. The distribution of the Ki-67 scores.

3.1. Histopathological Analysis

The periapical granuloma tissues were analyzed based on the diagnostic criteria of Omoregie et al. [29,30].

We classified the histological types of periapical granuloma into early, intermediate, and late stages based on the associated inflammatory cells (Figure 2a–d).

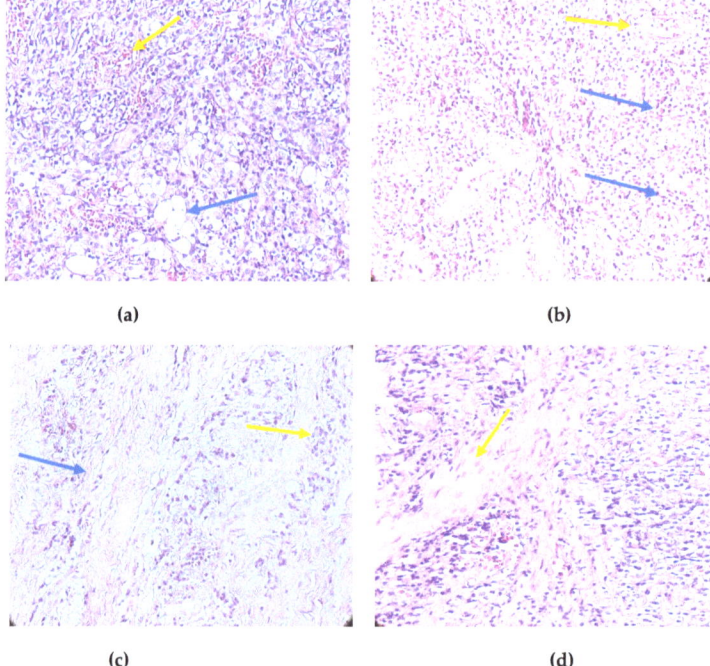

Figure 2. Histopathological aspects of periapical granulomas: (**a**) early periapical granuloma with numerous foamy macrophages (blue arrow) and blood vessels (yellow arrow); (**b**) intermediate periapical granuloma with mixed inflammatory infiltrate consisting of lymphocyte plasma cells and macrophages (blue arrows) and blood vessels (yellow arrow); (**c**) late periapical granuloma with rich connective stroma (blue arrow) and few inflammatory cells (yellow arrow); and (**d**) periapical granuloma (detail), inflammatory infiltrates, and fibrous stroma with prominent fibroblasts (yellow arrow). Hematoxylin–eosin staining, ×400 magnification.

3.2. Immunohistochemical Findings

During the immunohistochemical staining experiment, we observed the number of CD34-positive vessels and the number of Ki-67-positive cell nuclei. The positive expression of Ki-67 in the connective tissue resulted in a distinct nuclear brown staining that had a score of 0 to 3, as shown in Figure 3.

A positive reaction for the Ki-67 antibody was observed in 32 (86.5%) of the 35 cases of the periapical granulomas included in our study. A moderate expression (>10–50%) was the most frequently observed, as it was observed in 22 cases (59.5%). A light expression of Ki-67 (1–10%) was observed in 10 cases (27%), and in 3 cases (13.5%), Ki-67 expression was absent.

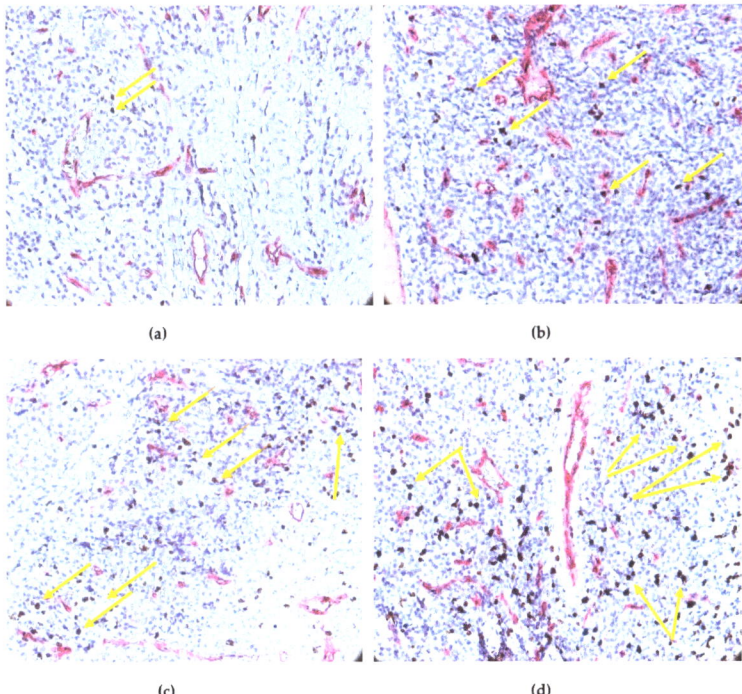

Figure 3. Ki-67 expression in periapical granulomas: (**a**) score 0 (1% positive nuclei, brown–yellow arrows); (**b**) score 1 (1–10% positive nuclei, brown–yellow arrows); (**c**) score 2 (>10–50% positive nuclei, brown–yellow arrows); and (**d**) score 3 (50% positive nuclei, brown–yellow arrows). Double CD34 Ki67 immunostaining, ×400 magnification.

As shown in Figure 4, we observed a high Ki-67 nuclear expression in the region of the inflammatory infiltrate, as well as in the epithelium's basal layer.

The positive expression of CD34 in the vascular endothelium resulted in cytoplasmic red staining. We noticed CD34-positive vessels in all the cases included in this study. The most numerous examples were observed in periapical granulomas classified as being in the intermediate stage with mixed inflammatory infiltrates. The vessels present in the area of the inflammatory infiltrate were heterogeneous in terms of morphology and size. Most of the immunohistochemically identified vessels were medium or small in size, though only some showed lumen. Small vessels with a narrow lumen bordered by proliferating endothelial cells were also present. We noted the CD34-positive vessels that formed compartments in the area of the inflammatory infiltrate. Numerous inflammatory cells were present in these vascular compartments.

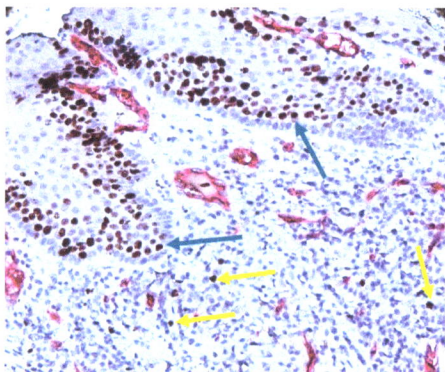

Figure 4. Stratified squamous epithelium with Ki-67-positive nuclei (brown, pointed to with blue arrow) in the basal area (positive control), a reduced number of Ki-67-positive nuclei in the area of the inflammatory infiltrate (brown, pointed to with the yellow arrows). CD34-Ki-67 double immunostaining, ×400 magnification.

CD34 and Ki-67 co-expression was noted in the vascular endothelium, which allowed for the quantification of the vascular microdensity in relation to endothelial proliferation, as shown in Figure 5a,b.

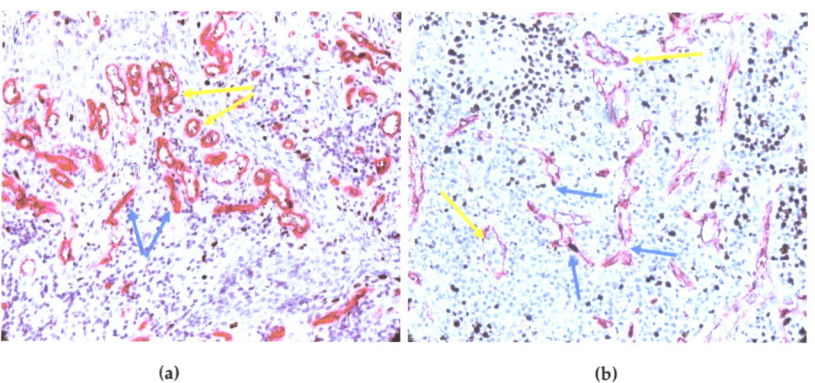

(a)   (b)

Figure 5. Vascular heterogeneity in periapical granulomas: (**a**) CD34-positive vessels varied in size and morphology, with both vessels without lumen (red–blue arrows) and small- and medium-sized vessels showing lumen (red–yellow arrows); and (**b**) CD34-Ki-67 co-expression at the level of the vascular endothelium, with vascular compartments. CD34-Ki-67 double immunostaining, ×400 magnification.

We also noted that, in some cases, intussusception characterized by the presence of vessels had a wide lumen, with protrusions noted towards the endothelium lumen. All the above aspects suggest the activation of angiogenesis in periapical granulomas.

The proliferative activity of periapical granulomas is an important indicator for evaluating the progression and proliferation potential of the lesion and the pathological tissue. Positive Ki-67 expression, being a consequence of a chronic irritation, can be an indicator of the lesion's evolution.

Thus, based on these results, our study is the only one to evaluate both Ki-67 and CD34 expression in periapical granulomas.

4. Discussion

Periapical granulomas are a consequence of a persistent bacterial infection localized in the roots of teeth, determining both the inflammatory response and the changes in the local environment triggered by the release of cytokines and growth factors [31]. They are histologically described as being rich granulation tissue, encapsulated by a fibrous membrane. Past studies discuss the cellular components of the granulation tissue, highlighting the presence of lymphocytes, monocytes, macrophages, and plasma cells resulting from chronic persistent inflammatory stimulus in the periapical space [32]. The reported humoral immune and cell-mediated reactions in periapical granulomas are involved in ongoing cellular proliferation [33]. The literature has reported these types of lesions in males and females [34]. In the present study, 51% of the samples belonged to males (18 patients), while the other studies reported a predominantly female population [35–37].

Comparing the prevalence between the different age groups, the literature reveals a higher incidence in the third and fourth decades of life [38]. However, there are studies that discuss the fact that inflammatory cysts are more commonly encountered in young adults, with this distribution most probably being determined by the oral and dental status of the studied population [39]. However, in the present research, the subjects had a median age of 43 years old. Regarding the localization of the periapical granulomas, the mandibular location was more common in our study, being similar to other existing data in the research field [37].

Studies have described the evolution of periapical inflammatory lesions as being directly dependent on the balance between cell proliferation and apoptosis [19]. Taking into consideration the fact that periapical granulomas are a response to bacterial stimuli that determine an inflammatory reaction, the release of inflammatory cytokines induces certain cellular stress that influences the immunoexpression of Ki-67 in periapical granulomas [22].

The Ki-67 antigen is a nuclear protein expressed by the cells that undergo a proliferating phase, with peak values in the phases G2 and M [40]. Taking this into consideration, researchers aimed to evaluate Ki-67 antibody expression in various malignancies [41]. Nevertheless, there are studies that focus on the presence of Ki-67 and PCNA in premalignant and malignant oral cavity lesions due to their implications for the proliferation process [42]. In addition, there is evidence related to the use of the immunoexpression of Ki-67 as a biological marker for the evaluation of a possible predisposition towards developing a cystic lesion [43]. The results of our study revealed positive Ki-67 immunoreactivity in the nuclei of the basal layers of the periapical granulomas compared to the low expression encountered in the nuclei of the inflammatory infiltrate. Indeed, similar results were reported by Sargozalei et al. [22]. In a study conducted by Slotweg et al. [44], it was noted that in the case of inflammatory periapical lesions, the expression of Ki-67 was higher in the basal layer compared to the odontogenic keratocysts, which exhibited a higher expression in the suprabasal layer. The results of the study performed by De Palma et al. [45] showed that the expression of Ki-67 in inflammatory keratocysts was higher compared to the non-inflammatory ones. These differences also influenced the different development pathways of these pathological entities [46]. The existing results show the importance of the odontogenic inflammatory entities and the evaluation of Ki-67 immunoexpression, offering a new perspective on the proliferative potential of a periapical lesion and, in some cases, its recurrence potential [46,47]. Chaturvedi et al. [47], in their study, identified the potential use of Ki-67 as a biomarker to evaluate the aggressiveness of benign odontogenic tumors. The results of their study indicated a positive correlation between the intensity of Ki-67-positive cells and the aggressive behaviors of the odontogenic tumor.

By targeting CD34 in periapical granulomas, we aimed to quantify angiogenesis in the pathological tissue. CD34 is defined as an adhesion molecule expressed in the endothelial and hematopoietic cells [48]. There are studies that show a positive correlation between CD34 and the intensity of the inflammatory infiltrate in pathological periapical tissue. In the present study, we reported similar results, identifying a higher immunoexpression of CD34 in the areas with a higher inflammatory infiltrate. In addition, by correlating the immunoexpression of CD34 with Ki-67, the results were positive, allowing us to identify a relationship between angiogenesis, the microvessel density, and the endothelial proliferation potential. The aggressive behavior of the periapical lesions was also linked to the intensity of CD34 expression, and the results of Mathiou et al. [49] describe the increases in the immunoexpression of CD34 and the microvessel density in the areas with an inflammatory infiltrate as increasing angiogenesis and influencing further development. Another study that focused on the presence of CD34 in periapical granulomas reported an increased expression of this molecule, determining the existence of an endothelial hyperplasia due to the increased angiogenesis [50].

The cellular and molecular mechanisms involved in granuloma progression and recurrence, particularly in terms of therapeutic interventions, could be used in future studies for the investigation of other osseous tumors like central giant cell granulomas. The etiology of this tumor type remains multifaceted and continues to be debated within the medical community, but early hypotheses have suggested an inflammatory, reactive reaction [51].

On the other hand, prophylaxis related to the occurrence of periapical granulomas must be studied further. Due to the implications of oral microbiota, the eubiotics administered to patients can help the local immune system of the oral cavity to stop the worsening of periapical injuries, as can the use of paraprobiotics (tyndallized probiotics) and postbiotics. Paraprobiotics are deactivated microbial cells that benefit the consumer without posing any health risks; they control the innate and adaptive immune systems, act as antagonists against pathogens, and have anti-inflammatory, antiproliferative, and antioxidant properties. Postbiotics, which comprise any material released or created by the metabolic activity of a microbe without including living bacteria themselves, should not be confused with probiotics and paraprobiotics [6]. Other factors that limit the formation and progression of a periapical granuloma can lead to good oral health, lowering the plaque index, ensuring the early detection and treatment of pulp inflammation and infection, and enabling the correct endodontic treatment of teeth with periapical symptoms.

Upon analyzing the expression of CD34 and Ki-67 in the samples, the results highlight the potential use of these proteins as biomarkers to evaluate the proliferative characteristics, inflammatory components, and future development of lesions.

One of the major limitations of this study is the number of samples. Our results should encourage new studies with larger samples to evaluate odontogenic periapical granulomas and improve the knowledge in this field. In addition, our findings and other potential studies could be the basis of antiangiogenic therapy.

5. Conclusions

Periapical granulomas are odontogenic pathologic entities that occur in response to chronic bacterial irritation. Pathological mechanisms and cellular interactions have an important influence on the evolution of lesions. In the present study, we identified the overexpression of Ki-67 and CD34 and calculated the Ki-67 index to evaluate and correlate the proliferation potential and angiogenesis in the presence of an inflammatory infiltrate. These findings suggest that the persistence of the inflammatory environment directly influences Ki-67 and CD34 expression, sustaining the proliferative capacity of the cells and abnormal angiogenesis.

Author Contributions: Conceptualization, C.R. and M.R. (Mircea Riviș); methodology, A.R. and M.R. (Marius Raica); software, A.C.M.; validation, R.A.C. and P.N.G.; formal analysis, M.R. (Mircea Riviș); investigation, A.R. and R.A.C.; resources, C.R. and M.R. (Marius Raica); data curation, A.C.M.; writing—original draft preparation, C.R.; writing—review and editing, M.R. (Marius Raica), A.R., and P.N.G.; visualization, P.N.G.; supervision, M.R. (Mircea Riviș); funding acquisition, C.R. All authors have read and agreed to the published version of the manuscript.

Funding: This research was funded by "Victor Babeș" University of Medicine and Pharmacy Timișoara, through the post-doctoral grant AN-API-DEN 2022–2023. We would also like to acknowledge "Victor Babeș" University of Medicine and Pharmacy Timișoara for their support in covering the costs of publication for this research paper.

Institutional Review Board Statement: This study was conducted in accordance with the Declaration of Helsinki and approved by the Ethics Committee of "Victor Babeș" University of Medicine and Pharmacy Timișoara (No. 39/19.04.2022).

Informed Consent Statement: Informed consent was obtained from all the subjects involved in this study.

Data Availability Statement: The data presented in this study are available on request from the corresponding author. The data are not publicly available due to restrictions related to the privacy of the funding protocol.

Conflicts of Interest: The authors declare no conflicts of interest.

References

1. Galler, K.M.; Weber, M.; Korkmaz, Y.; Widbiller, M.; Feuerer, M. Inflammatory Response Mechanisms of the Dentine-Pulp Complex and the periapical tissues. *J. Mol. Sci.* **2021**, *22*, 1480. [CrossRef] [PubMed] [PubMed Central]
2. Maia, L.M.; Espaladori, M.C.; Diniz, J.M.B.; Tavares, W.L.F.; de Brito, L.C.N.; Vieira, L.Q.; Sobrinho, A.P.R. Clinical endodontic procedures modulate periapical cytokine and chemokine gene expressions. *Clin. Oral Investig.* **2020**, *24*, 3691–3697. [CrossRef] [PubMed]
3. Tibúrcio-Machado, C.S.; Michelon, C.; Zanatta, F.B.; Gomes, M.S.; Marin, J.A.; Bier, C.A. The global prevalence of apical periodontitis: A systematic review and meta-analysis. *Int. Endod. J.* **2021**, *54*, 712–735. [CrossRef] [PubMed]
4. World Health Organization. *Application of the International Classification of Diseases to Dentistry and Stomatology: ICD-DA*, 3rd ed.; World Health Organization: Geneva, Switzerland, 1995; pp. 66–74.
5. Nair, P.N. Apical periodontitis: A dynamic encounter between root canal infection and host response. *Periodontol. 2000* **1997**, *13*, 121–148. [CrossRef] [PubMed]
6. Butera, A.; Gallo, S.; Pascadopoli, M.; Maiorani, C.; Milone, A.; Alovisi, M.; Scribante, A. Paraprobiotics in Non-Surgical Periodontal Therapy: Clinical and Microbiological Aspects in a 6-Month Follow-Up Domiciliary Protocol for Oral Hygiene. *Microorganisms* **2022**, *10*, 337. [CrossRef] [PubMed] [PubMed Central]
7. Graunaite, I.; Lodiene, G.; Maciulskiene, V. Pathogenesis of apical periodontitis: A literature review. *J. Oral Maxillofac. Res.* **2012**, *2*, e1. [CrossRef] [PubMed] [PubMed Central]
8. Malik, S.; Kamboj, M.; Narwal, A.; Devi, A. Immunohistochemical evaluation of cyclooxygenase-2 and mast cell density in periapical lesions. *Int. Endod. J.* **2023**, *56*, 980–990. [CrossRef] [PubMed]
9. Leonardi, R.; Caltabiano, M.; Pagano, M.; Pezzuto, V.; Loreto, C.; Palestro, G. Detection of vascular endothelial growth factor/vascular permeability factor in periapical lesions. *J. Endod.* **2003**, *29*, 180–183. [CrossRef] [PubMed]
10. Fonseca-Silva, T.; Santos, C.C.; Alves, L.R.; Dias, L.C.; Brito, M., Jr.; De Paula, A.M.; Guimarães, A.L. Detection and quantification of mast cell, vascular endothelial growth factor, and microvessel density in human inflammatory periapical cysts and granulomas. *Int. Endod. J.* **2012**, *45*, 859–864. [CrossRef] [PubMed]
11. Legorreta-Villegas, I.; Trejo-Remigio, D.A.; Ramírez-Martínez, C.M.; Portilla-Robertson, J.; Leyva-Huerta, E.R.; Jacinto-Alemán, L.F. Análisis de microdensidad vascular y factores de crecimiento en carcinoma oral de células escamosas. *Rev. ADM* **2020**, *77*, 287–294. [CrossRef]
12. Kademani, D.; Lewis, J.T.; Lamb, D.H.; Rallis, D.J.; Harrington, J.R. Angiogenesis and CD34 expression as a predictor of recurrence in oral squamous cell carcinoma. *J. Oral Maxillofac. Surg.* **2009**, *67*, 1800–1805. [CrossRef] [PubMed]
13. Pereira, T.; Dodal, S.; Tamgadge, A.; Bhalerao, S.; Tamgadge, S. Quantitative evaluation of microvessel density using CD34 in clinical variants of ameloblastoma: An immunohistochemical study. *J. Oral Maxillofac. Pathol.* **2016**, *20*, 51–58. [CrossRef] [PubMed] [PubMed Central]
14. Krause, D.S.; Fackler, M.J.; Civin, C.I.; May, W.S. CD34: Structure, biology, and clinical utility. *Blood* **1996**, *87*, 1–13. [CrossRef] [PubMed]
15. Rodrigues, C.R.; Moga, S.; Singh, B.; Aulakh, G.K. CD34 Protein: Its expression and function in inflammation. *Cell Tissue Res.* **2023**, *393*, 443–454. [CrossRef] [PubMed]
16. Lopes, C.B.; Armada, L.; Pires, F.R. Comparative Expression of CD34, Intercellular Adhesion Molecule-1, and Podoplanin and the Presence of Mast Cells in Periapical Granulomas, Cysts, and Residual Cysts. *J. Endod.* **2018**, *44*, 1105–1109. [CrossRef] [PubMed]
17. Kamal, N.M.; El Behairy, R.A. Evaluation of development and growth of peripheral giant cell granuloma using osteocalcin, cd68, cd34, and ki-67 markers. *Egypt. Dent. J.* **2017**, *63*, 3287–3300. [CrossRef]
18. El-Attar, R.H.M.; Wahba, O.M. Expression of Ki67, CD31, CD68 and P53 in Peripheral and Central Giant Cell Granuloma of the Jaws. *Arch. Cancer Res.* **2016**, *4*, 2. [CrossRef]
19. Martins, C.A.; Rivero, E.R.; Dufloth, R.M.; Figueiredo, C.P.; Vieira, D.S. Immunohistochemical detection of factors related to cellular proliferation and apoptosis in radicular and dentigerous cysts. *J. Endod.* **2011**, *37*, 36–39. [CrossRef] [PubMed]

20. Slootweg, P.J. p53 protein and Ki-67 reactivity in epithelial odontogenic lesions. An immunohistochemical study. *J. Oral Pathol. Med.* **1995**, *24*, 393–397. [CrossRef] [PubMed]
21. Nadalin, M.R.; Fregnani, E.R.; Silva-Sousa, Y.T.; Perez, D.E. Syndecan-1 (CD138) and Ki-67 expression in odontogenic cystic lesions. *Braz. Dent. J.* **2011**, *22*, 223–229. [CrossRef] [PubMed]
22. Sargolzaei, S.; Roufegarinejad, A.; Shamszadeh, S. Immunohistochemical Expression of PCNA and Ki-67 in Periapical Granuloma and Radicular. *J. Dent. Sch.* **2016**, *34*, 58–65.
23. Hamied, M.; Mohammad, S.; Ali, Z. Inflammatory Odontogenic Cysts. *Al-Kindy Coll. Med. J.* **2021**, *17*, 135–144. [CrossRef]
24. Hudson, J.D.; Shoaibi, M.A.; Maestro, R.; Carnero, A.; Hannon, G.J.; Beach, D.H. A proinflammatory cytokine inhibits p53 tumor suppressor activity. *J. Exp. Med.* **1999**, *190*, 1375–1382. [CrossRef] [PubMed] [PubMed Central]
25. Weidner, N. Chapter 14. Measuring intratumoral microvessel density. *Methods Enzymol.* **2008**, *444*, 305–323. [CrossRef] [PubMed]
26. Suciu, C.; Muresan, A.; Cornea, R.; Suciu, O.; Dema, A.; Raica, M. Semi-automated evaluation of Ki-67 index in invasive ductal carcinoma of the breast. *Oncol. Lett.* **2014**, *7*, 107–114. [CrossRef] [PubMed] [PubMed Central]
27. Kujan, O.; Al-Shawaf, A.Z.; Azzeghaiby, S.; AlManadille, A.; Aziz, K.; Raheel, S.A. Immunohistochemical comparison of p53, Ki-67, CD68, vimentin, α-smooth muscle actin and alpha-1-antichymotry-psin in oral peripheral and central giant cell granuloma. *J. Contemp. Dent. Pract.* **2015**, *16*, 20–24. [CrossRef] [PubMed]
28. Seleit, I.; Asaad, N.; Maree, A.; Wahed, M. Immunohistochemical Expression of p53 and Ki67 in Cutaneous Lupus Erythematosus. *J. Egypt. Women Dermatol. Soc. JEWDS* **2009**, *7*, 5–15.
29. Niemiec, B.A. Oral pathology. *Top. Companion Anim. Med.* **2008**, *23*, 59–71. [CrossRef] [PubMed]
30. Omoregie, F.O.; Ojo, M.A.; Saheeb, B.; Odukoya, O. Periapical granuloma associated with extracted teeth. *Niger. J. Clin. Pract.* **2011**, *14*, 293–296. [CrossRef] [PubMed]
31. Canassa, B.C.; Pavan, A.J. Inflammatory odontogenic cysts: A brief literature review. *J. Surg. Clin. Dent.-JSCD* **2014**, *2*, 20–28.
32. Piattelli, A.; Artese, L.; Rosini, S.; Quaranta, M.; Musiani, P. Immune cells in periapical granuloma: Morphological and immunohistochemical characterization. *J. Endod.* **1991**, *17*, 26–29. [CrossRef] [PubMed]
33. Tripi, T.R.; Bonaccorso, A.; Rapisarda, E.; Bartoloni, G. Proliferative activity in periapical lesions. *Aust. Endod. J.* **2003**, *29*, 31–33. [CrossRef] [PubMed]
34. Menditti, D.; Laino, L.; DI Domenico, M.; Troiano, G.; Guglielmotti, M.; Sava, S.; Mezzogiorno, A.; Baldi, A. Cysts and Pseudocysts of the Oral Cavity: Revision of the Literature and a New Proposed Classification. *In Vivo* **2018**, *32*, 999–1007. [CrossRef] [PubMed] [PubMed Central]
35. Rao, K.; Umadevi, H.S.; Priya, N.S. Clinicopathological study of 100 odontogenic cysts reported at VS dental college—A retrospective study. *J. Adv. Dent. Res.* **2011**, *2*, 51–58.
36. Saghravanian, N.; Zare-Mahmoodabadi, R.; Ghazi, N.; Hosseinpour, S. Odontogenic cysts: A 40-year retrospective clinicopathological study in an Iranian population. *Cumhur. Dent. J.* **2015**, *18*, 272–281.
37. Diatta, M.; Gadji, M.; Diémé, M.J.; Sarr, S.; Keita, M.; Kane, M.; Tine, S.D. Study of the cell proliferation index (Ki67) in inflammatory odontogenic cysts. *Adv. Oral Maxillofac. Surg.* **2023**, *11*, 100431. [CrossRef]
38. Manor, E.; Kachko, L.; Puterman, M.B.; Szabo, G.; Bodner, L. Cystic lesions of the jaws—A clinicopathological study of 322 cases and review of the literature. *Int. J. Med. Sci.* **2012**, *9*, 20–26. [CrossRef] [PubMed] [PubMed Central]
39. Monteiro, L.; Santiago, C.; Amaral, B.D.; Al-Mossallami, A.; Albuquerque, R.; Lopes, C. An observational retrospective study of odontogenic cyst's and tumours over an 18-year period in a Portuguese population according to the new WHO Head and Neck Tumour classification. *Med. Oral Patol. Oral Cir. Bucal* **2021**, *26*, e482–e493. [CrossRef] [PubMed] [PubMed Central]
40. Kreipe, H.; Heidebrecht, H.J.; Hansen, S.; Röhlk, W.; Kubbies, M.; Wacker, H.H.; Tiemann, M.; Radzun, H.J.; Parwaresch, R. A new proliferation-associated nuclear antigen detectable in paraffin-embedded tissues by the monoclonal antibody Ki-S1. *Am. J. Pathol.* **1993**, *142*, 3–9. [PubMed] [PubMed Central]
41. Scholzen, T.; Gerdes, J. The Ki-67 protein: From the known and the unknown. *J. Cell. Physiol.* **2000**, *182*, 311–322. [CrossRef] [PubMed]
42. Souza, P.E.; Mesquita, R.A.; Gomez, R.S. Evaluation of p53, PCNA, Ki-67, MDM2 and AgNOR in oral peripheral and central giant cell lesions. *Oral Dis.* **2000**, *6*, 35–39. [CrossRef] [PubMed]
43. Awni, S.; Conn, B. Decompression of keratocystic odontogenic tumors leading to increased fibrosis, but without any change in epithelial proliferation. *Oral Surg. Oral Med. Oral Pathol. Oral Radiol.* **2017**, *123*, 634–644. [CrossRef] [PubMed]
44. De Palma, G.D.; Masone, S.; Siciliano, F.; Maione, F.; Falletti, J.; Mansueto, G.; De Rosa, G.; Persico, G. Endocrine carcinoma of the major papilla: Report of two cases and review of the literature. *Surg. Oncol.* **2010**, *19*, 235–242. [CrossRef] [PubMed]
45. Ayoub, M.S.; Baghdadi, H.M.; El-Kholy, M. Immunohistochemical detection of laminin-1 and Ki-67 in radicular cysts and keratocystic odontogenic tumors. *BMC Clin. Pathol.* **2011**, *11*, 4. [CrossRef] [PubMed] [PubMed Central]
46. Amin, R.; Shenoy, R. Assessment of inflammatory domain on the proliferative activity of odontogenic Keratocyst in comparison with dentigerous cyst and perapical cyst. *J. Orofac. Sci.* **2021**, *13*, 148–154. [CrossRef]
47. Chaturvedi, T.P.; Gupta, K.; Agrawal, R.; Kumar, P.N.; Gupta, J. Immunohistochemical expression of Ki-67 and Glypican-3 to distinguish aggressive from nonaggressive benign odontogenic tumors. *J. Cancer Res. Ther.* **2022**, *18* (Suppl. S2), S205–S209. [CrossRef] [PubMed]

48. Zizzi, A.; Aspriello, S.D.; Ferrante, L.; Stramazzotti, D.; Colella, G.; Balercia, P.; Lo Muzio, L.; Piemontese, M.; Goteri, G.; Rubini, C. Immunohistochemical correlation between microvessel density and lymphoid infiltrate in radicular cysts. *Oral Dis.* **2013**, *19*, 92–99. [CrossRef] [PubMed]
49. Mathiou, V.; Tsiambas, E.; Maipas, S.; Thymara, I.; Peschos, D.; Lazaris, A.C.; Kavantzas, N. Impact of CD34-dependent Micro Vessel Density on Periapical Odontogenic Cysts. *Cancer Diagn. Progn.* **2023**, *3*, 189–193. [CrossRef] [PubMed] [PubMed Central]
50. Ajuz, N.C.; Antunes, H.; Mendonça, T.A.; Pires, F.R.; Siqueira, J.F., Jr.; Armada, L. Immunoexpression of interleukin 17 in apical periodontitis lesions. *J. Endod.* **2014**, *40*, 1400–1403. [CrossRef] [PubMed]
51. Aliu, F.; Shabani, D.B.; Aliu, I.; Qeli, E.D.; Kaçani, G.; Fiorillo, L.; Meto, A. Evaluating Treatment Modalities for Reducing Recurrence in Central Giant Cell Granuloma: A Narrative Review. *Dent. J.* **2024**, *12*, 295. [CrossRef]

Disclaimer/Publisher's Note: The statements, opinions and data contained in all publications are solely those of the individual author(s) and contributor(s) and not of MDPI and/or the editor(s). MDPI and/or the editor(s) disclaim responsibility for any injury to people or property resulting from any ideas, methods, instructions or products referred to in the content.

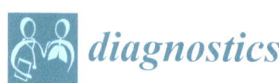

Article

Comparative Immunohistochemical Analysis of Craniopharyngioma and Ameloblastoma: Insights into Odontogenic Differentiation

Ban A. Salih * and Bashar H. Abdullah

College of Dentistry, University of Baghdad, Baghdad 10071, Iraq; bashar.hamid@codental.uobaghdad.edu.iq
* Correspondence: banoali929@gmail.com

Abstract: Background and objectives: Histopathological similarities between craniopharyngioma (CP) and ameloblastoma (AB) have long been recognized, particularly the shared features of palisading columnar epithelium and stellate reticulum-like areas. This study aimed to investigate potential odontogenic differentiation in CP akin to AB using immunohistochemical odontogenic markers. Methods: We analyzed AMELX, ODAM, and CK19 expression in 44 cases (20 CP and 24 AB). Results: While AMELX and ODAM showed diffuse strong positive expression in both tumors with no significant statistical differences, CK19 expression was notably higher in CP. Conclusion: The markers AMELX and ODAM associated with odontogenic differentiation exhibited similar profiles in both tumors due to shared similar embryological origins. Notably, CK19, a biomarker of odontogenic epithelium, showed even higher expression, suggesting distinct pathways. These findings offer insights into tumor biology and may aid in diagnostic and therapeutic approaches.

Keywords: craniopharyngioma; ameloblastoma; odontogenic differentiation; immunohistochemistry

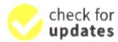

Citation: Salih, B.A.; Abdullah, B.H. Comparative Immunohistochemical Analysis of Craniopharyngioma and Ameloblastoma: Insights into Odontogenic Differentiation. *Diagnostics* **2024**, *14*, 2315. https:// doi.org/10.3390/diagnostics14202315

Academic Editor: Gustavo Baldassarre

Received: 30 August 2024
Revised: 10 October 2024
Accepted: 14 October 2024
Published: 17 October 2024

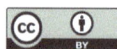

Copyright: © 2024 by the authors. Licensee MDPI, Basel, Switzerland. This article is an open access article distributed under the terms and conditions of the Creative Commons Attribution (CC BY) license (https:// creativecommons.org/licenses/by/ 4.0/).

1. Introduction

Craniopharyngiomas (CPs) are rare, histologically benign epithelial neoplasms that represent a significant challenge in neurosurgical practice. They constitute 1.2–4.6% of all primary intracranial tumors, where the incidence is estimated at 0.5–2 cases per million persons annually [1]. The first description of craniopharyngiomas was reported in 1857 by Zenker. This tumor was named craniopharyngioma by Cushing in 1932 and was widely established as a clinical entity [2]. CPs affect individuals across the lifespan, but their occurrence displays a distinct bimodal age distribution, peaking during childhood/early adolescence (5–15 years) and middle adulthood (44–56 years) [1]. While no clear gender predilection has been established, the anatomical location of these tumors, typically in the sellar/parasellar region, results in significant morbidity [2]. These tumors are generally diagnosed in patients who develop symptoms, including headaches or visual impairment (due to compression of the optic chiasm) and endocrine deficits from local mass effects on the hypothalamic–pituitary axis [2]. Management is further complicated by the fact that diagnosis of CP often has a long delay from symptom onset (up to 1–2 years) [2].

Craniopharyngiomas are rare in incidence, whereas ameloblastomas (ABs) were found to be the most common clinically significant odontogenic tumor; therefore, by itself, ameloblastoma equals all other odontogenic tumors except for limited cases of inside calcified composite [3,4]. Cusack first described ameloblastoma in 1827, which was later explained by Broca in 1868 [5,6]. Ameloblastoma was named adamantinoma by Baden in 1965 [7]. The term "ameloblastoma" was introduced in 1929 [7].

Although ABs can affect a wide age range, they are rarely observed in children younger than ten. The peak incidence is between the third and seventh decades of life, with no gender or ethnic predilection [3]. Most ABs (about 80%) arise from the mandible, especially in a molar/ramus location, and are manifested by an asymptomatic swelling [3].

Despite their distinct clinical presentations and sites of origin, CP and AB can pose diagnostic challenges due to their overlapping clinical and radiological features, particularly multilocular cystic formations [8]. The accurate differentiation of these tumors is crucial to guide appropriate treatment and management strategies.

Histopathologically, CPs are classified into two main subtypes: adamantinomatous (ACP) and papillary (PCP), with transitional or mixed forms also described [9]. The most prevalent subtype, ACP, typically presents as a large, multilobulated, solid cystic mass, often with calcifications and a characteristic "motor-oil"-like fluid content [9]. Microscopically, ACP shows islands of squamous epithelium in cords and trabeculae lined by palisading columnar cells [9]. Key diagnostic features include the presence of "stellate reticulum"-like areas, wet keratin, ghost cells, and reactive gliosis in surrounding brain tissue [9].

In contrast, PCP is almost exclusively observed in adults and tends to be a solid or mixed mass with viscous yellow cysts, rarely exhibiting calcifications [9]. Microscopically, PCP is composed of mature squamous epithelium forming pseudopapillae with an anastomosing fibrovascular stroma [9]. Notably, PCP lacks the peripheral palisading, stellate reticulum, and wet keratin characteristics of ACP [9].

Ameloblastomas also exhibit diverse histopathological patterns. Solid and multicystic ABs (which constitute approximately 75–86% of cases) are further subdivided into follicular, plexiform, acanthomatous, granular cell type, desmoplastic, and basal cell patterns [3]. The follicular type, which is the most common one, manifests leaf-like epithelial islands with peripheral columnar ameloblast-like cells and a central core of stellate reticulum-like cells [3]. The plexiform pattern consists of anastomosing cords or sheets of odontogenic epithelium bordered by ameloblast-like cells [3]. The other patterns are distinguished by varying degrees of squamous metaplasia, keratin formation, granular cell transformation, and desmoplasia [3].

The histopathological similarities between ACP and AB, particularly the shared features of palisading columnar epithelium and stellate reticulum-like areas, have long been recognized [8]. These resemblances are not mere coincidences but likely reflect their shared embryological origin from the oral ectoderm [8]. Both Rathke's pouch, the presumed origin of CPs, and the odontogenic epithelium, the source of ABs, arise from this common precursor tissue [8,10,11]. The process of tooth development, initiated by the thickening and invagination of the oral epithelium into ectomesenchyme, mirrors the early stages of Rathke's pouch development [10]. The shared developmental pathway provides a plausible explanation for the histological convergence of these tumors, prompting further investigation into their molecular underpinnings.

This study focuses on the comparative immunohistochemical analysis of three key markers: amelogenin (AMELX), odontogenic ameloblast-associated protein (ODAM), and cytokeratin 19 (CK19). These markers have been selected based on their well-established roles in tooth development and their potential relevance to the biology of CP and AB.

AMELX, a major enamel matrix protein, is crucial for enamel's structural organization and biomineralization [12,13]. It is expressed by ameloblast in the secretory stage [14]. Low-molecular-weight enamel matrix protein has been consistently shown in the enamel organ's inner enamel epithelium, stratum intermedium, and stellate reticulum [15]. While previously thought to be exclusive to enamel formation, AMELX expression has now been identified in other tissues, including bone and cartilage, suggesting a broader role in tissue development [13].

ODAM, another enamel protein, is vital in enamel maturation and mineralization [16]. Its expression has been detected in various epithelial neoplasms, including odontogenic tumors and cancers of the lung, breast, and stomach, suggesting a potential role in tumorigenesis [17]. Furthermore, ODAM has been proposed as a potential prognostic biomarker and therapeutic target for certain cancers [17].

CK19, a cytokeratin expressed in simple epithelia and various ductal tissues, is recognized as an essential biomarker of the odontogenic epithelium [18–20]. Its expression has been observed in several odontogenic tumors, including AB, highlighting its relevance to the study of these lesions [21,22]. Furthermore, CK19 was expressed in craniopharyngioma [9].

By comparing the expression profiles of AMELX, ODAM, and CK19 in CP and AB, this study aims to shed light on these tumors' potential shared embryological origins and divergent pathological mechanisms. The findings could contribute to a better understanding of tumor biology, enhance diagnostic accuracy, and open avenues for targeted therapies in the future.

2. Materials and Methods

This study comprised 44 formalin-fixed tissue blocks, including 20 cases of craniopharyngioma and 24 cases of ameloblastoma. The primary antibodies used in this study included anti-amelogenin (AMELX, MyBioSource, San Diego, CA, USA), anti-ODAM (Abbexa, Houston, TX, USA), and anti-CK19 (MyBioSource). All the primary antibodies were polyclonal. Positive tissue controls were included in each run following manufacturer data sheets (Figure 1). Negative tissue controls were prepared by adding phosphate-buffered saline (PBS) instead of primary antibodies to the slides. The immunohistochemical procedure was conducted according to the instructions provided in the data sheets of the Abcam secondary antibody detection kit (ab80436-EXPOSE Rabbit and Mouse Specific HRP/DAB Kit, Abcam, Cambridge, UK). The detection system kit and the primary antibodies were put in the refrigerator at 4 °C. Each solution was allowed to reach room temperature before each step.

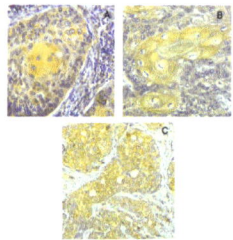

Figure 1. (**A**) Positive ODAM expression in the cytoplasm of the epithelioid cells and in the ghost cells of calcifying epithelial (Pindborg) odontogenic tumor that was used as a positive control for ODAM in the study (Immunohistochemistry, 400×). (**B**) Positive CK19 expression in the cytoplasm of the epithelial cells of the squamous cell carcinoma that was used as a positive control for CK19 in this study (Immunohistochemistry, 400×). (**C**) Breast carcinoma tissue used as a positive control for amelogenin in this study, with a positive cytoplasmic expression of amelogenin (Immunohistochemistry, 400×).

All tissue specimens (cases and control) were presumably fixed in 10% formalin before being processed into paraffin blocks, cut into 4-micron thick sections, and placed on slides with a positive charge. The slides were incubated at 60 °C for two hours in a hot air oven. Then, rehydration was performed by immersing the slides twice in xylene (5 min each), followed by a serial of ethanol dilutions (100%, 100%, 95%, 75%, 50%) for 3 min each and then distilled water. The retrieving procedure involved pretreatment with heat-mediated antigen retrieving solution (citrate buffer pH 6.0). After heating the water-filled water bath and the Kaplan jars with the retrieval solution to 90–95 °C, the slides were placed into the jars and cooked for 20 min at that same temperature. After that, the slides were cooled at room temperature for an additional 25 min. A protein block was added after applying a peroxidase block and incubating for 10 min at 37 °C to inhibit endogenous peroxidase activity. Next, each slide received at least 100 μL of diluted primary antibody and was incubated for an hour, and they were then put in the refrigerator at 4 °C overnight. The next day, secondary antibody and HRP conjugate were applied. The slides were then incubated in a humid chamber for 15 min in the incubator, followed by two rinses with PBS for 5 min each. Chromogen and DAB (Diamino Benzidine) substrates were applied to each slide, and the slides were placed away from light for 10 min. Hematoxylin counterstaining was performed by rinsing the slides for 30 s and then washing the slides with running water. Dehydration was performed to remove the water contained in the tissue by immersing the slides in a series of ethanol dilutions (50%, 75%, 95%, 100%- 100%), followed by immersion twice in xylene (5 min each) and covering with DPX mounting media.

Evaluation of the immunohistochemistry involved examining positive slides by counting the positive cells of ameloblasts and stellate reticulum in 5 high-power fields (400×). For amelogenin staining, the assessment was categorized as follows: "−" indicated no positive cells; "+", less than 10%; "++", 10–50%; "+++", over 50% positivity [10]. Similar to this, the proportion of positive cells was used to determine the score for ODAM staining, which ranged from "−" (0–4%) to "+++" (>75%) [23]. According to the following criteria, CK19 staining was assessed: "−" indicated fewer than 10% positive cells; "+", 10% to 50% positive cells; "2+", more than 50% positive cells [24].

Given the nature of our data and the study's sample size, we carefully chose acceptable statistical tests for comparing categorical data. The primary consideration was the distribution and expected frequency of data points within each category of our contingency tables.

The Chi-squared test is frequently utilized with larger sample sizes and when the expected frequencies in each category of the contingency table exceed 5. This condition ensures that the approximations used to calculate the p-values are valid.

However, in our study, several categories had expected frequencies of less than five due to the small sample size in each group (20 cases of craniopharyngioma and 24 cases of ameloblastoma). This circumstance often leads to a significant chance of type I errors (incorrectly rejecting the null hypothesis) when employing the Chi-squared test.

As a result, we chose Fisher's exact test, specifically developed for small sample sizes and robust to data distribution within the contingency table. Unlike the Chi-squared test, Fisher's exact test does not rely on large sample assumptions and is more appropriate for our study, where the cell counts are low. This test yields an exact p-value based on the hypergeometric distribution, making it a better choice for our comparative investigation of immunohistochemical marker expression in craniopharyngioma and ameloblastoma. Using Fisher's exact test ensures the accuracy of our findings, reducing the risk of statistical error caused by small, uneven sample numbers across the compared groups.

By employing Fisher's exact test, we adhere to statistical best practices, providing a strong analytical framework that supports our findings' validity and thereby improves our study's scientific rigor.

3. Results

In total, 44 cases were examined, comprising 20 cases of craniopharyngioma and 24 cases of ameloblastoma. Among the craniopharyngioma cases, 18 were of the adamantinomatous subtype (nine cystic, eight follicular, and one plexiform-like) while 2 were papillary. Fourteen cases of the adamantinomatous type exhibited ghost cells. Regarding ameloblastoma, 7 cases were cystic, 5 were plexiform, and 12 were follicular.

The immunohistochemical analysis of AMELX, ODAM, and CK19 across the 44 cases revealed distinct expression patterns between craniopharyngioma and ameloblastoma. The results are summarized in Table 1, which includes frequencies, percentages, and confidence intervals for each marker expression category. However, the expression patterns varied considerably among the cases. Some cases exhibited only ameloblast or stellate reticulum expression, while others showed both.

Regarding amelogenin expression, there were no significant differences between craniopharyngioma and ameloblastoma (p = 0.320) (Figure 2A–C). Most cases of both diagnoses demonstrated strong amelogenin positivity (+3). Notably, 90% of adamantinomatous craniopharyngioma cases with ghost cells showed strong amelogenin expression in these cells.

Table 1. Comparison of AMELX, ODAM, and CK19 expression between craniopharyngioma and ameloblastoma using Fisher's exact test.

Marker	Diagnosis	Score 1 (n, %, 95% CI)	Score 2 (n, %, 95% CI)	Score 3 (n, %, 95% CI)	p-Value
AMELX	Craniopharyngioma	2 (9.1%, 2.3–29.0%)	1 (4.5%, 0.8–20.4%)	17 (77.3%, 58.9–89.6%)	0.32
	Ameloblastoma	2 (8.3%, 2.1–27.0%)	5 (20.8%, 9.1–41.7%)	17 (70.8%, 52.8–84.7%)	
ODAM	Craniopharyngioma	2 (9.1%, 2.3–29.0%)	2 (9.1%, 2.3–29.0%)	16 (72.7%, 54.3–85.4%)	0.209
	Ameloblastoma	4 (16.7%, 6.6–36.6%)	7 (29.2%, 15.3–48.7%)	13 (54.2%, 34.2–73.0%)	
CK19	Craniopharyngioma	2 (9.1%, 2.3–29.0%)	18 (81.8%, 63.6–92.3%)	0 (0%, 0–15.4%)	0.008
	Ameloblastoma	12 (50.0%, 30.7–69.3%)	12 (50.0%, 30.7–69.3%)	0 (0%, 0–15.4%)	

Note: Confidence intervals (CI) for percentages are based on the Wilson score method. AMELX—amelogenin; ODAM—odontogenic ameloblast-associated protein; CK19—cytokeratin19.

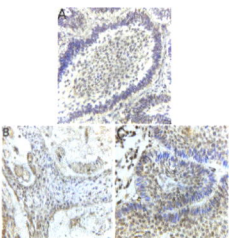

Figure 2. (A) Follicular ameloblastoma with cytoplasmic expression of amelogenin antibody in the stellate reticulum and peripheral layer resembling ameloblast (Immunohistochemistry, 400×). (B) Papillary craniopharyngioma positive cytoplasmic expression of amelogenin antibody in the squamous epithelial cells (Immunohistochemistry, 400×). (C) Adamantinomatous craniopharyngioma with a cytoplasmic expression of amelogenin antibody in both stellate-like area and peripheral ameloblast (Immunohistochemistry, 400×).

ODAM expression also did not significantly differ between craniopharyngioma and ameloblastoma ($p = 0.209$), with the majority of cases showing strong positive expression (+3) (Figure 3A–C). Notably, ODAM expression was observed in both ameloblast-like cells and stellate reticulum in 61% of cases. In comparison, it was observed solely in stellate reticulum in 30% of cases and ameloblast-like cells in four cases. Ghost cells in adamantinomatous craniopharyngioma cases also exhibited strong ODAM expression.

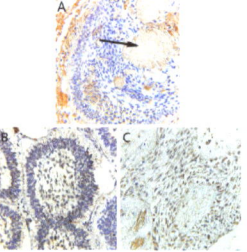

Figure 3. (A) Adamantinomatous craniopharyngioma with cytoplasmic expression of ODAM antibody in both ameloblast and stellate-like area, with positive expression of ODAM in the ghost cells (black arrow) (Immunohistochemistry, 400×). (B) Follicular ameloblastoma with cytoplasmic expression of ODAM antibody in both stellate reticulum and ameloblast (Immunohistochemistry, 400×). (C) Papillary craniopharyngioma with membranous expression of ODAM antibody in the squamous epithelial cells (Immunohistochemistry, 400×).

The expression of CK19 was significantly higher in craniopharyngioma compared to ameloblastoma ($p = 0.008$), with most craniopharyngioma cases showing strong positivity

(+2) (Figure 4A–C). The effect size calculated (phi coefficient = 0.42) indicates a moderate association. Notably, strong CK19 expression was observed in the stellate reticulum, with 54.5% of cases showing expression solely in the stellate reticulum and 38.5% showing expression in both ameloblast-like cells and stellate reticulum. Only 7% of cases exhibited CK19 expression solely in ameloblast-like cells. Ghost cells also demonstrated strong CK19 expression.

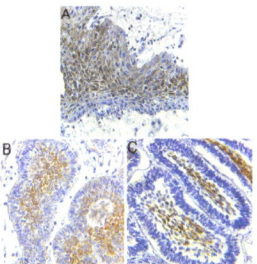

Figure 4. (**A**) Papillary craniopharyngioma with cytoplasmic expression of CK19 antibody in the squamous epithelial cells (Immunohistochemistry, 400×). (**B**) Adamantinomatous craniopharyngioma with membranous expression of CK19 antibody in the stellate-like area (Immunohistochemistry, 400×). (**C**) Follicular ameloblastoma with cytoplasmic expression of CK19 antibody in the stellate reticulum-like area (Immunohistochemistry, 400×).

Figures 2–4 illustrate the expression patterns of AMELX, ODAM, and CK19, respectively, visually comparing the two types of tumors. Figure 5 includes bar graphs that represent the percentage of cases showing each marker's expression level, enhancing the interpretability of the results. These figures visually demonstrate the differences and similarities in marker expression between craniopharyngioma and ameloblastoma, highlighting the unique immunohistochemical profiles observed.

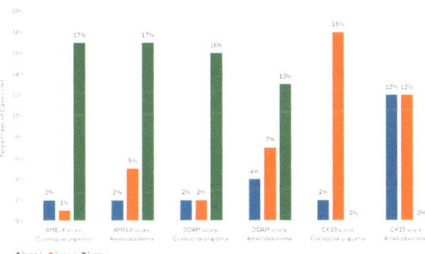

Figure 5. Comparison of AMELX, ODAM, and CK19 expression levels between craniopharyngioma and ameloblastoma.

In summary, while amelogenin and ODAM expression did not significantly differ between craniopharyngioma and ameloblastoma, CK19 expression was significantly higher in craniopharyngioma. These findings underscore the varied immunohistochemical profiles between the two tumor types and may provide insights into their underlying molecular characteristics and developmental pathways.

4. Discussion

This study investigated the immunohistochemical expression of amelogenin (AMELX), odontogenic ameloblast-associated protein (ODAM), and cytokeratin 19 (CK19) in craniopharyngioma and ameloblastoma, aiming to shed light on their potential shared embryological origins and divergent pathological mechanisms. Our findings revealed similarities in AMELX and ODAM expression between these two tumor types, supporting the hypothesis of a shared embryological origin from the oral ectoderm. This aligns with previous research indicating the role of amelogenin, an enamel protein synthesized by ameloblasts [10], as an indication of the development of epithelial cells in odontogenic lesions [25] and a predictor of histological behavior. Amelogenin's utility as a definitive marker for identifying and differentiating odontogenic lesions from other epithelial lesions in the oral and maxillofacial regions has been well-established [15].

Similarly, ODAM, a developmental antigen crucial for tooth maturation, plays a role in the pathogenesis of various odontogenic and epithelial neoplasms [17]. Its expression in ameloblast differentiation and enamel mineralization [19] further supports the odontogenic differentiation of ameloblastoma.

The similarities in AMELX and ODAM expression between these tumors support the hypothesis of a shared embryological origin. Craniopharyngiomas are thought to arise from epithelial remnants of Rathke's pouch [8], while ameloblastomas originate from oral epithelium and odontogenic cells [7]. Both Rathke's pouch and odontogenic epithelium are derived from the stomodeal ectoderm, a process involving the thickening and invagination of the oral epithelium into ectomesenchyme [10]. This common embryological origin may explain the shared ODAM and AMELX expression between these intracranial and intraosseous tumors.

However, despite these shared characteristics, our study revealed a key difference in the expression of CK19. The significantly higher expression of CK19 in craniopharyngioma compared to ameloblastoma suggests a potentially distinct pathway in its odontogenic differentiation. This finding is particularly intriguing considering the role of CK19 as a marker of odontogenic epithelium, as previously established [24,26]. CK19 is known to be upregulated during the conversion of inner enamel epithelium to ameloblasts and is considered a stem cell marker for understanding the pathogenesis of odontogenic cysts and tumors [26]. The expression of CK19 in craniopharyngioma has also been reported by Campanini et al. [9]. Reduced enamel epithelium with overexpressed CK19 indicates the immaturity of the tumor cell lineage, may interfere with terminal differentiation, and may show the capacity of cells to proliferate [26]. These findings, along with the hypothesis of the shared embryological origin of these two tumors, further support the odontogenic differentiation of craniopharyngioma.

Further, the significantly higher CK19 expression in craniopharyngioma holds exciting implications for the diagnosis and prognosis of these tumors, since CK19 was considered a strong epithelial tumor marker used to diagnose and evaluate the prognosis of various tumors of epithelial origin [27]. Additionally, CK19 serves as a useful research tool in the prognosis, diagnosis, and management of both tumors owing to its overexpression in several tumors [28]. In other studies, associations between reduced CK19 expression and some unfavorable phenotypic tumor features and poor patient prognosis were discovered [29].

The differential expression of CK19 may reflect variations in the underlying signaling pathways driving tumor development in craniopharyngioma and ameloblastoma. While both tumors exhibit dysregulation of the Wnt signaling pathway, a key player in tooth development [30], the specific downstream effectors and their influence on CK19 expression may differ. This divergence could be attributed to the distinct microenvironments and cellular contexts in which these tumors arise. Craniopharyngiomas develop in the sellar/suprasellar region, which is surrounded by pituitary tissue and influenced by hormonal factors. At the same time, ameloblastomas arise within the jawbones, interacting with a different set of surrounding cells and signaling molecules. These distinct environments could lead to variations in signaling pathways' activation and downstream effects, ultimately impacting CK19 expression.

While our study provides valuable insights, it is important to acknowledge its limitations. The retrospective design and relatively small sample size limit the ability to control for potential confounding factors and generalize the findings to all populations. The inherent heterogeneity of craniopharyngiomas and ameloblastomas, with their diverse histological subtypes, might also have influenced the observed marker expression patterns.

Technical variations inherent to immunohistochemical staining, such as differences in tissue fixation, processing, and antibody incubation times, could also have contributed to variability in the results.

Future studies with larger, well-characterized cohorts are warranted to validate these findings. These studies should include detailed analyses of different histological subtypes and correlate marker expression with clinical outcomes, such as tumor recurrence and overall survival. Further investigation into the specific molecular mechanisms underlying the differential expression of CK19 and its role in tumor development is also crucial. This could involve examining the expression and activity of downstream effectors of the Wnt signaling pathway and exploring potential interactions with other signaling pathways.

5. Conclusions

In conclusion, our study demonstrates similarities in AMELX and ODAM expression between craniopharyngioma and ameloblastoma, supporting their shared embryological origins. However, the significantly higher expression of CK19 in craniopharyngioma suggests a distinct pathway in its odontogenic differentiation. This finding highlights CK19 as a potential diagnostic marker and therapeutic target for craniopharyngioma. By advancing our understanding of these tumors' immunohistochemical profiles, we contribute to the broader efforts in refining diagnostic accuracy and exploring new treatment options.

Author Contributions: Conceptualization, B.H.A.; methodology, B.A.S.; investigation, B.A.S.; resources, B.A.S.; data curation, B.A.S.; writing—original draft preparation, B.A.S.; writing—review and editing, B.H.A.; supervision, B.H.A.; project administration, B.H.A. All authors have read and agreed to the published version of the manuscript.

Funding: This research received no external funding.

Institutional Review Board Statement: The research was approved by the research ethics committee of the College of Dentistry, University of Baghdad (protocol code 697), on 1 December 2022.

Informed Consent Statement: Informed consent was obtained from all subjects involved in the study.

Data Availability Statement: The data supporting this study's findings are available from the corresponding author upon reasonable request.

Conflicts of Interest: There are no conflicts of interest to declare.

References

1. Muller, H.L.; Merchant, T.E.; Warmuth-Metz, M.; Martinez-Barbera, J.P.; Puget, S. Craniopharyngioma. *Nat. Rev. Dis. Primers* **2019**, *5*, 75. [CrossRef]
2. Garnett, M.R.; Puget, S.; Grill, J.; Sainte-Rose, C. Craniopharyngioma. *Orphanet. J. Rare Dis.* **2007**, *2*, 18. [CrossRef]
3. Neville, B.W.; Damm, D.D.; Allen, C.M.; Chi, A.C. *Oral and Maxillofacial Pathology*; Elsevier Health Sciences: Amsterdam, The Netherlands, 2023.
4. Waheed, S.A.; Zaidan, T.F.; Abdullah, B.H. Odontogenic Cysts and Tumors of Maxilla and Maxillary Sinus (A Clinicopathological Analysis). *J. Bagh. Coll. Dent.* **2021**, *33*, 38–43. [CrossRef]
5. McClary, A.C.; West, R.B.; McClary, A.C.; Pollack, J.R.; Fischbein, N.J.; Holsinger, C.F.; Sunwoo, J.; Colevas, A.D.; Sirjani, D. Ameloblastoma: A clinical review and trends in management. *Eur. Arch. Otorhinolaryngol.* **2016**, *273*, 1649–1661. [CrossRef] [PubMed]
6. Hendra, F.N.; Van Cann, E.M.; Helder, M.N.; Ruslin, M.; de Visscher, J.G.; Forouzanfar, T.; de Vet, H.C.W. Global incidence and profile of ameloblastoma: A systematic review and meta-analysis. *Oral Dis.* **2020**, *26*, 12–21. [CrossRef] [PubMed]
7. Kreppel, M.; Zöller, J. Ameloblastoma—Clinical, radiological, and therapeutic findings. *Oral Dis.* **2018**, *24*, 63–66. [CrossRef]
8. Da Silva, L.A.M.; Filho, S.R.C.; Saraiva, M.J.D.; Maia, C.R.; Santos, C.D.F.D.P.; Santos, P.P.A. Clinical, Radiographic and Histopathological Analysis of Craniopharyngiomas and Ameloblastomas: A Systematic Review. *Head Neck Pathol.* **2022**, *16*, 1195–1222. [CrossRef] [PubMed] [PubMed Central]
9. Campanini, M.L.; Almeida, J.P.; Martins, C.S.; de Castro, M. The molecular pathogenesis of craniopharyngiomas. *Arch. Endocrinol. Metab.* **2023**, *67*, 266–275. [CrossRef]
10. Sekine, S.; Takata, T.; Shibata, T.; Mori, M.; Morishita, Y.; Noguchi, M.; Uchida, T.; Kanai, Y.; Hirohashi, S. Expression of enamel proteins and LEF1 in adamantinomatous craniopharyngioma: Evidence for its odontogenic epithelial differentiation. *Histopathology* **2004**, *45*, 573–579. [CrossRef] [PubMed]

11. Al-Qazzaz, H.H.; Abdullah, B.H.; Jany, S.J. A clinicopathological analysis of 151 odontogenic tumors based on new WHO classification 2022: A retrospective cross-sectional study. *J. Bagh. Coll. Dent.* **2024**, *36*, 27–33. [CrossRef]
12. Shin, N.Y.; Yamazaki, H.; Beniash, E.; Yang, X.; Margolis, S.S.; Pugach, M.K.; Simmer, J.P.; Margolis, H.C. Amelogenin phosphorylation regulates tooth enamel formation by stabilizing a transient amorphous mineral precursor. *J. Biol. Chem.* **2020**, *295*, 1943–1959. [CrossRef]
13. Bansal, A.K.; Shetty, D.C.; Bindal, R.; Pathak, A. Amelogenin: A novel protein with diverse applications in genetic and molecular profiling. *J. Oral Maxillofac. Pathol.* **2012**, *16*, 395–399. [CrossRef]
14. Al-Qazzaz, H.H.; Abdullah, B.H.; Museedi, O.S. Correlation of amyloid and ameloblast-associated proteins to odontogenic cysts and tumors: A cross-sectional study. *Health Sci. Rep.* **2023**, *6*, e1061. [CrossRef]
15. Zakaraia, S.; Almohareb, M.; Zaid, K.; Doumani, M.; Seirawan, M.Y. Amelogenin is a Potential Biomarker for the Aggressiveness in Odontogenic Tumors. *Asian Pac. J. Cancer Prev. APJCP* **2018**, *19*, 1375–1379. [CrossRef]
16. Ikeda, Y.; Neshatian, M.; Holcroft, J.; Ganss, B. The enamel protein ODAM promotes mineralization in a collagen matrix. *Connect. Tissue Res.* **2018**, *59* (Suppl. S1), 62–66. [CrossRef]
17. Kestler, D.P.; Foster, J.S.; Macy, S.D.; Murphy, C.L.; Weiss, D.T.; Solomon, A. Expression of Odontogenic Ameloblast-Associated Protein (ODAM) in Dental and Other Epithelial Neoplasms. *Mol. Med.* **2008**, *14*, 318–326. [CrossRef]
18. Song, D.; Yang, S.; Tan, T.; Wang, R.; Ma, Z.; Wang, Y.; Wang, L. ODAM promotes junctional epithelium-related gene expression via activation of WNT1 signaling pathway in an ameloblast-like cell line, ALC. *J. Periodontal Res.* **2021**, *56*, 482–491. [CrossRef] [PubMed]
19. Heikinheimo, K.; Kurppa, K.J.; Laiho, A.; Peltonen, S.; Berdal, A.; Bouattour, A.; Ruhin, B.; Catón, J.; Thesleff, I.; Leivo, I.; et al. Early dental epithelial transcription factors distinguish ameloblastoma from keratocystic odontogenic tumor. *J. Dent. Res.* **2015**, *94*, 101–111. [CrossRef] [PubMed]
20. Hadi, M.T.; Yas, L.S. A comparative immunohistochemical expression of cytokeratin 19 in odontogenic keratocyst, dentigerous, and radicular cysts. *J. Emerg. Med. Trauma Acute Care* **2024**, *2024*, 3. [CrossRef]
21. Kumamoto, H.; Yoshida, M.; Ooya, K. Immunohistochemical detection of amelogenin and cytokeratin 19 in epithelial odontogenic tumors. *Oral Dis.* **2001**, *7*, 171–176. [CrossRef]
22. Martínez-Martínez, M.; Mosqueda-Taylor, A.; Carlos-Bregni, R.; Pires, F.R.; Delgado-Azanero, W.; Neves-Silva, R.; Aldape-Barrios, B.; Paes-de Almeida, O. Comparative histological and immunohistochemical study of ameloblastomas and ameloblastic carcinomas. *Med. Oral Patol. Oral Cir. Bucal.* **2017**, *22*, e324–e332. [CrossRef] [PubMed] [PubMed Central]
23. Delaney, M.A.; Singh, K.; Murphy, C.L.; Solomon, A.; Nel, S.; Boy, S.C. Immunohistochemical and biochemical evidence of amelo-blastic origin of amyloid-producing odontogenic tumors in cats. *Vet. Pathol.* **2013**, *50*, 238–242. [CrossRef]
24. Tsuji, K.; Wato, M.; Hayashi, T.; Yasuda, N.; Matsushita, T.; Ito, T.; Gamoh, S.; Yoshida, H.; Tanaka, A.; Morita, S. The expression of cytokeratin in keratocystic odontogenic tumor, orthokeratinized odontogenic cyst, dentigerous cyst, radicular cyst and dermoid cyst. *Med. Mol. Morphol.* **2014**, *47*, 156–161. [CrossRef]
25. Anigol, P.; Kamath, V.V.; Satelur, K.; Anand, N.; Yerlagudda, K. Amelogenin in odontogenic cysts and tumors: An immunohistochemical study. *Natl. J. Maxillofac. Surg.* **2014**, *5*, 172–179.
26. Akhila, C.N.V.; Sreenath, G.; Prakash, A.R.; Rajini Kanth, M.; Reddy, A.V.S.; Kumar, S.N. Expression of stem cell marker cytokeratin 19 in reduced enamel epithelium, dentigerous cyst and unicystic ameloblastoma—A comparative analysis. *J. Oral Maxillofac. Pathol.* **2021**, *25*, 136–140. [CrossRef]
27. Abdelaziz, L.A.; Ebian, H.F.; Harb, O.A.; Nosery, Y.; Taha, H.F.; Nawar, N. Clinical significance of cytokeratin 19 and OCT4 as survival markers in non-metastatic and metastatic breast cancer patients. *Contemp. Oncol.* **2022**, *26*, 78–87. [CrossRef]
28. Mehrpouya, M.; Pourhashem, Z.; Yardehnavi, N.; Oladnabi, M. Evaluation of cytokeratin 19 as a prognostic tumoral and metastatic marker with focus on improved detection methods. *J. Cell Physiol.* **2019**, *234*, 21425–21435. [CrossRef]
29. Menz, A.; Bauer, R.; Kluth, M.; von Bargen, C.M.; Gorbokon, N.; Viehweger, F.; Lennartz, M.; Völkl, C.; Fraune, C.; Uhlig, R.; et al. Diagnostic and prognostic impact of cytokeratin 19 expression analysis in human tumors: A tissue microarray study of 13,172 tumors. *Hum. Pathol.* **2021**, *115*, 19–36. [CrossRef]
30. Reya, T.; Clevers, H. Wnt signalling in stem cells and cancer. *Nature* **2005**, *434*, 843–850. [CrossRef]

Disclaimer/Publisher's Note: The statements, opinions and data contained in all publications are solely those of the individual author(s) and contributor(s) and not of MDPI and/or the editor(s). MDPI and/or the editor(s) disclaim responsibility for any injury to people or property resulting from any ideas, methods, instructions or products referred to in the content.

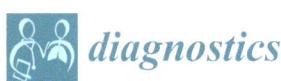

Article

Frequency and Demographic Analysis of Odontogenic Tumors in Three Tertiary Institutions: An 11-Year Retrospective Study

Asma Almazyad [1,2,3,*], Mohammed Alamro [1], Nasser Almadan [4,5], Marzouq Almutairi [1] and Turki S. AlQuwayz [4]

1. Maxillofacial Surgery and Diagnostic Sciences Department, College of Dentistry, King Saud bin Abdulaziz University for Health Sciences, Riyadh 11481, Saudi Arabia; alamro679@ksau-hs.edu.sa (M.A.); marzouqalmutairy@gmail.com (M.A.)
2. King Abdullah International Medical Research Center, Riyadh 11481, Saudi Arabia
3. Department of Pathology and Laboratory Medicine, King Abdulaziz Medical City, Ministry of National Guard Health Affair, Riyadh 11426, Saudi Arabia
4. Prince Sultan Military Medical Center, Riyadh 11159, Saudi Arabia; nmalmadan@gmail.com (N.A.); turkisaad1@hotmail.com (T.S.A.)
5. Dental Specialist Center, Hafar AlBaten 39953, Saudi Arabia
* Correspondence: mazyadas@ksau-hs.edu.sa; Tel.: +966-555210048

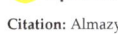

Citation: Almazyad, A.; Alamro, M.; Almadan, N.; Almutairi, M.; AlQuwayz, T.S. Frequency and Demographic Analysis of Odontogenic Tumors in Three Tertiary Institutions: An 11-Year Retrospective Study. *Diagnostics* **2024**, *14*, 910. https://doi.org/10.3390/diagnostics14090910

Academic Editor: Luis Eduardo Almeida

Received: 8 April 2024
Revised: 22 April 2024
Accepted: 23 April 2024
Published: 26 April 2024

Copyright: © 2024 by the authors. Licensee MDPI, Basel, Switzerland. This article is an open access article distributed under the terms and conditions of the Creative Commons Attribution (CC BY) license (https://creativecommons.org/licenses/by/4.0/).

Abstract: Odontogenic tumors (OTs) are distinct conditions that develop in the jawbones, exhibiting diverse histopathological features and variable clinical behaviors. Unfortunately, the literature on this subject in Saudi Arabia remains sparse, indicating a pressing need for more comprehensive data concerning the frequency, demographics, treatment modalities, and outcomes of OTs. Objectives: The study aims to evaluate the frequency, demographic features, treatment, and outcomes of OTs across three tertiary medical centers. Methods and Material: OT cases were identified in King Abdulaziz Medical City (KAMC), King Fahad Medical City (KFMC), and Prince Sultan Military Medical City (PSMMC) from January 2010 to December 2021. Results: Ninety-two OT cases were identified from the anatomical pathology laboratories of three tertiary hospitals. KFMC contributed the highest number of cases (43.5%), followed by KAMC (30.4%) and PSMMC (26.1%). The median age of OT patients was 29 years (range: 5–83), with males representing more than half of the patients (56.5%). The mandible was the most frequent site of OT occurrence (72.5%), with ameloblastoma being the predominant OT (63.0%), followed by odontoma (19.5%). Among the treatment modalities, bone resection was employed the most (51.0%), followed by enucleation (25.6%). Notably, 11.5% of OT cases with available follow-up data exhibited recurrence, with ameloblastoma accounting for eight recurrent cases. Conclusions: Although OTs are relatively common in the jaws, they are rare in anatomical pathology laboratories and the general population. This study contributes valuable insights into the epidemiology characteristics, treatment trends, and recurrence rates of OTs in Saudi Arabia.

Keywords: ameloblastoma; biopsy; odontoma; odontogenic tumors; odontogenic myxoma; tertiary hospitals

1. Introduction

Odontogenic tumors (OTs) constitute a significant category of lesions primarily occurring in the jawbone, with occasional occurrence in the gingiva. These tumors originate from abnormal odontogenesis processes or the proliferation of odontogenic epithelial and odontogenic ectomesenchyme remnants [1,2]. Histologically, OTs display features reminiscent of various odontogenic tissues and development stages. The World Health Organization (WHO) categorizes OTs based on tissue type, with the latest 2022 classification featuring six purely epithelial, four purely mesenchymal, and four mixed tumors. Many OTs have clinical or histological subtypes reviewed and summarized in Table 1 [2]. While the existing literature and systematic reviews offer insight into the frequency and demographics of OTs, with reported rates ranging from 1.8% to 9.6% across various geographic locations [3–7], a notable research gap exists regarding OTs in Saudi Arabia. Only three published papers [8–10], including a study from Riyadh, Saudi Arabia, by Alsheddi et al. [10], reviewed 188 cases in a single oral pathology laboratory over twenty-six years. Among the commonly reported OTs, ameloblastoma (AM) was the most prevalent, followed by odontoma (OD), while less common tumors included cementoblastoma (CB) and central odontogenic fibroma (OF) [11]. A primordial odontogenic tumor (POT), a rare OT, was not included in most OT series as it was only described in 2014 and subsequently incorporated by the WHO classification in 2017 [12].

Table 1. The 5th edition of the WHO classification of odontogenic tumors, 2022 [2].

	Abbreviation	Definition	Clinical Presentation	Radiographic Presentation
		Epithelial Odontogenic Tumors		
Ameloblastoma	AM			
Conventional ameloblastoma	cAM	A locally invasive and benign odontogenic tumor, most commonly in the posterior mandible.	Painless, slowly increasing swelling in the jaw, seen in the 4th to 5th decade, often asymptomatic with potential facial asymmetry and noticeable in cases in larger lesions.	Unilocular or multilocular radiolucency located in the posterior mandible. The multilocular type exhibits a soap bubble or honeycomb appearance, and root resorption of the adjacent teeth is frequent.
Unicystic ameloblastoma	UniAM	A distinct cystic variant constituting up to 25% of intraosseous AM.	Painless swelling is typically observed in the 2nd to 3rd decade, associated with the impacted 3rd molar in the posterior mandible.	Unilocular radiolucent area surrounding the crown of an impacted third molar.
Extraosseous/peripheral ameloblastoma	PeriAM	A rare variant comprising 1% of Ams; it arises either from the remnants of dental lamina within the oral mucosa or the basal cells of the surface epithelium.	Painless sessile nodule of the gingiva, occurring in the 5th to 6th decade and located in the premolar–molar region of the mandible.	N/A
Adenoid ameloblastoma	AdenoAM	Rare epithelial OT characterized by cribriform growth pattern, duct-like structures, and an occasional dentinoid, displaying aggressive behavior with a 70% recurrence rate.	Asymptomatic swelling with no site predilection; it may exhibit occasional pain and paresthesia.	The unilocular or multilocular with internal calcifications, cortical perforations, or root resorption.
Metastasizing ameloblastoma	MetAM	A histologically benign AM exhibiting metastasis to distant organs, commonly in the lungs.	Variable presentation and pulmonary metastasis may include a dry cough, hemoptysis, or dyspnea.	Similar to cAM in the jawbone
Adenomatoid odontogenic tumor	AOT	Uncommon, encapsulated OT with indolent behavior.	Known as two-thirds of a tumor because 2/3 occur in the 2nd decade, 2/3 occur in females, and 2/3 are associated with an impacted maxillary canine.	Unilocular radiolucency with variable radiopaque flecks (resembling snowflakes) is typically observed around the crown of an unerupted tooth, commonly the canine.

Table 1. Cont.

	Abbreviation	Definition	Clinical Presentation	Radiographic Presentation
Squamous odontogenic tumor	SOT	Uncommon benign OT with squamous differentiation.	Painless swelling in the 4th decade, occasionally seen lateral to the roots of the teeth. Multiple or peripheral SOT has been reported.	Triangular or semicircular corticated radiolucency along the teeth roots. Tooth displacement occasionally seen.
Calcifying epithelial odontogenic tumor (Pindborg tumor)	CEOT	Uncommon benign epithelial OT with amyloid deposition and calcifications.	An asymptomatic, slowly growing mass occurring in the 4th decade and commonly in the posterior mandible.	Unilocular or multilocular radiolucency with variable radiodensity. Half of the cases were associated with an impacted tooth.
		Epithelial and Mesenchymal Odontogenic Tumors		
Odontoma	OD	Hamartomatous growth exhibits different dental hard and soft tissues in various development stages.	Asymptomatic, slowly growing mass typically observed in the 2nd and 3rd decade, located in the anterior maxilla (compound) or posterior mandible (complex).	Compound: several tooth-like structures of varying sizes and shapes with a radiolucent rim. Complex: a calcified mass exhibiting radiodensity akin to the tooth structure, surrounded by a radiolucent rim.
Ameloblastic fibroma	AF	Benign-mixed OT without hard tissue deposition.	Asymptomatic, slowly growing lesion was seen in the second decade, most commonly in the mandible.	Unilocular or multilocular and corticated radiolucent lesion, 80% associated with an unerupted tooth.
Dentinogenic ghost cell tumor	DGCT	Rare benign OT displaying locally aggressive behavior, characterized by the abundance of ghost cells and dentinoid deposition.	Asymptomatic, slowly increasing swelling identified in the 3rd to 5th decade, typically localized in the posterior region of either jaw.	Well-defined, unilocular or multilocular-mixed radiolucent lesion. Tooth displacement or resorption is occasionally seen.
Primordial odontogenic tumor	POT	Recently described mixed POT exhibiting primitive dental tissue with occasional hard tissue deposition.	Slowly growing lesion in the first two decades and always associated with an unerupted tooth, commonly the third molar.	Well-demarcated, unilocular, bilocular, or multilocular radiolucency associated with an unerupted tooth.
		Mesenchymal Odontogenic Tumors		
Odontogenic fibroma	OF	Rare OT consists mainly of mature fibrous tissue and inactive odontogenic epithelium with a peripheral variant (the most common peripheral odontogenic tumor).	Asymptomatic, slowly growing lesion seen in the fourth decade occurring commonly in the anterior maxilla and posterior mandible. Anterior maxillary lesions may cause soft tissue depression or dimpling.	Central OF: Unilocular or multilocular well-defined radiolucency is often seen intimately around the roots of teeth.
Cementoblastoma	CB	Benign neoplasm of cementoblasts, representing less than 3% of all OTs.	Slowly increasing painful swelling associated with teeth roots, most commonly the mandibular first molar.	The tumor appears as a radiopaque mass fused to one or more tooth roots and is surrounded by a thin radiolucent rim and resorption of the associated root is common.

Table 1. Cont.

	Abbreviation	Definition	Clinical Presentation	Radiographic Presentation
Cemento-ossifying fibroma	COF	OT is derived from mesenchymal stem cells with differentiation towards periodontal structures, such as bone and cementum-like material.	Asymptomatic bony expansion in the posterior mandible mostly in the 3rd and 4th decades.	Well-demarcated radiolucency with a sclerotic rim in the tooth-bearing area of the jaws, accompanied by variable radiopacities. Bowing of the inferior border of the mandible may be evident.
Odontogenic myxoma	OM	The most common mesenchymal OT is composed of mainly myxoid stroma and occasional inactive odontogenic epithelium.	Painless swelling of the posterior mandible seen in the 2nd and 3rd decades.	Unilocular multilocular "honeycomb" or "tennis racket" radiolucency with diffuse borders and teeth displacement or resorption.

N/A: not applicable.

The existing literature primarily focuses on demographics, clinical characteristics, and histological examination, lacking substantial information on clinical behavior and treatment options. In response to this gap, our study aims to report OT frequency, demographic data, treatment modalities, and follow-up information, drawing from three tertiary hospitals in Riyadh, Saudi Arabia.

2. Methods and Materials

This retrospective study aimed to analyze the frequency, demographic data, and biological features of patients diagnosed with OTs at three tertiary medical hospitals in Riyadh, Saudi Arabia, King Abdulaziz Medical City (KAMC), King Fahad Medical City (KFMC), and Prince Sultan Military Medical City (PSMMC) from January 2010 to December 2021. The study adhered to the principles of the Declaration of Helsinki. The authors obtained institutional review board approval from the King Abdullah International Medical Research Center (IRB# NRC21R/222/06) and King Fahad Medical City (IRB# 00010471).

All relevant data, including patient age, sex, tumor site, treatment modalities, and follow-up information, were extrapolated from medical records. Hematoxylin and eosin-stained slides from all cases were retrieved and cross-examined by a certified oral pathologist (AA) to confirm the histopathologic diagnosis based on the 2022 WHO classification of odontogenic and maxillofacial bone tumors. In cases of uncertainty, another oral pathologist (NM) conducted a secondary review to reach a consensus. Figures 1 and 2 show representative histopathological photomicrographs of each observed OT in this series.

The inclusion criteria are as follows:
1. Tumors with histopathological features compatible with an OT diagnosis.
2. Patients with available demographic and clinical information, pathological reports, and histological slides.

The exclusion criteria are as follows:
1. Patients with incomplete demographic and clinical data.
2. Patients with missing histological slides.

Descriptive analysis of patient age, sex, site, OT type, treatment, and follow-up information was performed using STATA 14.2 software (StataCorp.), College Station, TX, USA. The correlation between age, gender, location, and OT type among different tertiary hospitals was assessed using the chi-square test for categorical data and the Kruskal–Wallis test for continuous data since the data failed the normal distribution test. A p-value less than 0.05 was considered statistically significant. Graphs were generated using STATA 14.2 software (StataCorp.), College Station, TX, USA.

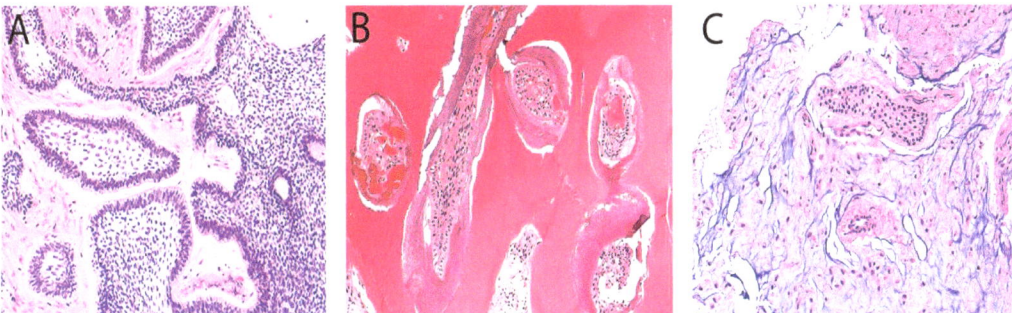

Figure 1. Representative histological images of the most common OTs: AM (**A**), OD (**B**), and OM (**C**). (**A**) AM displays multiple follicular islands with central stellate reticulum cells and peripheral basophilic columnar cells with reverse polarity. (**B**) OD exhibits multiple hard dental structures, such as the dentinal tubules and enamel matrix, with a fish-scale appearance. (**C**) OM shows multiple odontogenic rests with peripheral hyalinization and a paracellular myoxid background.

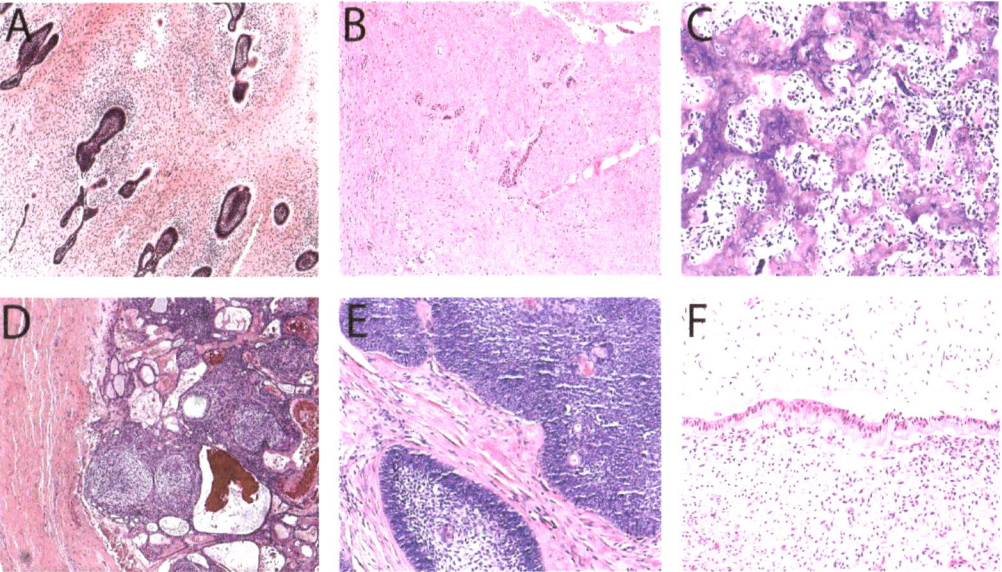

Figure 2. Representative histological images of other OTs seen in the current series: AF (**A**), OF (**B**), CB (**C**), AOT (**D**), AM carcinoma (**E**), and POT (**F**). (**A**) AF shows multiple ameloblastic islands within primitive ectomesenchymal stroma. (**B**) OF exhibits diffuse fibrotic stroma with scattered odontogenic epithelial rests. (**C**) CB shows hard tissue deposits similar to the cementum lined by multiple layers of cementoblasts and multinucleated giant cells. (**D**) AOT exhibits a fibrous capsule with nodular growth of epithelial and spindle cells with a whirling pattern and duct formation. (**E**) AM carcinoma displays ameloblastic islands with high cellularity, hyperchromasia, and keratin pearls. (**F**) POT consists of primitive ectomesenchymal tissue lined by a single layer of columnar epithelium with reverse nuclear polarity.

3. Results

In 11 years, ninety-two cases of OTs were identified in the archives of three different tertiary hospitals in Riyadh, Saudi Arabia. The retrospective analysis revealed that forty

(43.5%) and twenty-eight (30.4%) tumors originated from KFMC and KAMC, respectively. Additionally, twenty-four tumors were retrieved from PSMMC (Figure 3A). The distribution of cases per year in each hospital is illustrated in Figure 3B, highlighting peak occurrence in 2014, 2016, and 2021. Overall, OTs affected 52 (56.5%) males and 40 (43.5%) females, resulting in a male-to-female ratio of 1.3:1. Notably, KAMC exhibited a higher ratio of 1.54:1. At the same time, PSMMC showed an equal distribution between genders (Figure 3C and Table 2). The median age of the patients was 29 years, with most OT cases diagnosed in the second-to-fourth decades, constituting 63.0% (Figure 3D). No significant age differences were observed among the three hospitals, with a p-value of 0.40 (Table 2 and Figure 4A). Mandible involvement was predominant, accounting for almost two-thirds (72.5%) of the OT cases, with consistent site distribution across all hospitals (Figures 3E and 4B and Table 2).

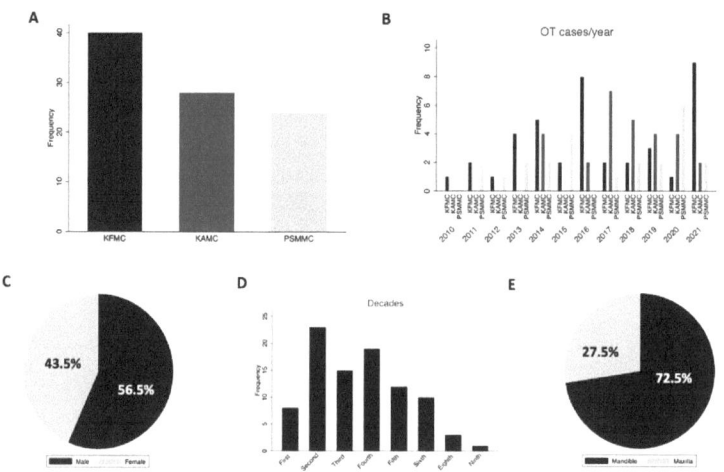

Figure 3. (**A**) OT distribution in each center. (**B**) OTs are distributed in each center per year. KFMC had the highest frequency in 2016 and 2021. (**C**) Gender distribution of OTs. (**D**) Age distribution of OTs. (**E**) Location distribution of OTs.

Table 2. Summary of demographics in the three tertiary centers.

	All Three Centers	KFMC	KAMC	PSMMC	p-Value
Cases	92	40 (43.5%)	28 (30.4%)	24 (26.1%)	
Age median (range)	29 (5–83)	33 (6–76)	22 (5–83)	26 (7–56)	0.4020
Gender					
Male	52	23	17	12	
Female	40	17	11	12	
Male/female ratio	1.27:1	1.16:1	1.54:1	1:1	0.6031
Mandible/maxilla ratio	2.64:1	2.25:1	2.8:1	3:1	0.884

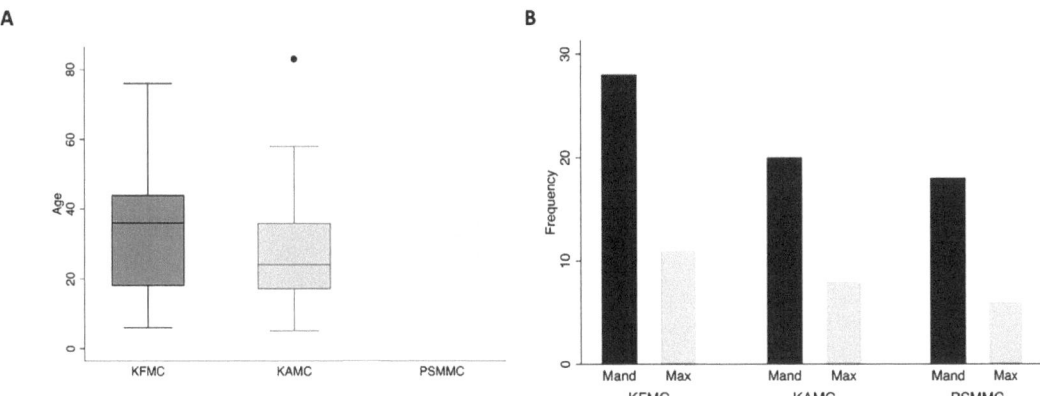

Figure 4. (**A**) The mean age of OTs is similar in all hospitals, with a *p*-value of 0.40. (**B**) Site distribution of OTs in each hospital, with a *p*-value of 0.89.

AM represented most cases across all centers, accounting for 63.0% (58 cases), making it the most prevalent OT. OD was the second most common OT, constituting 19.5% of the cases (Figure 5). Other OTs included four cases of OM (4.3%) and three cases of AF (3.3%). Only two COF, two AOT, and two CB cases were identified in the cohort. Additionally, there was one POT case from KFMC. PSMMC reported the sole case of malignant OT within the cohort. The distribution of OTs differed significantly among the hospitals, with a *p*-value of 0.01. At KFMC and PSMMC, AM predominated, while KAMC exhibited a more balanced distribution between AM and OD. KFMC also had the most OM and OF cases (Table 3).

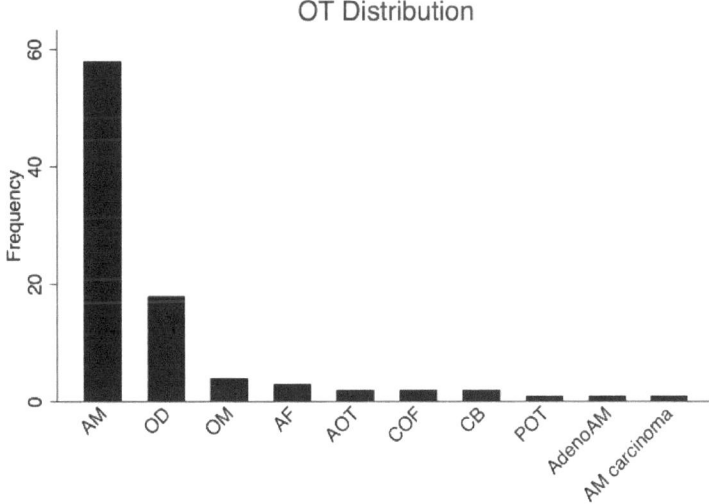

Figure 5. OT frequency in the three tertiary hospitals.

Table 3. Distribution of OT among three different tertiary hospitals.

	All Three Centers	KFMC	KAMC	PSMMC
Epithelial Odontogenic Tumors				
Ameloblastoma	58 (63.0%)	27 (46.6%)	12 (20.7%)	19 (32.7%)
Adenoid ameloblastoma	1 (1.1%)	1 (100%)	0	0
Adenomatoid odontogenic tumor	2 (2.2%)	1 (50%)	0	1 (50%)
Ameloblastic carcinoma	1 (1.1%)	0	0	1 (100%)
Mixed Epithelial–Mesenchymal Odontogenic Tumors				
Odontoma	18 (19.5%)	3 (16.7%)	12 (66.6%)	3 (16.7%)
Ameloblastic fibroma	3 (3.3%)	3 (100%)	0	0
Primordial odontogenic tumor	1 (1.1%)	1 (100%)	0	0
Mesenchymal Odontogenic Tumors				
Odontogenic myxoma	4 (4.3%)	3 (75.0%)	0	1 (25.0%)
Central odontogenic fibroma	2 (2.2%)	1 (50%)	1 (50%)	0
Cementoblastoma	2 (2.2%)	0	2 (100%)	0
Total	92 (100%)	40 (43.5%)	28 (30.4%)	24 (26.1%)

Table 4 provides an overview of the clinicopathological characteristics of OTs. Among 82 patients with available treatment information, resection was the most common treatment modality (51.0%), followed by enucleation (25.6%), as outlined in Table 5. Additionally, follow-up data for 73 cases revealed recurrence in 11 (15.1%) cases (Table 6).

Table 4. Summary of the clinicopathological features of odontogenic tumors.

	Number of Case	Age Median (Range)	Gender		Location *	
			M	F	Mandible	Maxilla
Epithelial Odontogenic Tumors						
Ameloblastoma	58 (63.0%)	36 (6–83)	34 (58.6%)	24 (41.4%)	47 (81.0%)	11 (19.0%)
Conventional ameloblastoma	54 (93.1%)	38 (6–83)	33 (61.1%)	21 (38.9%)	44 (81.5%)	10 (18.5%)
Unicystic ameloblastoma	4 (6.9%)	20 (16–51)	1 (25.0%)	3 (75.0%)	3 (75.0%)	1 (25.0%)
Adenoid ameloblastoma	1 (1.1%)	14 (N/A)	0	1 (100%)	0	1 (100%)
Adenomatoid odontogenic tumor	2 (2.2%)	17 (15–19)	1 (50.0%)	1 (50.0%)	1 (50.0%)	1 (50.0%)
Ameloblastic carcinoma	1 (1.1%)	31 (N/A)	1 (100%)	0	1 (100%)	0
Mixed Epithelial–Mesenchymal Odontogenic Tumors						
Odontoma	18 (19.5%)	20 (5–50)	10 (55.6%)	8 (44.4%)	8 (47.1%)	9 (52.9%)
Complex	10 (55.6%)	17 (5–50)	5 (50.0%)	5 (50.0%)	8 (80.0%)	2 (20.0%)
Compound	8 (44.4%)	17 (9–37)	5 (62.5%)	3 (37.5%)	0	7 (100%)
Ameloblastic fibroma	3 (3.3%)	13 (6–26)	1 (25.0%)	2 (27.5%)	2 (75.0%)	1 (25.0%)
Primordial odontogenic tumor	1 (1.1%)	16 (N/A)	1 (100%)	0	1 (100%)	0
Mesenchymal Odontogenic Tumors						
Odontogenic myxoma	4 (4.3%)	31 (27–36)	3 (75.0%)	1 (25.0%)	2 (50.0%)	2 (50.0%)
Central odontogenic fibroma	2 (2.2%)	30 (15–45)	1 (50.0%)	1 (50.0%)	2 (100%)	0
Cementoblastoma	2 (2.2%)	32 (17–48)	0	2 (100%)	2 (100%)	0
Total	92 (100%)		52 (56.5%)	40 (43.5%)	66 (72.5%)	25 (27.5%)

* The location of one case of odontoma was not reported.

Table 5. Summary of the treatment modalities of each odontogenic tumor.

	Number of Cases	Treatment		
		Enucleation	Excision	Resection
Epithelial Odontogenic Tumors				
Ameloblastoma	52 (63.4%)	6 (11.5%)	12 (23.1%)	34 (65.4%)
Conventional ameloblastoma	48 (92.3%)	4 (8.3%)	12 (25.0%)	32 (66.7%)
Unicystic ameloblastoma	4 (7.7%)	2 (50.0%)	0	2 (50%)
Adenoid ameloblastoma	1 (1.2%)	0	0	1 (100%)
Adenomatoid odontogenic tumor	1 (1.2%)	1 (100%)	0	0
Ameloblastic carcinoma	1 (1.2%)	0	0	1 (100%)
Mixed Epithelial–Mesenchymal Odontogenic Tumors				
Odontoma	17 (20.8%)	12 (70.6%)	4 (23.5%)	1 (5.9%)
Ameloblastic fibroma	2 (2.4%)	1 (50.0%)	0	1 (50.0%)
Primordial odontogenic tumor	1 (1.2%)	0	0	1 (100%)
Mesenchymal Odontogenic Tumors				
Odontogenic myxoma	4 (5.0%)	0	1 (25.0%)	3 (75.0%)
Central odontogenic fibroma	1 (1.2%)	1 (100%)	0	0
Cementoblastoma	2 (2.4%)	2 (100%)	0	0
Total	82 (100%)	23 (25.6%)	17 (21.0%)	42 (51.0%)

Table 6. Summary of the follow-up information for odontogenic tumors that showed recurrence.

	Number of Cases	Recurrence	No Recurrence	Follow-Up Period
Ameloblastoma	50	8 (16.0%)	42 (84.0%)	1 year–6 years
Odontoma	17	1 (5.9%)	16 (94.1%)	1 year–3 years
Odontogenic myxoma	4	1 (25.0%)	3 (75.0%)	7 months–4 years
Ameloblastic fibroma	2	1 (50.0%) *	1 (50.0%)	1 year
Total	73	11 (15.1%)	62 (84.9%)	N/A

* Recurrence after one year of ameloblastic fibrosarcoma and succumbing to the disease due to liver and lung metastasis after six years.

Fifty-eight cases (63.0%) of AMs were identified, with a median age of 36, of which 34 (58.6%) were males. The mandible was the most common location (81.0%). Primary treatment modalities for AM included resection (66.7%) and excision (25.0%) (Table 5). Follow-up data for fifty cases revealed that only eight patients showed recurrence (Figure 6). Recurrence rates did not show any notable variation across the various treatment choices. Most AMs were of the conventional clinical subtype, with only four unicystic cases. No peripheral AM cases were reported. The main clinicopathological difference between conventional and unicystic AM was the median age and gender distribution, with unicystic AM tending to occur in females in their second decade.

There were 18 (19.5%) cases of OD with a median age of 20, of which 10 (55.6%) were males. Similar to AM, ODs showed almost equal site predilection with a ratio of 0.88:1 for the mandible-to-maxilla (Table 4). For OD, the primary treatment modality was enucleation (70.6%), with only one case treated with resection (Table 5). Seventeen patients with OD were followed up after treatment, and only one patient showed recurrence (Table 6).

OM ranked as the third most common OT, with only four cases (4.4%) reported in the cohort. The median age of patients was 31, and 3 (75%) were male. There was an equal preference for location between the mandible and maxilla (Table 4). Additionally, two-thirds of the cases were treated with resection. All cases were followed-up, and the case treated with excision showed recurrence (Tables 5 and 6). The limited number of other OTs precluded extracting meaningful insight regarding clinicopathological information and treatment options.

Interestingly, the series had one case of AdenoAM in a 14-year-old female with a history of familial adenomatoid polyposis who died after six years due to encephalopathy. It is worth noting that there was only one case of malignant OT, histologically diagnosed as ameloblastic carcinoma in a 31-year-old male in the mandible, and it was resected. However, this patient was lost to follow-up.

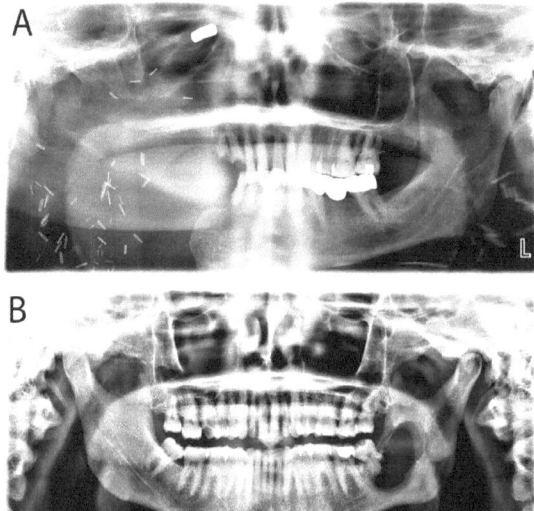

Figure 6. Examples of radiographic presentations of recurrent ameloblastoma. (**A**) Recurrent ameloblastoma on the right posterior mandible post-resection. (**B**) Recurrent ameloblastoma on the right posterior mandible post-excision.

4. Discussion

The present study marks a significant advancement in understanding OTs within Riyadh, Saudi Arabia. This retrospective multicenter series draws data from three leading tertiary hospitals in Riyadh, Saudi Arabia. It is the second-largest series of OT cases documented within the Kingdom and the wider Gulf region. Traditionally, studies on the frequency and prevalence of OTs have been confined to single institutions, potentially skewing the perception of their actual occurrence within a given geographic area. In addition, our prior examination of odontogenic cysts from these same hospitals yielded 372 cases, shedding light on their prevalence in this region [13]. Our findings reveal a notable contrast as follows: odontogenic cysts (OCs) are observed to be four times more frequent than OTs in Riyadh, Saudi Arabia, which is a significantly higher ratio than previously reported figures (OCs were reported to be 2.2 times more common than OTs) [11]. One possible explanation for this notable difference is that the previously reported ratio included the odontogenic keratocyst as an OT, which has since been reclassified as a cyst. This highlights the importance of comprehensive, multicenter studies in accurately capturing the epidemiological landscape of OTs within specific regions. Moreover, while the majority of studies on the frequency of OTs have concentrated on demographic and clinicopathological data, our current investigation aims to delve deeper. Specifically, we illuminate the landscape of treatment options and provide insights into the follow-up information regarding OTs.

Three primary studies investigated the frequency of OTs in the Gulf region, covering Kuwait, Saudi Arabia, and the United Arab Emirates (Table 7) [8–10]. However, comparing our series to these studies presents challenges due to variations in time periods and sample sizes. Another complicating factor is the evolution of OT classification over time and the identification of new entities, such as POT [2]. Only Alsheddi M et al. provided the mean age of their cohort (29 years old), which closely aligns with the mean age of our cohort

(30 years old) [10]. However, the mean age was not mentioned in the other two studies, making it difficult to extract this information from their data [8,9].

Table 7. Comparison of OT distribution in the current study and other Saudi and Gulf countries.

	Current Study (Three Centers), Riyadh, SA	Ali MA et al., Kuwait University, Jabriya, Kuwait [8]	Alsheddi M et al., King Saud University, Riyadh, KSA [10]	Al-Rawi N et al., Tawam Hospital, Abu Dhabi, UAE [9]
Sample size	92	27	108 *	22
Period	11 years	6 years	26 years	20 years
Mean age	30	N/R	29	N/R
Male/female ratio	1.3:1	1.25:1	1.4:1	1:1
Mandible/maxilla ratio	2.64:1	3.5:1	2.1:1	1.62:1
Epithelial Odontogenic Tumors				
Ameloblastoma	58 (63.0%)	17 (63.0%)	47 (43.5%)	4 (18.1%)
Adenoid ameloblastoma	1 (1.1%)	N/R	N/R	N/R
Adenomatoid odontogenic tumor	2 (2.2%)	N/R	8 (7.4%)	N/R
Calcifying epithelial odontogenic tumor	N/R	1 (3.7%)	2 (1.8%)	N/R
Ameloblastic carcinoma	1 (1.1%)	N/R	1 (0.9%)	0 (0%)
Clear cell odontogenic carcinoma	N/R	N/R	1 (0.9%)	N/R
Mixed Epithelial–Mesenchymal Odontogenic Tumors				
Odontoma	18 (19.5%)	9 (33.3%)	28 (26.0%)	17 (77.8%)
Ameloblastic fibroma	3 (3.3%)	N/R	4 (3.7%)	N/R
Primordial odontogenic tumor	1 (1.1%)	N/R	N/R	N/R
Dentinogenic ghost cell tumor	N/R	N/R	N/R	N/R
Mesenchymal Odontogenic Tumors				
Odontogenic myxoma	4 (4.3%)	N/R	12 (11.1%)	N/R
Central odontogenic fibroma	2 (2.2%)	N/R	1 (0.9%)	N/R
Cementoblastoma	2 (2.2%)	N/R	4 (3.7%)	N/R
Total	92 (100%)	27 (100%)	108 (100%)	22 (100%)

* The total number of cases reported in this series was 188, but we excluded keratocystic odontogenic tumors and calcifying cystic odontogenic tumors since they are reclassified as cysts. N/R; not reported.

Nonetheless, OTs were consistently prevalent among males and in the mandibular site across all studies. Additionally, AM was the most common OT in Kuwait, and a previous study in Riyadh mirrored our findings [8,10]. Conversely, OD was found to be the most common OT in the United Arab Emirates [9]. It is worth mentioning that the paper by Al-Rawi N et al. [9] from the United Arab Emirates reported only AM and OD as OTs occurring in the maxillofacial regions in their series, raising the possibility that they did not capture all OTs present in their archive. None of the papers reported POT, which is a rare entity only described in 2014. Similar to our study, malignant OTs were rare, with only Alsheddi M et al. [10] reporting two cases (ameloblastic carcinoma and clear cell odontogenic carcinoma). The other two studies did not report any malignancies of odontogenic origin [8,9].

The mean age of patients diagnosed with OTs in the present study was 30, aligning with the mean age of the OT series reported from Tokyo, Japan; Nagpur, India; Cairo, Egypt; and a multicenter study in Nigeria [3,14–16]. However, certain studies have reported notably higher mean ages, such as Mascitti M et al. [17] from the Marche region, Italy, and Chrysomali E et al. [18] from Athens, Greece. OTs in the Riyadh population were more common in males, like most papers on the frequency of OT [3,14,16–19]. However, two different papers from Brazil reported a slight female predominance [20,21]. Conversely, a balanced male-to-female ratio was reported in some regions, such as Cairo, Egypt [15]. Mandible predilection was consistent with all published data [3,14–22].

In our series, AM accounted for more than half of the cases (63.0%); this observation was similar in Italy, Brazil, and India [14,17,21]. However, AM is still the most common OT in other regions with variable frequency (13.5% to 80.1%) [11]. Other studies found OD to be the most common OT [3,22,23] and the second most common OT in our series. OM was consistently the third most common OT in most OT series [11]. It is expected to find no POT records in the OT series published before the description of POT in 2014. Interestingly, POT has still not been reported in recent papers, emphasizing the rarity and lack of awareness of such an entity [3,23,24]. We speculate that a few POTs in some of the series are reported under OM [25,26]. Additionally, odontogenic malignancy appears rare across regions worldwide, ranging from 0.2% to 4.0% [3,14–18,20–22]. Our data are consistent with the reported percentage, with only 1.1% of the current series being malignant OT. However, Kebede et al. [27] reported a higher rate of 19.6%. The variation in frequency may be attributed to the lack of well-established diagnostic criteria for odontogenic malignancy. Hence, there is a need for stringent diagnostic protocols to reduce the frequency range and ensure accurate diagnosis (Table 8).

Table 8. Comparison of OT distribution in the current study and selected international studies.

	Current Study (Three Centers), Riyadh, SA	Kokubun K et al. Tokyo, Japan [3]	de Medeiros WK et al. Natal, Northeastern Brazil [20]	Mascitti M et al. Ancona, Italy [17]
Sample size	92	1089	247	100
Period	11 years	45 years	22 years	25 years
Mean age	30	29	28	49.7
Male/female ratio	1.3:1	1.2:1	1:1.2	1.78:1
Mandible/maxilla ratio	2.64:1	2.1:1	2:1	2.1:1
Epithelial Odontogenic Tumors				
Ameloblastoma	58 (63.0%)	456 (41.9%)	112 (45.4%)	56 (56%)
Adenoid ameloblastoma	1 (1.1%)	N/R	N/R	N/R
Adenomatoid odontogenic tumor	2 (2.2%)	17 (1.6%)	10 (4.0%)	2 (2.0%)
Squamous odontogenic tumor	N/R	2 (0.2%)	N/R	1 (1.0%)
Calcifying epithelial odontogenic tumor	N/R	8 (1.6%)	5 (2.0%)	4 (4.0%)
Ameloblastic carcinoma	1 (1.1%)	1 (0.1)	1 (0.4%)	2 (2.0%)
Primary intra-osseous carcinoma	N/R	8 (0.7%)	N/R	N/R
Clear cell odontogenic carcinoma	N/R	N/R	1 (0.4%)	1 (1.0%)
Mixed Epithelial–Mesenchymal Odontogenic Tumors				
Odontoma	18 (19.5%)	463 (42.5%)	89 (36.1%)	17 (17.0%)
Ameloblastic fibroma	3 (3.3%)	17 (1.6%)	4 (1.6%)	3 (3.0%)
Primordial odontogenic tumor	1 (1.1%)	N/R	N/R	N/R
Dentinogenic ghost cell tumor	N/R	7 (0.6%)	1 (0.4%)	2 (2.0%)
Mesenchymal Odontogenic Tumors				
Odontogenic myxoma	4 (4.3%)	41 (3.8%)	17 (6.9%)	4 (4.0%)
Central odontogenic fibroma	2 (2.2%)	22 (2.0%)	3 (1.2%)	1 (1.0%)
Cementoblastoma	2 (2.2%)	8 (0.7%)	4 (1.6%)	2 (2.0%)
Cemento-ossifying fibroma	N/R	38 (3.5%)	N/R	4 (4.0%)
Odontogenic sarcoma	N/R	1 (0.1%)	N/R	1 (1.0%)
Total	92 (100%)	1089 (100%)	247 (100%)	100 (100%)

N/R; not reported.

AM is a benign odontogenic tumor with aggressive behavior and a high recurrence rate if treated conservatively [28]. In our study, bone resection was the most used treatment option for AM, accounting for 66.7% of cases. Other treatment modalities included enucleation and excision. The recurrence rate of AM in this study was approximately 16.0%, with no significant difference among treatment modalities used. This recurrence rate is consistent with the rates reported in pooled data from 20 studies, which found a recurrence rate of 20%. However, radical treatment showed a significantly lower recurrence of 8.0%, compared to conservative treatment options such as enucleation or curettage, which had a recurrence rate of 41% [29]. In our case series, we observed recurrences in one case of OM and one OD. OM has a recurrence rate of 13.0% regardless of treatment, while it increases to 19.0% if treated conservatively [30]. The OM case in our series was treated conservatively with excision, which confirms the need for a more radical treatment of OM. On the other hand, OD recurrence is rare and poorly documented in the literature. It is likely due to incomplete removal or the presence of another OT in the affected area.

Our retrospective study is subject to inherent limitations arising from its dependence on existing medical records. We faced challenges concerning incomplete data, leading to data attrition and compromises in data validity. While retrospective studies provide valuable insights into past events, treatment practices, and outcomes, their findings may lack generalizability and applicability to broader populations. Therefore, the data presented require careful interpretation when drawing conclusions.

5. Conclusions

Our research offers valuable information on the epidemiology, demographic features, treatment trends, and recurrence rates of OTs in Riyadh, Saudi Arabia, supported by data collected from three prominent tertiary hospitals. Our findings underscore the predominance of AM as the most common OT and highlight the frequent occurrence of OTs in the mandible. Moreover, our observations regarding treatment modalities, with bone resection being the most prevalent approach, contribute to understanding current clinical practices. The documented recurrence rate, particularly among ameloblastoma cases, emphasizes the importance of long-term follow-up and underscores the need for further research to optimize management strategies and improve patient outcomes. Importantly, to the best of our knowledge, this study represents the only comprehensive investigation on OTs in Saudi Arabia, highlighting the necessity for similar studies across different regions to gain a more thorough understanding of these conditions nationwide.

Author Contributions: Conceptualization, A.A., M.A. (Mohammed Alamro) and M.A. (Marzouq Almutairi); Methodology, A.A., M.A. (Mohammed Alamro) and M.A. (Marzouq Almutairi); Formal Analysis, A.A. and N.A.; Investigation, M.A. (Mohammed Alamro), M.A. (Marzouq Almutairi), N.A. and T.S.A.; Resources, M.A. (Mohammed Alamro), N.A. and T.S.A.; Data Curation, M.A. (Mohammed Alamro) and M.A. (Marzouq Almutairi), T.S.A. and N.A.; Writing—Original Draft Preparation, A.A. and M.A. (Mohammed Alamro), Writing—Review and Editing, A.A., M.A. (Mohammed Alamro) and N.A.; Visualization, A.A. and N.A.; Supervision, A.A. All authors have read and agreed to the published version of the manuscript.

Funding: This research received no external funding.

Institutional Review Board Statement: The study was conducted according to the guidelines of the Declaration of Helsinki and approved by the Institutional Review Board from King Abdullah International Medical Research Center (IRB# NRC21R/222/06) on 20 June 2021, and King Fahad Medical City (IRB# 00010471) on 19 October 2022.

Informed Consent Statement: Not applicable.

Data Availability Statement: The data presented in this study are available on request from the corresponding author. The data are not publicly available due to the hospital policies.

Conflicts of Interest: The authors declare no conflicts of interest.

References

1. Vered, M.; Wright, J.M. Update from the 5th Edition of the World Health Organization Classification of Head and Neck Tumors: Odontogenic and Maxillofacial Bone Tumours. *Head Neck Pathol.* **2022**, *16*, 63–75. [CrossRef] [PubMed]
2. Bishop, J.A.C.; John, K.C.; Gale, N.; Helliwell, T.; Hyrcza, M.D.; Lewis, J.S., Jr.; Loney, E.L.; Mehortra, R.; Nete, O.; Muller, S.; et al. *WHO Classification of Tumors of Head and Neck Tumours*, 5th ed.; WHO Classification of Tumours Series; WHO: Lyon, France, 2022; Volume 9.
3. Kokubun, K.; Yamamoto, K.; Nakajima, K.; Akashi, Y.; Chujo, T.; Takano, M.; Katakura, A.; Matsuzaka, K. Frequency of Odontogenic Tumors: A Single Center Study of 1089 Cases in Japan and Literature Review. *Head Neck Pathol.* **2022**, *16*, 494–502. [CrossRef] [PubMed]
4. Siriwardena, B.; Tennakoon, T.; Tilakaratne, W. Relative frequency of odontogenic tumors in Sri Lanka: Analysis of 1677 cases. *Pathol.-Res. Pract.* **2012**, *208*, 225–230. [CrossRef] [PubMed]
5. Mamabolo, M.; Noffke, C.; Raubenheimer, E. Odontogenic tumours manifesting in the first two decades of life in a rural African population sample: A 26 year retrospective analysis. *Dentomaxillofac. Radiol.* **2011**, *40*, 331–337. [CrossRef] [PubMed]
6. Luo, H.Y.; Li, T.J. Odontogenic tumors: A study of 1309 cases in a Chinese population. *Oral Oncol.* **2009**, *45*, 706–711. [CrossRef] [PubMed]
7. Jing, W.; Xuan, M.; Lin, Y.; Wu, L.; Liu, L.; Zheng, X.; Tang, W.; Qiao, J.; Tian, W. Odontogenic tumours: A retrospective study of 1642 cases in a Chinese population. *Int. J. Oral Maxillofac. Surg.* **2007**, *36*, 20–25. [CrossRef] [PubMed]
8. Ali, M.A. Biopsied jaw lesions in Kuwait: A six-year retrospective analysis. *Med. Princ. Pract.* **2011**, *20*, 550–555. [CrossRef]
9. Al-Rawi, N.H.; Awad, M.; Al-Zuebi, I.E.; Hariri, R.A.; Salah, E.W. Prevalence of odontogenic cysts and tumors among UAE population. *J. Orofac. Sci.* **2013**, *5*, 95–100. [CrossRef]
10. AlSheddi, M.A.; AlSenani, M.A.; AlDosarib, A.W. Odontogenic tumors: Analysis of 188 cases from Saudi Arabia. *Ann. Saudi Med.* **2015**, *35*, 146–150. [CrossRef] [PubMed]
11. Johnson, N.R.; Gannon, O.M.; Savage, N.W.; Batstone, M.D. Frequency of odontogenic cysts and tumors: A systematic review. *J. Investig. Clin. Dent.* **2014**, *5*, 9–14. [CrossRef] [PubMed]
12. Mosqueda-Taylor, A.; Pires, F.R.; Aguirre-Urízar, J.M.; Carlos-Bregni, R.; de la Piedra-Garza, J.M.; Martínez-Conde, R.; Martínez-Mata, G.; Carreño-Álvarez, S.J.; da Silveira, H.M.; Dias, B.S.d.B.; et al. Primordial odontogenic tumour: Clinicopathological analysis of six cases of a previously undescribed entity. *Histopathology* **2014**, *65*, 606–612. [CrossRef] [PubMed]
13. Almazyad, A.; Almutairi, M.; Almadan, N.; Alamro, M.; Maki, F.; AlQuwayz, T.S.; Alrumeh, A.S. Frequency and Demographic Profile of Odontogenic Cysts in Riyadh, Saudi Arabia: Retrospective Multicenter Study. *Diagnostics* **2023**, *13*, 355. [CrossRef] [PubMed]
14. Kaur, H.; Gosavi, S.; Hazarey, V.K.; Gupta, V.; Bhadauria, U.S.; Kherde, P. Impact of changing classification systems on prevalence and frequency distribution of odontogenic tumors in tertiary care center of Nagpur. *Braz. J. Otorhinolaryngol.* **2022**, *88* (Suppl. S1), S3–S13. [CrossRef] [PubMed]
15. Al-Aroomy, L.; Wali, M.; Alwadeai, M.; Desouky, E.; Amer, H. Odontogenic tumors: A Retrospective Study in Egyptian population using WHO 2017 classification. *Med. Oral Patol. Oral Cir. Bucal* **2022**, *27*, e198–e204. [CrossRef]
16. Aregbesola, B.; Soyele, O.; Effiom, O.; Gbotolorun, O.; Taiwo, A.; Amole, I. Odontogenic tumours in Nigeria: A multicentre study of 582 cases and review of the literature. *Med. Oral Patol. Oral Cir. Bucal* **2018**, *23*, e761–e766. [CrossRef] [PubMed]
17. Mascitti, M.; Togni, L.; Troiano, G.; Caponio, V.C.A.; Sabatucci, A.; Balercia, A.; Rubini, C.; Muzio, L.L.; Santarelli, A. Odontogenic tumours: A 25-year epidemiological study in the Marche region of Italy. *Eur. Arch. Otorhinolaryngol.* **2020**, *277*, 527–538. [CrossRef] [PubMed]
18. Chrysomali, E.; Leventis, M.; Titsinides, S.; Kyriakopoulos, V.; Sklavounou, A. Odontogenic tumors. *J. Craniofac. Surg.* **2013**, *24*, 1521–1525. [CrossRef] [PubMed]
19. Bianco, B.C.F.; Sperandio, F.F.; Hanemann, J.A.C.; Pereira, A.A.C. New WHO odontogenic tumor classification: Impact on prevalence in a population. *J. Appl. Oral Sci.* **2020**, *28*, e20190067. [CrossRef] [PubMed]
20. de Medeiros, W.K.; da Silva, L.P.; Pinto, L.P.; de Souza, L.B. Clinicopathological analysis of odontogenic tumors over 22 years period: Experience of a single center in northeastern Brazil. *Med. Oral Patol. Oral Cir. Bucal* **2018**, *23*, e664–e671.
21. Lima-Verde-Osterne, R.; Turatti, E.; Cordeiro-Teixeira, R.; Barroso-Cavalcante, R. The relative frequency of odontogenic tumors: A study of 376 cases in a Brazilian population. *Med. Oral Patol. Oral Cir. Bucal* **2017**, *22*, e193–e200. [CrossRef] [PubMed]
22. Jaeger, F.; de Noronha, M.S.; Silva, M.L.V.; Amaral, M.B.F.; Grossmann, S.d.M.C.; Horta, M.C.R.; de Souza, P.E.A.; de Aguiar, M.C.F.; Mesquita, R.A. Prevalence profile of odontogenic cysts and tumors on Brazilian sample after the reclassification of odontogenic keratocyst. *J. Craniomaxillofac. Surg.* **2017**, *45*, 267–270. [CrossRef] [PubMed]
23. Izgi, E.; Mollaoglu, N.; Simsek, M. Prevalence of odontogenic cysts and tumors on turkish sample according to latest classification of world health organization: A 10-year retrospective study. *Niger. J. Clin. Pract.* **2021**, *24*, 355–361. [CrossRef]
24. Mello, F.W.; Melo, G.; Kammer, P.V.; Speight, P.M.; Rivero, E.R.C. Prevalence of odontogenic cysts and tumors associated with impacted third molars: A systematic review and meta-analysis. *J. Craniomaxillofac. Surg.* **2019**, *47*, 996–1002. [CrossRef] [PubMed]
25. Ranjbar, M.; Khiavi, M.M.; Ghazi, M.; Derakhshan, S. Primordial Odontogenic Tumor; Archival Review of 19380 Cases in a 55-Year Retrospective Study. *Asian Pac. J. Cancer Prev.* **2023**, *24*, 2845–2853. [CrossRef] [PubMed]
26. Poomsawat, S.; Ngamsom, S.; Nonpassopon, N. Primordial odontogenic tumor with prominent calcifications: A rare case report. *J. Clin. Exp. Dent.* **2019**, *11*, e952–e956. [CrossRef] [PubMed]

27. Kebede, B.; Tare, D.; Bogale, B.; Alemseged, F. Odontogenic tumors in Ethiopia: Eight years retrospective study. *BMC Oral Health* **2017**, *17*, 54. [CrossRef] [PubMed]
28. Kreppel, M.; Zoller, J. Ameloblastoma-Clinical, radiological, and therapeutic findings. *Oral Dis.* **2018**, *24*, 63–66. [CrossRef] [PubMed]
29. Hendra, F.N.; Kalla, D.S.N.; Van Cann, E.M.; de Vet, H.C.W.; Helder, M.N.; Forouzanfar, T. Radical vs conservative treatment of intraosseous ameloblastoma: Systematic review and meta-analysis. *Oral Dis.* **2019**, *25*, 1683–1696. [CrossRef] [PubMed]
30. Saalim, M.; Sansare, K.; Karjodkar, F.; Farman, A.; Goyal, S.; Sharma, S. Recurrence rate of odontogenic myxoma after different treatments: A systematic review. *Br. J. Oral Maxillofac. Surg.* **2019**, *57*, 985–991. [CrossRef] [PubMed]

Disclaimer/Publisher's Note: The statements, opinions and data contained in all publications are solely those of the individual author(s) and contributor(s) and not of MDPI and/or the editor(s). MDPI and/or the editor(s) disclaim responsibility for any injury to people or property resulting from any ideas, methods, instructions or products referred to in the content.

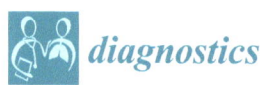 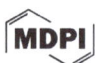

Review

Circulating HPV Tumor DNA and Molecular Residual Disease in HPV-Positive Oropharyngeal Cancers: A Scoping Review

Andrea Migliorelli, Andrea Ciorba *, Marianna Manuelli, Francesco Stomeo, Stefano Pelucchi and Chiara Bianchini

ENT & Audiology Unit, Department of Neurosciences, University Hospital of Ferrara, 44100 Ferrara, Italy
* Correspondence: andrea.ciorba@unife.it; Tel.: +39-0532-239745

Abstract: The aim of this review is to assess the utility of circulating HPV tumor DNA (ctHPVDNA) clearance in the monitoring of molecular residual disease in HPV-related oropharyngeal squamous cell carcinoma (OPSCC) patients. Recently, ctHPVDNA in patient plasma was found to be a promising biomarker for HPV OPSCC. Changes in this biomarker appear to be associated with treatment response and may be useful for identifying molecular residual disease. A review of the literature was performed using PubMed/MEDLINE, EMBASE, and Cochrane Library databases according to the PRISMA criteria for scoping reviews (from 2017 to July 2024). A total of 5 articles and 562 patients have been included. Three studies examine the role of ctHPVDNA clearance in CRT, while the remaining two studies consider surgery as a treatment option. The results of this scoping review indicate that ctHPVDNA has a potential role to serve as a valuable biomarker in the assessment of molecular residual disease. Further studies are required to confirm the efficacy of this marker for stratifying this group of patients.

Keywords: ctHPVDNA; OPSCC; liquid biopsy

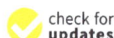

Citation: Migliorelli, A.; Ciorba, A.; Manuelli, M.; Stomeo, F.; Pelucchi, S.; Bianchini, C. Circulating HPV Tumor DNA and Molecular Residual Disease in HPV-Positive Oropharyngeal Cancers: A Scoping Review. *Diagnostics* **2024**, *14*, 2662. https://doi.org/10.3390/diagnostics14232662

Academic Editor: Luis Eduardo Almeida

Received: 30 September 2024
Revised: 24 November 2024
Accepted: 25 November 2024
Published: 26 November 2024

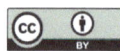

Copyright: © 2024 by the authors. Licensee MDPI, Basel, Switzerland. This article is an open access article distributed under the terms and conditions of the Creative Commons Attribution (CC BY) license (https://creativecommons.org/licenses/by/4.0/).

1. Introduction

Human papillomavirus (HPV) infection is a sexually transmitted disease that is a major cause of numerous cancers, with cervical cancer being the most common. The estimated prevalence of HPV infection among American citizens in 2018 exceeded 80 million, with 14 million new cases being documented in that year [1]. The oncogenic role of HPV in cancer pathogenesis is well established based on studies of cervical carcinoma in women.

HPV represents a large family of undeveloped double-stranded DNA viruses. The virus's circular genome of approximately 8000 base pairs encodes two structural genes necessary for the assembly of the viral capsid, as well as six non-structural genes (E1, E2, and E4) involved in viral replication and regulation. The remaining three genes, E5, E6, and E7, are associated with HPV-mediated cellular transformation. The E6 and E7 genes represent the most definitive markers as they are the only viral genes that are consistently maintained and expressed in HPV-positive tumor cells [2–8].

The precise role of HPV infection in the pathogenesis of head and neck squamous cell carcinoma is not clearly defined yet [9]. Head and neck cancers represent the sixth most common form of cancer worldwide. As reported by the Surveillance, Epidemiology, and End Results (SEER) program, there are more than 430,000 new cases of head and neck cancer annually [10]. Over 90% of head and neck cancers are squamous cell carcinomas (HNSCCs) [11]. Patients with HPV-positive oropharyngeal cancers (OPSCCs) exhibit distinct clinical, demographic, and prognostic characteristics compared with those with HPV-negative oropharyngeal cancers. This notable distinction has led to the introduction of a staging differentiation in the eighth edition of the American Joint Committee on Cancer (AJCC) staging system [12]. HPV OPSCCs predominantly affect non-smoking white males and have a significantly superior overall prognosis in comparison with their HPV-negative counterparts. The discrepancy in risk factors, incidence, and prognosis has led to the classification of HPV OPSCC as a distinct entity from HPV-negative OPSCCs [1,12].

HPV OPSCC has a significantly superior prognosis in comparison with HPV-negative OPSCC. The patient population is younger and healthier, which theoretically allows for a longer survival period. Consequently, the impact of treatment on long-term quality of life is more pronounced.

In light of these considerations, the scientific community has recently devoted considerable effort to the implementation of deintensification strategies in therapeutic regimens, with the objective of avoiding overtreatment and enhancing patient quality of life [13,14]. In particular, an increasing number of studies have investigated the potential of liquid biopsy and circulating HPV tumor DNA biomarker (ctHPVDNA) for the diagnosis and follow-up of HPV OPSCC [15–17]. The ctHPVDNA is a fragment of the HPV genome and is specific only for patients with HPV-related cancer [18]. Quantitative real-time PCR (q-PCR) is the simplest and most widely used technology to detect HPV DNA; however, in 2020, a kit was approved in the United States that allows for the assay of ctHPVDNA in a standard procedure [19].

The aim of this review is to assess the utility of ctHPVDNA clearance in the monitoring of molecular residual disease in HPV-related OPSCC. To the best of our knowledge, this is the first review analyzing ctHPVDNA accuracy in assessing molecular residual disease in HPV OPSCC patients.

2. Materials and Methods

A detailed review of the English-language literature on ctHPVDNA in HPV-related OPSCC was performed using PubMed/MEDLINE, EMBASE, and Cochrane Library databases. The search period was from 2017 to July 2024, conducted with the aim of selecting the most recent studies. The terms used were "oropharyngeal cancer", "HPV related oropharyngeal cancer" or "HPV-OPSCC" and "ctHPVDNA", "circulating tumor", "liquid biopsy" or "molecular residual disease". The search yielded 954 candidate articles. The search was performed according to the "Preferred Reporting Items for Systematic Reviews and Meta-Analyses" (PRISMA) guidelines for scoping reviews (Figure 1) [20]. The inclusion criteria applied were: (i) prospective study; (ii) publication date after 2017; (iii) studies that assessed molecular residual disease by ctHPVDNA in patients with HPV + OPSCC; (iv) clearly defined methods of detection of viral DNA; and (v) English language. Conference abstracts, case reports, retrospective studies, and publications written in a language different from English have been excluded. Two authors (A.M. and M.M.) have independently evaluated all titles, and relevant articles have been individuated according to inclusion/exclusion criteria; a senior author (A.C.) resolved any disagreements. At the end of the full-text review, only 5 articles met the inclusion criteria [21–26].

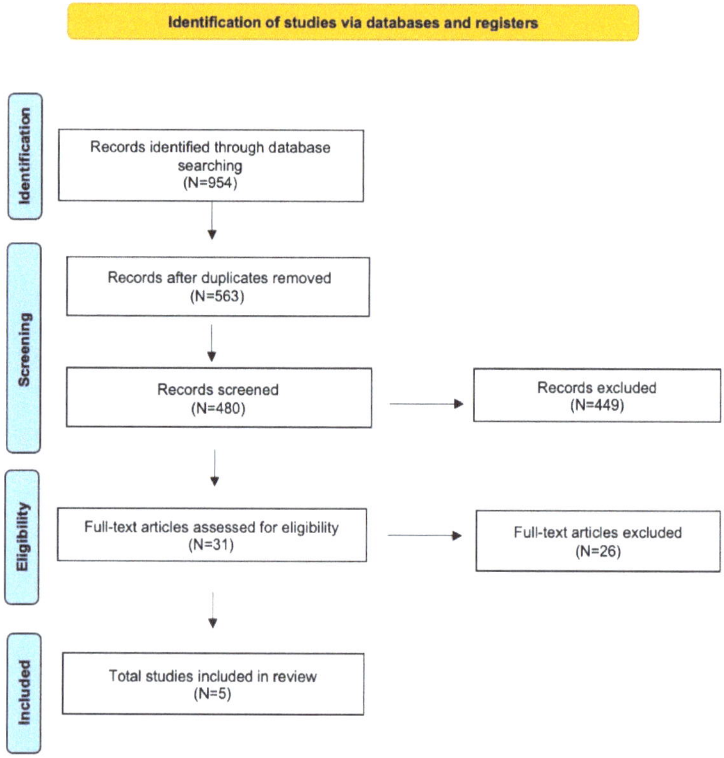

Figure 1. The literature review performed using the PRISMA guidelines for scoping reviews.

3. Results

ctHPVDNA was employed for the assessment of therapeutic efficacy and residual disease in a total of 562 patients. The results of the review process are summarized in Table 1.

Table 1. Literature review.

Author (yrs)	Nop	Mean Age	T	N	Treatment	Primers/Probes	Methods	Positive Liquid Biopsy at Diagnosis	Test Timing	Mean Copies/mL Before Treatment (Range)
Chera (2019) [21]	103	60	0: 5 1: 15 2: 69 3: 7 4: 7	0: 5 1: 16 2: 82 3: 0	CRT	HPV: 16, 18, 31, 33, 35	ddPCR	92 (89%)	Before treatment Weekly during treatment Each post-treatment follow-up visit	419 copies/mL (8–22,579)
Cao (2022) [22]	34	64	0: 1 3: 3 4: 29	0: 2 1: 28 2: 2 3: 2	CRT	HPV: 16, 18	ddPCR	28 (82%)	Before treatment At weeks 2, 4, and 7 of treatment At 3–6–12 months after the end of treatment	460 copies/mL (0–34,714)

Table 1. Cont.

Author (yrs)	Nop	Mean Age	T	N	Treatment	Primers/Probes	Methods	Positive Liquid Biopsy at Diagnosis	Test Timing	Mean Copies/mL Before Treatment (Range)
O'Boyle (2022) [23]	49	62	0: 1 1: 23 2: 22 3: 2 4: 1	0: 4 1: 38 2: 3 3: 4	S: 34 CRT: 15	E7 from HPV: 16, 18, 33, 35, 45	ddPCR	48 (98%)	S: pre-treatment; 1 day, 7 days, 30 days, 3 months, and 12 months post-treatment CRT: pre-treatment; weekly during, 3-, and 12-months post-treatment	2076 copies/mL (0–37,350)
Adrian (2023) [24]	136	60	1: 22 2: 60 3: 17 4:37	0: 5 1:10 2:114 3: 7	CRT	Hpv: 6, 11, 16, 18, 11, 16, 18, 26, 30, 31, 33, 35, 39, 40, 42, 43, 45, 51, 52, 53, 54, 56, 58, 59, 61, 62, 66, 67, 68 (a e b), 69, 70, 73, 74, 81, 82, 83, 85, 86, 87, 89, 90, 91, 114	qPCR + Luminex test	124 (91%)	Before and after treatment	67.5 copies/mL
Souza (2024) [25]	240	62.5	0: 44 1/2: 155 3/4: 41	0: 25 1: 171 2: 27 3: 17	S + adjuvant CRT: 60 S: 61 CRT: 100 C: 1 RT: 17	HPV: 16, 18, 31, 33, 35	ddPCR	N/A	Before and after treatment	N/A
Rosenberg (2024) [26]	31	N/A	N/A	N/A	CI Neoadjuvant + S/CT/RT	HPV: 16, 18	HPV-SEQ	31 (100%)	Before and 6–9 weeks after neoadjuvant treatment	N/A

Abbreviation: C: chemotherapy; CI: chemoimmunotherapy; CRT: chemoradiotherapy; ddPCR: digital drop PCR; N: nodes; N/A: not available; Nop: Number of patients; qPCR: quantified by real-time PCR; RT: radiotherapy; S: surgery; SEQ: next-generation sequencing-based safe-sequencing system; T: primary tumor; Yrs: years.

The earliest study emerging from the review is that of Chera et al. (2019) [21], in which the authors attempted to perform a risk stratification by studying baseline ctHPVDNA levels and clearance kinetics. The study demonstrated that ctHPVDNA levels at baseline exceeding 200 copies/mL are indicative of genomic tumor biomarkers and, consequently, a more favorable prognosis. Furthermore, patients with a favorable clearance profile, defined as the clearance of more than 95% of the baseline ctHPVDNA values at week four of chemoradiotherapy (CRT), have a more favorable prognosis. In contrast, patients with unfavorable clearance exhibited a higher frequency of disease persistence at the conclusion of therapy.

Subsequently, Cao and colleagues [22] examined ctHPVDNA values in patients with OPSCC p16+ stage III AJCC 8 who had undergone radiochemotherapy. The findings indicate that the alteration in values during the initial two weeks of therapy is a predictor of subsequent therapeutic outcomes. Following a two-week period, the patients were divided into two groups based on whether their ctHPVDNA values had increased or decreased compared with their baseline levels. In particular, a reduction in ctHPVDNA at the two-week mark of CRT in comparison with pre-treatment levels was linked to an increased likelihood of treatment failure or tumor progression within the 12-month period following TR. Furthermore, clearance of ctHPVDNA at weeks 4 or 7 of therapy was not predictive of progression.

In the same year, O'Boyle et al. [23] investigated whether the kinetics of ctHPVDNA clearance following surgical treatment of HPV OPSCC may be associated with the risk of residual disease. The findings were that ctHPVDNA levels below 1 copy/mL on the first postoperative day correlated with no residual disease, patients with levels between 1 and

100 copies/mL with possible microscopic residual disease, and those with levels above 100 copies/mL with macroscopic residual disease.

In 2023, the role of ctHPVDNA at baseline and at the end of treatment was evaluated in patients enrolled in the ARTSCAN III study [24]. The authors discovered that low ctHPVDNA values at the outset of treatment are indicative of a favorable prognostic index for disease-free survival and overall survival. However, no correlation was observed between these values and locoregional control.

In 2024, Souza et al. [25] conducted an evaluation of ctHPVDNA as a tool for the surveillance and assessment of treatment response in patients with HPV OPSCC. The high negative predictive value (98.9% for patients undergoing surgery + adjuvant treatment and 100% for patients undergoing surgery alone) is therefore of importance in the evaluation of definitive treatment. In the event of a positive post-treatment test, further investigation with imaging and closer follow-up is recommended.

Recently, the phase 2 OPTIMAII study, which was conducted in advance-stage patients to evaluate the role of neoadjuvant chemoimmunotherapy, used ctHPV DNA analysis in a subgroup to assess response to neoadjuvant therapy.

Samples were collected from 31 patients before therapy and 6–9 weeks after the start of adjuvant therapy. All patients had detectable levels of HPV DNA at baseline. The 26 patients with complete clearance had a significantly better two-year progression-free survival than those with detectable ctHPV DNA [26].

In summary, all authors have studied the kinetics of ctHPVDNA following treatment. Threshold values are scarcely comparable because of the use of non-standardized measurement methods; at present, it is still not possible to establish an unambiguous cut-off level. However, these studies demonstrate the importance of investigating the kinetics of ctHPVDNA following treatment.

4. Discussion

At present, the follow-up protocol for patients with OPSCC is based on imaging and clinical examination. However, the low accuracy and poor diagnostic value of follow-up methods can result in the patient undergoing unnecessary imaging and surgery, leading to overtreatments with a significant negative impact on the patient's quality of life [27–29]. A multitude of deintensification strategies have been the subject of recent studies [30–35]. In particular, researchers have investigated the clinical applications of ctHPVDNA in biological fluids for the monitoring of HPV OPSCC patients [15–17,36]. The progression of tumors is associated with the expression of oncogenic viral DNA and proteins. It is noteworthy that the circulating EBV DNA load is currently regarded as a novel biomarker that reflects prognosis and changes in response to treatment in nasopharyngeal cancer [37]. Similarly, ctHPVDNA may have a comparable impact and diagnostic efficacy for HPV OPSCC cancers, as proposed by several authors. In fact, a 2023 meta-analysis has demonstrated that droplet digital polymerase chain reaction (ddPCR) for ctDNA has favorable accuracy, sensitivity, and specificity in the diagnosis of HPV-related OPSCC. These authors conducted an analysis of 729 patients with HPV-related OPSCC and ctHPVDNA emerges as a crucial biomarker for diagnosing these patients [16]. Also, another meta-analysis conducted by Campo et al. [15] demonstrated that ctHPVDNA may also be a valuable tool for monitoring patient outcomes; a sensitivity of 86% (95% CI: 78–91%) and a specificity of 96% (95% CI: 91–99%) has been observed in the analysis of 1311 patients with HPV OPSCC.

The present review examines a further feature: the application of ctHPVDNA in the detection of molecular residual disease, thus anticipating findings that can be detected by imaging. To date, there only are a few studies in the literature regarding the use of ctHPVDNA as a biomarker to monitor molecular residual disease, and to the best of our knowledge, this is the first review analyzing the accuracy of ctHPVDNA in assessing molecular residual disease for HPV OPSCC patients. In particular, this scoping review examined the treatment results of 562 patients with HPV-related OPSCC. The mean age of the patients included in the study is consistent, ranging from 60 to 64 years. Three studies have examined the role of ctHPVDNA clearance in CRT, two studies have investigated its role in surgery as a treatment option, and a recent study has considered its role in neoadjuvant chemoimmunotherapy. According to the data of the present review, the positivity rate for liquid biopsy in patients with a confirmed diagnosis of HPV OPSCC via biopsy exhibits considerable variability, with reported rates ranging from 100 to 82%. This can be attributed to the utilization of disparate primers; an increased number of HPV types tested is associated with a heightened probability of obtaining a positive liquid biopsy result, as previously discussed, given that not all HPV-related cancers are determined by the presence of types 16 or 18.

Furthermore, the present review indicates that the timing of sampling for liquid biopsy varies considerably between studies, emphasizing the necessity of a standard protocol. Moreover, the included studies employed disparate kits and primers. The initial studies were conducted to analyze alterations in ctHPVDNA clearance in patients undergoing CRT. The results on the effectiveness of ctHPVDNA clearance in monitoring CRT efficacy and molecular residual disease can be difficult to evaluate. The results of the studies reviewed indicate that the biomarker has significant potential and may become a crucial tool for risk stratification in the future. However, further studies are necessary to establish standardized protocols for its use in clinical practice.

Interestingly, the analysis of ctHPVDNA clearance for monitoring residual disease in patients undergoing surgical treatment could offer significant findings. O'Boyle et al. [23] developed a risk stratification system for macroscopic, microscopic, and nonmolecular residual disease based on the number of copies/mL of ctHPVDNA present as early as the first postoperative day. Consequently, ctHPVDNA levels on the first postoperative day have been correlated with the risk of residual disease. These findings have illustrated the potential utility of ctHPVDNA as a biomarker for personalized treatment in patients with HPV-positive squamous cell carcinoma undergoing surgery.

It is likely that the role of ctHPVDNA in stratifying the risk of molecular residual disease in surgically treated patients is of great importance. At present, the standard post-treatment evaluation is performed with PET at three months; however, this procedure can still retain a high number of false positives and a relatively low positive predictive value of 30% in 12-week surveillance for HPV OPSCC [38–40]. Thus, ctHPVDNA could represent a sensitive and effective method for the detection of residual disease. In the near future, it may be used as a complementary technique alongside PET in order to enhance patient follow-up.

Recently, other molecular techniques have been proposed in the literature, aiming to perform targeted follow-up and early detection of residual disease, with a view of enabling personalized and tailored treatments. (i) Some studies have evaluated the presence of HPVDNA in saliva, but these findings, although promising, are still at an early stage, and for the present time, saliva sampling with HPVDNA assay is proposed as a complement to ctHPVDNA and not as its replacement [41–43]. Furthermore, recent evidence suggests that it has good potential for assessing treatment response [44]. (ii) MicroRNAs could have the potential to serve as biomarkers for the early detection of patients with residual disease following treatment for HPV OPSCC. Currently, the literature has primarily focused on their use for early detection; however, they may also have a role in the early assessment of treatment response in the future [44]. (iii) Tumor-derived extracellular vesicles (exosomes) are nanometric particles with DNA, RNA, proteins and lipids inside, which are derived from both normal and cancer cells [45]. They have recently been proposed as biomarkers for the evaluation of patients with HPV OPSCC.

In summary, PET is currently the gold standard for assessing response to treatment, but it has many limitations and a high false-positive rate. For the assessment of molecular residual disease, ctHPVDNA represents the most studied and established technique available to date, with promising results. However, micro-RNA and exosome analysis are emerging as possible complementary methods that may improve the results of liquid biopsy by allowing for more personalized treatment of these patients.

ctHPVDNA has demonstrated high specificity and sensitivity in the diagnosis and identification of HPV OPSCC recurrence. The present review has illustrated that ctHPVDNA may be of pivotal importance in surgically treated patients and also following neoadjuvant chemoimmunotherapy. This illustrates the potential role of ctHPVDNA when considering a de-escalation treatment [24]. In our opinion, perioperative ctHPVDNA monitoring will provide useful information for identifying residual disease and for personalizing treatments.

The major drawbacks of this study are (i) the small number of studies available in the literature so far, and therefore those included within this review; (ii) the heterogeneity of the timing of sampling to assess ctHPVDNA clearance; and (iii) the use of different assay kits and primers within the selected studies.

5. Conclusions

In conclusion, the results of this scoping review indicate that ctHPVDNA has a potential role to serve as a valuable biomarker in the assessment of molecular residual disease, but the results, although encouraging, are still preliminary.

Data from the literature are poorly comparable due to the different methods and timings of measuring ctHPVDNA, so at present, it is not possible to describe a practical universal procedure (i.e., standard cut-off levels or time of sampling). This technique could eventually be incorporated within the management protocols for patients with HPV OPSCC in the future, aiming (i) to stratify the risk of molecular residual disease and thus (ii) evaluate the most appropriate therapeutic strategy for the treatment of these patients. The objective of this methodology is to minimize overtreatment and improve the quality of life of the patients.

Further prospective, multicenter studies are required to (i) standardize the procedure, (ii) determine the optimal timing for samplings, and (iii) confirm the efficacy of this technique.

Author Contributions: Conceptualization, A.M., M.M., A.C. and C.B.; methodology, A.M., M.M. and A.C.; formal analysis, A.M., M.M. and A.C.; investigation and data curation, A.M., M.M. and A.C.; writing—original draft preparation, A.M., M.M. and A.C.; writing—review and editing, F.S., S.P. and C.B.; supervision, A.C. and C.B. All authors have read and agreed to the published version of the manuscript.

Funding: This research received no external funding.

Institutional Review Board Statement: Not applicable.

Informed Consent Statement: Not applicable.

Data Availability Statement: No new data were created or analyzed in this study.

Conflicts of Interest: The authors declare no conflicts of interest.

References

1. Roman, B.R.; Aragones, A. Epidemiology and incidence of HPV-related cancers of the head and neck. *J. Surg. Oncol.* **2021**, *124*, 920–922. [CrossRef] [PubMed]
2. Schwarz, E.; Freese, U.K.; Gissmann, L.; Mayer, W.; Roggenbuck, B.; Stremlau, A.; Hausen, H.Z. Structure and transcription of human papillomavirus sequences in cervical carcinoma cells. *Nature* **1985**, *314*, 111–114. [CrossRef] [PubMed]
3. Economopoulou, P.; Kotsantis, I.; Psyrri, A. Special Issue about Head and Neck Cancers: HPV Positive Cancers. *Int. J. Mol. Sci.* **2020**, *21*, 3388. [CrossRef] [PubMed]
4. Shah, M.; Anwar, M.A.; Park, S.; Jafri, S.S.; Choi, S. In silico mechanistic analysis of IRF3 inactivation and high-risk HPV E6 species-dependent drug response. *Sci. Rep.* **2015**, *5*, 13446. [CrossRef]
5. Rampias, T.; Sasaki, C.; Psyrri, A. Molecular mechanisms of HPV induced carcinogenesis in head and neck. *Oral Oncol.* **2014**, *50*, 356–363. [CrossRef]
6. Tumban, E. A current update on human papillomavirus-associated head and neck cancers. *Viruses* **2019**, *11*, 922. [CrossRef]
7. Weinberger, P.M.; Yu, Z.; Haffty, B.G.; Kowalski, D.; Harigopal, M.; Brandsma, J.; Sasaki, C.; Joe, J.; Camp, R.L.; Rimm, D.L.; et al. Molecular classification identifies a subset of human papillomavirus–associated oropharyngeal cancers with favorable prognosis. *J. Clin. Oncol.* **2006**, *24*, 736–747. [CrossRef]

8. Seiwert, T.Y.; Zuo, Z.; Keck, M.K.; Khattri, A.; Pedamallu, C.S.; Stricker, T.; Brown, C.; Pugh, T.J.; Stojanov, P.; Cho, J.; et al. Integrative and comparative genomic analysis of HPV-positive and HPV-negative head and neck squamous cell carcinomas. *Clin. Cancer Res.* **2015**, *21*, 632–641. [CrossRef]
9. Shah, J.P.; Patel, S.G.; Singh, B.; Wong, R. *Jatin Shah's Head and Neck Surgery and Oncology*; Elsevier—Health Sciences Division: Amsterdam, The Netherlands, 2020.
10. Head and Neck Squamous Cell Carcinoma. Available online: https://www.sciencedirect.com/topics/medicine-and-dentistry/head-and-neck-squamous-cell-carcinoma (accessed on 26 November 2020).
11. Tagliabue, M.; Mena, M.; Maffini, F.; Gheit, T.; Blasco, B.Q.; Holzinger, D.; Tous, S.; Scelsi, D.; Riva, D.; Grosso, E.; et al. Role of Human Papillomavirus Infection in Head and Neck Cancer in Italy: The HPV-AHEAD Study. *Cancers* **2020**, *12*, 3567. [CrossRef]
12. Zanoni, D.K.; Patel, S.G.; Shah, J.P. Changes in the 8th Edition of the American Joint Committee on Cancer (AJCC) Staging of Head and Neck Cancer: Rationale and Implications. *Curr. Oncol. Rep.* **2019**, *21*, 52. [CrossRef]
13. Migliorelli, A.; Manuelli, M.; Ciorba, A.; Pelucchi, S.; Bianchini, C. The Role of HPV in Head and Neck Cancer. In *Handbook of Cancer and Immunology*; Rezaei, N., Ed.; Springer: Cham, Switzerland, 2024.
14. Fakhry, C.; Zhang, Q.; Nguyen-Tan, P.F.; Rosenthal, D.; El-Naggar, A.; Garden, A.S.; Soulieres, D.; Trotti, A.; Avizonis, V.; Ridge, J.A.; et al. Human papillomavirus and overall survival after progression of oropharyngeal squamous cell carcinoma. *J. Clin. Oncol.* **2014**, *32*, 3365–3373. [CrossRef] [PubMed]
15. Campo, F.; Iocca, O.; Paolini, F.; Manciocco, V.; Moretto, S.; De Virgilio, A.; Moretti, C.; Vidiri, A.; Venuti, A.; Bossi, P.; et al. The landscape of circulating tumor HPV DNA and TTMV-HPVDNA for surveillance of HPV-oropharyngeal carcinoma: Systematic review and meta-analysis. *J. Exp. Clin. Cancer Res.* **2024**, *43*, 215. [CrossRef] [PubMed]
16. Paolini, F.; Campo, F.; Iocca, O.; Manciocco, V.; De Virgilio, A.; De Pascale, V.; Moretto, S.; Dalfino, G.; Vidiri, A.; Blandino, G.; et al. Is it time to improve the diagnostic workup of oropharyngeal cancer with circulating tumor HPV DNA: Systematic review and meta-analysis. *Head Neck* **2023**, *45*, 2945–2954. [CrossRef]
17. Andrioaie, I.M.; Luchian, I.; Dămian, C.; Nichitean, G.; Andrese, E.P.; Pantilimonescu, T.F.; Trandabăț, B.; Prisacariu, L.J.; Budală, D.G.; Dimitriu, D.C.; et al. The Clinical Utility of Circulating HPV DNA Biomarker in Oropharyngeal, Cervical, Anal, and Skin HPV-Related Cancers: A Review. *Pathogens* **2023**, *12*, 908. [CrossRef]
18. Sivars, L.; Palsdottir, K.; Crona Guterstam, Y.; Falconer, H.; Hellman, K.; Tham, E. The current status of cell-free human papillomavirus DNA as a biomarker in cervical cancer and other HPV-associated tumors: A review. *Int. J. Cancer* **2022**, *152*, 2232–2242. [CrossRef] [PubMed]
19. Lang Kuhs, K.A.; Brenner, J.C.; Holsinger, F.C.; Rettig, E.M. Circulating Tumor HPV DNA for Surveillance of HPV-Positive Oropharyngeal Squamous Cell Carcinoma: A Narrative Review. *JAMA Oncol.* **2023**, *9*, 1716–1724. [CrossRef]
20. Tricco, A.C.; Lillie, E.; Zarin, W.; O'Brien, K.K.; Colquhoun, H.; Levac, D.; Moher, D.; Peters, M.D.J.; Horsley, T.; Straus, S.E.; et al. PRISMA Extension for Scoping Reviews (PRISMA-ScR): Checklist and Explanation. *Ann. Intern. Med.* **2018**, *169*, 467–473. [CrossRef]
21. Chera, B.S.; Kumar, S.; Beaty, B.T.; Marron, D.; Jefferys, S.; Green, R.; Goldman, E.C.; Amdur, R.; Sheets, N.; Dagan, R.; et al. Rapid Clearance Profile of Plasma Circulating Tumor HPV Type 16 DNA during Chemoradiotherapy Correlates with Disease Control in HPV-Associated Oropharyngeal Cancer. *Clin. Cancer Res.* **2019**, *25*, 4682–4690. [CrossRef] [PubMed]
22. Cao, Y.; Haring, C.T.; Brummel, C.; Bhambhani, C.; Aryal, M.; Lee, C.; Neal, M.H.; Bhangale, A.; Gu, W.; Casper, K.; et al. Early HPV ctDNA Kinetics and Imaging Biomarkers Predict Therapeutic Response in p16+ Oropharyngeal Squamous Cell Carcinoma. *Clin. Cancer Res.* **2022**, *28*, 350–359. [CrossRef]
23. O'Boyle, C.J.; Siravegna, G.; Varmeh, S.; Queenan, N.; Michel, A.; Pang, K.C.S.; Stein, J.; Thierauf, J.C.; Sadow, P.M.; Faquin, W.C.; et al. Cell-free human papillomavirus DNA kinetics after surgery for human papillomavirus-associated oropharyngeal cancer. *Cancer* **2022**, *128*, 2193–2204. [CrossRef]
24. Adrian, G.; Forslund, O.; Pedersen, L.; Sjövall, J.; Gebre-Medhin, M. Circulating tumour HPV16 DNA quantification—A prognostic tool for progression-free survival in patients with HPV-related oropharyngeal carcinoma. *Radiother. Oncol.* **2023**, *186*, 109773. [CrossRef] [PubMed]
25. Souza, S.S.; Stephens, E.M.; Bourdillon, A.T.; Bhethanabotla, R.; Farzal, Z.; Plonowska-Hirschfeld, K.; Qualliotine, J.R.; Heaton, C.M.; Ha, P.K.; Ryan, W.R. Circulating tumor HPV DNA assessments after surgery for human papilloma virus-associated oropharynx carcinoma. *Am. J. Otolaryngol.* **2024**, *45*, 104184. [CrossRef]
26. Rosenberg, A.J.; Agrawal, N.; Juloori, A.; Cursio, J.; Gooi, Z.; Blair, E.; Chin, J.; Ginat, D.; Pasternak-Wise, O.; Hasina, R.; et al. Neoadjuvant Nivolumab Plus Chemotherapy Followed By Response-Adaptive Therapy for HPV+ Oropharyngeal Cancer: OPTIMA II Phase 2 Open-Label Nonrandomized Clinical Trial. *JAMA Oncol.* **2024**, *10*, 923–931. [CrossRef]
27. Campo, F.; Zocchi, J.; Moretto, S.; Mazzola, F.; Petruzzi, G.; Donà, M.G.; Benevolo, M.; Iocca, O.; De Virgilio, A.; Pichi, B.; et al. Cell-free human papillomavirus-DNA for monitoring treatment response of head and neck squamous cell carcinoma: Systematic review and meta-analysis. *Laryngoscope* **2021**, *132*, 560–568. [CrossRef] [PubMed]
28. Pellini, R.; Manciocco, V.; Turri-Zanoni, M.; Vidiri, A.; Sanguineti, G.; Marucci, L.; Sciuto, R.; Covello, R.; Sperduti, I.; Kayal, R.; et al. Planned neck dissection after chemoradiotherapy in advanced oropharyngeal squamous cell cancer: The role of US, MRI and FDG-PET/TC scans to assess residual neck disease. *J. Craniomaxillofac. Surg.* **2014**, *42*, 1834–1839. [CrossRef] [PubMed]
29. Harish, K. Neck dissections: Radical to conservative. *World J. Surg. Oncol.* **2005**, *3*, 21. [CrossRef]

30. Marur, S.; Li, S.; Cmelak, A.J.; Gillison, M.L.; Zhao, W.J.; Ferris, R.L.; Westra, W.H.; Gilbert, J.; Bauman, J.E.; Wagner, L.I.; et al. Phase II trial of induction chemotherapy followed by reduced-dose radiation and weekly cetuximab in patients with HPV-associated resectable squamous cell carcinoma of the oropharynx—ECOG-ACRIN Cancer Research Group. *J. Clin. Oncol.* 2017, *35*, 490–497. [CrossRef]
31. Yom, S.; Torres-Saavedra, P.; Caudell, J.; Waldron, J.; Gillison, M.; Truong, M.; Jordan, R.; Subramaniam, R.; Yao, M.; Chung, C.; et al. NRG-HN002: A Randomized Phase II Trial for Patients with p16-Positive, Non-Smoking-Associated, Locoregionally Advanced Oropharyngeal Cancer. *Int. J. Radiat. Oncol. Biol. Phys.* 2019, *105*, S684. [CrossRef]
32. ECOG-ACRIN. Transoral Surgery Followed by Low-Dose or Standard-Dose Radiation Therapy with or without Chemotherapy in Treating Patients with HPV Positive Stage III-IVA Oropharyngeal Cancer. Available online: https://www.clinicaltrials.gov/study/NCT01898494#study-record-dates (accessed on 13 March 2024).
33. Nichols, A.C.; Yoo, J.; Hammond, J.A.; Fung, K.; Winquist, E.; Read, N.; Venkatesan, V.; MacNeil, S.D.; Ernst, D.S.; Palma, D.A.; et al. Early-stage squamous cell carcinoma of the oropharynx: Radiotherapy vs. trans-oral robotic surgery (ORATOR)—Study protocol for a randomized phase II trial. *BMC Cancer* 2013, *13*, 133. [CrossRef]
34. Nichols, A.C.; Lang, P.; Prisman, E.; Berthelet, E.; Tran, E.; Hamilton, S.; Wu, J.; Fung, K.; De Almeida, J.R.; Bayley, A.; et al. Treatment de-escalation for HPV-associated oropharyngeal squamous cell carcinoma with radiotherapy vs. trans-oral surgery (ORATOR2): Study protocol for a randomized phase II trial. *BMC Cancer*, 2020; *20*, 125.
35. Owadally, W.; Hurt, C.; Timmins, H.; Parsons, E.; Townsend, S.; Patterson, J.; Hutcheson, K.; Powell, N.; Beasley, M.; Palaniappan, N.; et al. PATHOS: A phase II/III trial of risk-stratified, reduced intensity adjuvant treatment in patients undergoing transoral surgery for Human papillomavirus (HPV) positive oropharyngeal cancer. *BMC Cancer* 2015, *15*, 602. [CrossRef]
36. Campo, F.; Paolini, F.; Manciocco, V.; Moretto, S.; Pichi, B.; Moretti, C.; Blandino, G.; De Pascale, V.; Benevolo, M.; Pimpinelli, F.; et al. Circulating tumor HPV DNA in the management of HPV+ oropharyngeal cancer and its correlation with MRI. *Head Neck* 2024, *46*, 2206–2213. [CrossRef] [PubMed]
37. Xie, X.; Ren, Y.; Wang, K.; Yi, B. Molecular prognostic value of circulating Epstein-Barr viral DNA in nasopharyngeal carcinoma: A meta-analysis of 27,235 cases in the endemic area of Southeast Asia. *Genet. Test. Mol. Biomark.* 2019, *23*, 448–459. [CrossRef] [PubMed]
38. Rulach, R.; Zhou, S.; Hendry, F.; Stobo, D.; James, A.; Dempsey, M.-F.; Grose, D.; Lamb, C.; Schipani, S.; Rizwanullah, M.; et al. 12-Week PET-CT Has Low Positive Predictive Value for Nodal Residual Disease in Human Papillomavirus-Positive Oropharyngeal Cancers. *Oral Oncol.* 2019, *97*, 76–81. [CrossRef] [PubMed]
39. Yu, Y.; Mabray, M.; Silveira, W.; Shen, P.Y.; Ryan, W.R.; Uzelac, A.; Yom, S.S. Earlier and More Specific Detection of Persistent Neck Disease with Diffusion-Weighted MRI versus Subsequent PET/CT after Definitive Chemoradiation for Oropharyngeal Squamous Cell Carcinoma. *Head Neck* 2017, *39*, 432–438. [CrossRef] [PubMed]
40. Zhou, S.; Chan, C.; Rulach, R.; Dyab, H.; Hendry, F.; Maxfield, C.; Dempsey, M.-F.; James, A.; Grose, D.; Lamb, C.; et al. Long-Term Survival in Patients with Human Papillomavirus-Positive Oropharyngeal Cancer and Equivocal Response on 12-Week PET-CT Is Not Compromised by the Omission of Neck Dissection. *Oral Oncol.* 2022, *128*, 105870. [CrossRef]
41. Motegi, A.; Kageyama, S.I.; Kashima, Y.; Hirata, H.; Hojo, H.; Nakamura, M.; Fujisawa, T.; Enokida, T.; Tahara, M.; Matsuura, K.; et al. Detection of HPV DNA in Saliva of Patients with HPV-Associated Oropharyngeal Cancer Treated with Radiotherapy. *Curr. Oncol.* 2024, *31*, 4397–4405. [CrossRef]
42. Tang, K.D.; Wan, Y.; Zhang, X.; Bozyk, N.; Vasani, S.; Kenny, L.; Punyadeera, C. Proteomic Alterations in Salivary Exosomes Derived from Human Papillomavirus-Driven Oropharyngeal Cancer. *Mol. Diagn. Ther.* 2021, *25*, 505–515. [CrossRef]
43. Nguyen, B.; Meehan, K.; Pereira, M.R.; Mirzai, B.; Lim, S.H.; Leslie, C.; Clark, M.; Sader, C.; Friedland, P.; Lindsay, A.; et al. A Comparative Study of Extracellular Vesicle-Associated and Cell-Free DNA and RNA for HPV Detection in Oropharyngeal Squamous Cell Carcinoma. *Sci. Rep.* 2020, *10*, 6083. [CrossRef]
44. Mayne, G.C.; Woods, C.M.; Dharmawardana, N.; Wang, T.; Krishnan, S.; Hodge, J.C.; Foreman, A.; Boase, S.; Carney, A.S.; Sigston, E.A.W.; et al. Cross Validated Serum Small Extracellular Vesicle microRNAs for the Detection of Oropharyngeal Squamous Cell Carcinoma. *J. Transl. Med.* 2020, *18*, 280. [CrossRef]
45. Allevato, M.M.; Smith, J.D.; Brenner, M.J.; Chinn, S.B. Tumor-Derived Exosomes and the Role of Liquid Biopsy in Human Papillomavirus Oropharyngeal Squamous Cell Carcinoma. *Cancer J.* 2023, *29*, 230–237. [CrossRef]

Disclaimer/Publisher's Note: The statements, opinions and data contained in all publications are solely those of the individual author(s) and contributor(s) and not of MDPI and/or the editor(s). MDPI and/or the editor(s) disclaim responsibility for any injury to people or property resulting from any ideas, methods, instructions or products referred to in the content.

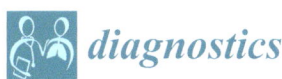

Article

In Vivo Regulation of Active Matrix Metalloproteinase-8 (aMMP-8) in Periodontitis: From Transcriptomics to Real-Time Online Diagnostics and Treatment Monitoring

Nur Rahman Ahmad Seno Aji [1,2], Tülay Yucel-Lindberg [3], Ismo T. Räisänen [1,*], Heidi Kuula [1], Mikko T. Nieminen [1,4], Maelíosa T. C. Mc Crudden [5], Dyah Listyarifah [6], Anna Lundmark [3], Fionnuala T. Lundy [5], Shipra Gupta [7] and Timo Sorsa [1,8]

[1] Department of Oral and Maxillofacial Diseases, Head and Neck Center, University of Helsinki and Helsinki University Hospital, 00290 Helsinki, Finland
[2] Department of Periodontics, Faculty of Dentistry, Universitas Gadjah Mada, Jalan Denta No. 1 Sekip Utara, 10 Sleman, Yogyakarta 55281, Indonesia
[3] Division of Pediatric Dentistry, Department of Dental Medicine, Karolinska Institutet, 171 77 Huddinge, Sweden
[4] Department of Otorhinolaryngology—Head and Neck Surgery, Helsinki University Hospital and University of Helsinki, 00290 Helsinki, Finland
[5] Wellcome-Wolfson Institute for Experimental Medicine, School of Medicine Dentistry and Biomedical Science, Queen's University Belfast, Belfast BT9 7BL, UK
[6] Department of Dental Biomedical Sciences, Faculty of Dentistry, Universitas Gadjah Mada, Jl. Denta Sekip Utara No 1, Yogyakarta 55281, Indonesia
[7] Oral Health Sciences Centre, Post Graduate Institute of Medical Education & Research, Chandigarh 160012, India
[8] Division of Oral Diseases, Department of Dental Medicine, Karolinska Institutet, 171 77 Stockholm, Sweden
* Correspondence: ismo.raisanen@helsinki.fi

Citation: Aji, N.R.A.S.; Yucel-Lindberg, T.; Räisänen, I.T.; Kuula, H.; Nieminen, M.T.; Mc Crudden, M.T.C.; Listyarifah, D.; Lundmark, A.; Lundy, F.T.; Gupta, S.; et al. In Vivo Regulation of Active Matrix Metalloproteinase-8 (aMMP-8) in Periodontitis: From Transcriptomics to Real-Time Online Diagnostics and Treatment Monitoring. *Diagnostics* **2024**, *14*, 1011. https://doi.org/10.3390/diagnostics14101011

Academic Editor: Gianna Dipalma

Received: 17 April 2024
Revised: 9 May 2024
Accepted: 12 May 2024
Published: 15 May 2024

Copyright: © 2024 by the authors. Licensee MDPI, Basel, Switzerland. This article is an open access article distributed under the terms and conditions of the Creative Commons Attribution (CC BY) license (https://creativecommons.org/licenses/by/4.0/).

Abstract: Background: This study investigated in vivo regulation and levels of active matrix metalloproteinase-8 (aMMP-8), a major collagenolytic protease, in periodontitis. Methods: Twenty-seven adults with chronic periodontitis (CP) and 30 periodontally healthy controls (HC) were enrolled in immunohistochemistry and transcriptomics analytics in order to assess *Treponema denticola* (Td) dentilisin and MMP-8 immunoexpression, mRNA expression of MMP-8 and its regulators (IL-1β, MMP-2, MMP-7, TIMP-1). Furthermore, the periodontal anti-infective treatment effect was monitored by four different MMP-8 assays (aMMP-8-IFMA, aMMP-8-Oralyzer, MMP-8-activity [RFU/minute], and total MMP-8 by ELISA) among 12 CP (compared to 25 HC). Results: Immunohistochemistry revealed significantly more *Td*-dentilisin and MMP-8 immunoreactivities in CP vs. HC. Transcriptomics revealed significantly elevated IL-1β and MMP-7 RNA expressions, and MMP-2 RNA was slightly reduced. No significant differences were recorded in the relatively low or barely detectable levels of MMP-8 mRNAs. Periodontal treatment significantly decreased all MMP-8 assay levels accompanied by the assessed clinical indices (periodontal probing depths, bleeding-on-probing, and visual plaque levels). However, active but not total MMP-8 levels persisted higher in CP than in periodontally healthy controls. Conclusion: In periodontal health, there are low aMMP-8 levels. The presence of *Td*-dentilisin in CP gingivae is associated with elevated aMMP-8 levels, potentially contributing to a higher risk of active periodontal tissue collagenolysis and progression of periodontitis. This can be detected by aMMP-8-specific assays and online/real-time aMMP-8 chair-side testing.

Keywords: active matrix metalloproteinase-8; aMMP-8; *Td*-dentilisin; periodontitis; transcriptomic; proteomic

1. Introduction

Periodontitis is a host-mediated, chronic inflammatory disease induced by dysbiotic bacterial biofilms and is characterized by progressive collagenolytic destruction and loss of the periodontal attachment and alveolar bone [1]. Within the bacterial biofilm, *Treponema denticola* (*Td*), an obligate anaerobe, is among the most well-characterized and frequently isolated spirochaetes associated with periodontitis [2]. One of its key virulence factors responsible for its high invasiveness is its cell surface-bound chymotrypsin-like proteinase (CTLP), also known as dentilisin [2]. *Td*-dentilisin can modulate host immunity and facilitate apoptosis in various cell types [2]. *Td*-dentilisin also degrades multiple host extracellular matrix and basement membrane (BM) proteins, hydrolyses non-matrix bioactive peptides and mediators, enhances *Td* penetration into the epithelium, activates pro-matrix metalloproteinases, and promotes its integration into biofilm communities [2]. Virulence factors of *Td* can trigger inflammatory and adaptive immune responses and increase the release and activation of MMP-8 [2–4]. This is mediated by the binding of pathogen-associated molecular patterns to pattern recognition receptors (toll-like receptors) of host inflammatory and resident cells [3]. The inflammatory cells (mainly neutrophils), resident fibroblasts, and epithelial cells in the periodontal tissues release proinflammatory mediators (interleukin-1β, tumor necrosis factor-alpha, prostaglandin E2, RANKL, etc.) and proteolytic enzymes, including MMPs, which can initiate the periodontal tissue destruction [3,5,6].

MMPs regulate the cell-matrix composition and hydrolyze the components of the ECM and BM, which are also potentially degraded to a lesser extent by microbial proteases [2–4]. MMPs also modify immune responses [4,7,8]. MMPs' activities are mainly regulated by endogenous tissue inhibitors of matrix metalloproteinases (TIMPs), and the MMP/TIMP ratio frequently determines the extent of ECM protein degradation and tissue remodeling [3,4,7,8]. An imbalance in the MMPs/TIMP ratio is considered to tilt the balance toward pathological tissue destruction in periodontitis [3,4,7,8].

MMP-8 is the major collagenolytic protease present in both gingival crevicular fluid (GCF) and gingival tissue and is implicated in the inflammatory and immunological cascades in periodontitis [4,9–14]. MMP-8 can additionally process various non-matrix bioactive proteins such as cytokines, complement components, and insulin receptors [4,7]. The active form of MMP-8 (aMMP-8) is elevated in a diseased mouth rinse, gingival crevicular fluid, and peri-implant sulcular fluid samples and is potentially useful to diagnose, predict the stage and grade periodontitis/periimplantitis. Furthermore, it can act as a biomarker to differentiate periodontitis from gingivitis and a healthy state [9,14–16].

MMP-8 gene expression is regulated primarily at the transcriptional level during neutrophil development and maturation in the bone marrow [17–21], and the de novo up-regulation of its and other MMP's mRNAs, in response to growth factors and cytokines in periodontitis and arthritis, has often been demonstrated [8,19,22]. Overexpression of MMPs necessitates the tight regulation of the collagenolytic and tissue-destructive MMP genes and proteins in periodontitis [4,8].

Recently, the activation of the host proMMP-8 by *Td*-dentilisin in patients with periodontitis and periimpantitis was reported [2,20]. Therefore, we hypothesized that increased *Td*-dentilisin could eventually invade and up-regulate aMMP-8 levels in periodontitis-affected tissues and oral fluids.

In this study, we aimed to (i) detect *Td*-dentilisin and MMP-8 immunoexpression levels in gingival tissue samples of patients with periodontitis compared with periodontally healthy gingivae to (ii) assess the MMP-8, MMP-2, MMP-7, TIMP-1, and IL-1β mRNA expressions in the diseased vs. healthy gingiva. In addition, (iii) determine aMMP-8 and total MMP-8 levels before and after non-antibiotic anti-infective scaling and root planing treatment in chronic periodontitis (CP) in relation to healthy controls (HC), using independent aMMP-8 immuno—and catalytic activity assays.

2. Materials and Methods

2.1. Patients and Tissue Samples

The gingival tissue specimens were collected from stage III/IV grade B/C periodontitis (CP) patients ($n = 27$) and from periodontally healthy control (HC) patients ($n = 30$).

The clinical dental examination and gingival tissue sample collection were approved by the Regional Ethics Board in Stockholm (number 2008/1935-31/3) and the local ethical committee of the Helsinki University Hospital, Finland (106§/26.06.2019; dnro HUS/1271/2019) and Regionala etikprövingsnämnden i Stockholm, (EPN) (2016-08-24/2016/1:8 and 2016-1-24; Dnr 2016/1410-31/1) in accordance with the Helsinki Declaration. All participants provided signed informed consent before enrolling in this study. The periodontitis tissue specimens were obtained from patients with generalized stage III/IV adult CP as diagnosed by a clinical assessment of pocket depths, loss of attachment, bone loss, and bleeding on probing [10]. The patients had radiographic alveolar bone loss in 30%-50% of teeth, loss of attachments between 5 and 7 mm, and elevated aMMP-8 (22–38 ng/mL) levels [10]. The patients had not received any antimicrobial or MMP-8 inhibitory low-dose doxycycline, bisphosphonate, chlorhexidine medication [3,4,7,8,19], or professional periodontal treatment of the sampling area prior to the participation of this study. Gingivitis or initial/early developing stage I periodontitis was defined clinically as the occurrence of redness, swelling of the gingiva, bleeding on probing, and aMMP-8 test positivity [1,9,10,15,16,23]. Gingivitis samples for this study were obtained from patients with gingival index < 2 and probing depth $\leq$ 3 mm without supporting soft and bone tissue destruction and recovered during gingivectomy in the case of gingival enlargement in the incisor, canine, or premolar sites [9,10,15,16,23].

Periodontitis-affected gingival tissue samples were collected during periodontal flap surgery and of gingivitis during gingivectomy. Healthy control tissue specimens from clinically non-inflamed gingiva were taken during the odontectomy of a fully embedded third molar. Although there were no clinically apparent signs of inflammation or pericoronitis, we cannot fully exclude the possibility that some control tissues might have been histologically slightly inflamed, as shown by the presence of some inflammatory cell infiltrates in the lamina propria [24]. The tissue sections were evaluated by an oral pathologist. The periodontitis tissue samples contained the oral, sulcular, and junctional epithelium and lamina propria beneath the epithelium, while healthy control tissues only contained oral epithelium and the lamina propria (since it was impossible to have the sulcular epithelium in this healthy tissue). Thus, we used sulcular epithelium and its lamina propria for periodontitis, while for the healthy tissues, we used its oral epithelium and lamina propria. Additionally, 5 periodontitis-affected gingival tissue samples contained dental plaque biofilm adjacent to the tissue, and the immunoexpression of Td-dentilisin in this plaque was evaluated in addition to the gingival tissue. The biopsy samples were carefully selected according to specific criteria, followed by an evaluation based on histological findings.

2.2. Immunohistochemical Analysis

From the collected gingival tissue samples, periodontitis-affected (n = 9) and healthy (n = 10) tissue specimens were formaldehyde-fixed, processed, and paraffin-embedded for immunohistochemistry. Histological staining was performed on the paraffin-embedded gingival tissue biopsies. Serial sections (4 µm) were deparaffinized using xylene and rehydrated through ethanol series. Sections of each biopsy were histologically stained with hematoxylin and eosin in order to assess the orientation of the tissue structures. Immunoexpression of Td-dentilisin and MMP-8 in the gingival tissue sections was determined by immunohistochemical staining with Td-dentilisin (1:1500 rabbit polyclonal IgG, as described by Al-Samadi et al. [24] and 6 µg/mL MMP-8 rabbit polyclonal antibody [25], respectively. Sections for MMP-8 and Td-dentilisin immunostainings were subject to antigen retrieval using the same following procedure. After deparaffinization, the antigens were retrieved in a citrate buffer using microwaves (MicroMED T/T Mega Histoprocessing Labstation; Milestone Srl, Sorisole, Italy). Endogenous peroxidase activity was inhibited with 3% H_2O_2 in PBS for 15 min. To inhibit non-specific staining, slides were incubated for 1 h at room temperature in normal goat serum from the Vectastain® kit 1:10 in 0.1% BSA-PBS. Slides were then incubated with primary Ab (anti-MMP-8 and Td-dentilisin [1:3000] antibodies) overnight at +4 °C. Biotinylated anti-rabbit IgG from Vectastain® kit

(Vector Laboratories, Burlingame, CA, USA) was used as a secondary antibody (1:200 dilutions in 0.1% BSA-PBS. Slides were then incubated in avidin–biotin–peroxidase complexes. The color was developed in 0.006% H_2O_2 containing 0.023% 3,3′-diaminobenzidine tetrahy-drochloride (DAB) chromogen for 10 min. Slides were washed in PBS three times, with 5 min between each step [24]. The staining of Td-dentilisin was graded as 0 (negative, [9,10,15,16,23]), 0,5 (very low, [+/−]), 1 (low, [+]), 2 (moderate, [++]), and 3 (strong, [+++]). MMP-8 was scored as 0 (negative, [9,10,15,16,23]), 1 (low, [+]), 2 (moderate, [++]), and 3 (strong, [+++]).

2.3. RNA Sequencing and Transcriptomics of Gingival Tissue Biopsies

The gingival tissue samples collected from patients with adult chronic stage III/IV grade B/C CP (n = 18) and the healthy controls (HC, n = 20) were processed for transcriptomic analysis (TRNSCRMS). For periodontitis, the classification and inclusion criteria were radiographic bone resorption, clinical attachment level 5–7 mm, tooth sites with probing depth (PPD) $\geq$6 mm, and enhanced bleeding on probing representing stage III/IV-grade B/C-periodontitis [1,10,11]. For healthy control subjects, the inclusion criteria were no sign of periodontal disease, no gingival/periodontal inflammation, probing depth $\leq$ 3.0 mm, clinical attachment level $\leq$ 3.0 mm, and no bleeding on probing [1,10]. This study was approved by the Regional Ethics Board in Stockholm (number 2008/1935-31/3).

Total RNA was isolated using the Qiagen RNeasy kit (VWR, Stockholm, Sweden). The quality of RNA was assessed using the RNA 6000 NanoLabChip kit of the Bioanalyzer system from Agilent Technologies (Santa Clara, CA, USA). The RNA libraries were prepared and sequenced using the Illumina stranded TruSeq protocol. This involved capturing polyA-RNA with polyT-coated magnetic beads, RNA fragmentation, reverse transcription, second strand synthesis with dUTP incorporation, ligation of sequencing adapters, and PCR amplification of adapter-ligated fragments, following Illumina's provided instructions. The sequence alignment and analysis were performed, as previously described [26].

The RNA-seq data for the selected genes, including MMP-8, MMP-7, MMP-2, TIMP-1, and IL-1β, were further analyzed for differential expressions in CP and HC samples. Additionally, the housekeeping genes glyceraldehyde 3-phosphate-dehydrogenase (GAPDH) was included in the analysis [26]. A flow chart of transcriptomic and immunohistochemical analysis is provided in Figure 1.

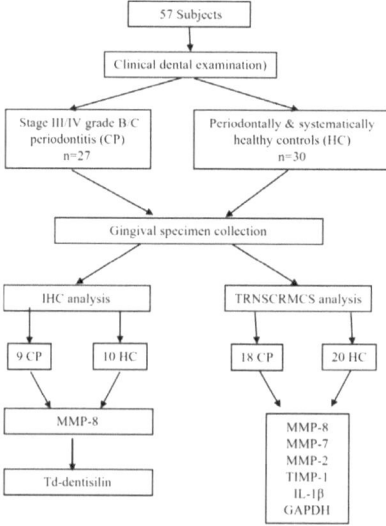

Figure 1. Flow chart of immunohistochemical (IHC) and transcriptomic (TRNSCRMS) analyses.

2.4. Periodontal Anti-Infective Scaling and Root Planing Treatment

Comprehensive periodontal examination, non-antibiotic anti-infective scaling, and root planing periodontal treatment were carried out by a single periodontist. After aMMP-8 POCT test and clinical full mouth recordings at baseline (t0), anti-infective full-mouth scaling and root planing treatment procedures were performed along with oral hygiene instructions for 12 CP patients stage III/IV-grade B/C, a separate set of CP patients [1,9,10]. At 5 (t1) and 10 (t2) weeks after the aMMP-8 POCT testing and the full-mouth clinical examination, anti-infective periodontal treatment was carried out again. The 23–25-year-old systemically and periodontally healthy dental students, who were enrolled as healthy controls (HC, had an aMMP-8 POCT test and full-mouth clinical examination.

1. Chairside PoC and quantitative aMMP-8 analyses;
2. aMMP-8 levels were measured online and in real time quantitatively by a rapid PoC chairside aMMP-8 kits (Periosafe®, Dentognostics GmbH, Solingen, Germany) and a quantitative reader (Oralyzer®, Dentognostics GmbH, Solingen, Germany) from the collected mouth rinse samples from both the periodontitis patient group ($n = 12$) and the healthy control group of 25 systemically and periodontally healthy dental students. Any remaining oral mouth rinse fluid was transferred to Eppendorf tubes and stored at $-70\ °C$ for further laboratory analysis [9,10];
3. Measurement of the aMMP-8 Levels by Immunofluorometric Assay (IFMA)

The aMMP-8 levels from mouth rinse samples were also determined by a time-resolved immunofluorescence assay (IFMA), as described previously [9]. Briefly, aMMP-8-specific monoclonal antibodies 8708 and 8706 (Actim Oy, Espoo, Finland) were used in the analysis as capture and tracer antibodies, respectively. In this protocol, the diluted samples were allowed to incubate for 1 h with the Europium-labeled tracer antibody. The fluorescence was measured using an EnVision 2015 multimode reader (PerkinElmer, Turku, Finland) [10].

2.5. MMP-8 Activity Assay Using Relative Fluorescence Units/Min (RFU)

An MMP-8 activity assay was adapted from the protocol of McCrudden et al. (2017) with slight modifications [27]. The wells of Greiner® 96-well black high binding plates (Merck, Darmstadt, Germany) were coated with 100 µL/well MMP-8 capture antibody (Merck Millipore, Watford, UK), at a concentration of 2 µg/mL in 0.05 M carbonate buffer, pH 9.6. The plate was covered and incubated at $4\ °C$ overnight. The contents of the wells were discarded the following day, and plates were washed three times with phosphate-buffered saline (PBS, pH 7.4) containing 0.05% (v/v) Tween-20 (PBST). A blocking step was then carried out with 200 µL of PBST containing 1% (w/v) bovine serum albumin (BSA) at room temperature for 1 h. Wells were washed three times with PBST and incubated at room temperature for 2 h with 100 µL/well GCF samples or recombinant MMP-8 standard (Bio-Techne, Abingdon, UK). Recombinant MMP-8, supplied in its proform, was activated (as directed by manufacturers) by pre-treatment with 1 mM 4-aminophenylmercuric acetate (APMA) for 1 h at $37\ °C$ prior to use in the MMP-8 activity assay. All GCF samples (prepared at a dilution factor of 1:4), as well as the APMA-activated MMP-8 standards (3.125–100 ng/mL), were diluted in AnaSpec MMP assay buffer (AnaSpec, Fremont, CA, USA) prior to analysis in the MMP-8 activity assay. Duplicate preparations of all samples and standards were carried out in the assay. Following this incubation step, plates were washed three times with PBST. To each well, 45 µL AnaSpec MMP assay buffer was added, followed by 45 µL of 10 µM AnaSpec 520 MMP fluorescence resonance energy transfer (FRET) substrate SB-XIV (AnaSpec, Fremont, CA, USA). Prior to use, the FRET substrate was reconstituted to 1 mM in dimethyl sulfoxide (DMSO) and diluted to 100 µM in MMP Assay Buffer (AnaSpec, Fremont, CA, USA). The substrate was then stored in aliquots at $-20\ °C$. Following the addition of the MMP Assay Buffer and FRET substrate to the wells of the plate, fluorescence measurements were recorded immediately at excitation and emission wavelengths of 485 nm and 525 nm, respectively. Measurements were recorded over a 70 min period, at 5 min intervals, on a microtitre plate reader (Genios, Tecan, Reading, UK) using Magellan software Version 7.2 (Tecan, Reading, UK), and the results were displayed as relative fluorescence units (RFU) per minute (RFU/min) [27].

2.6. Statistical Analysis

MMP-8 and *Td*-dentilisin immunoexpressions (IHC) and transcriptomic (TRNSCRMS) analysis of MMP-8, MMP-7, MMP-2, TIMP-1, IL-1β parameters were calculated by an independent samples *t*-test was performed to assess the significance of differences between CP and HC group in all recorded parameters. The periodontal anti-infective treatment effect, i.e., differences in the levels of the four different MMP-8 assays (aMMP-8 IFMA, aMMP-8 Oralyzer, MMP-8 activity [RFU/minute], and total MMP-8 by ELISA) and the clinical parameters between t0, t1, and t2 were tested with Friedman's test (asymptotic, 2-sided), followed by pairwise post hoc comparisons by Dunn–Bonferroni test. A two-tailed *p*-value < 0.05 was considered statistically significant. Data management and statistical analysis were performed by utilizing spreadsheet software (Microsoft Excel for Mac 16.78) and the SPSS version 29.0 (IBM SPSS Statistics for Windows, IBM Corp., Armonk, NY, USA).

3. Results

Ex Vivo Immunoexpression of Td-Dentilisin and MMP-8 in Human Periodontitis-Affected vs. Healthy Gingival Tissues

Gingival tissue specimens were stained with antibodies to *Td*-dentilisin and MMP-8 to visualize immunoexpressions in CP gingiva compared with HC gingiva. The immunostainings of the *Td*-dentilisin and MMP-8 are shown in Figures 2 and 3, respectively. *Td*-dentilisin could be detected most clearly and intracellularly intensively in the gingival epithelium relative to lamina propria. *Td*-dentilisin immunoexpressions increased according to the severity of periodontitis (stages and grades), indicating the evident invasion route of *Td* and its dentilisin–protease from the superficial dental plaque biofilm into deeper periodontal tissues in vivo. The immunoexpressions of *Td*-dentilisin were significantly stronger in CP-affected tissues than in HC-gingivae ($p < 0.05$) (Figure 2, Table 1). The majority of CP-affected tissues expressed low to moderate *Td*-dentilisin immunopositivity along with the increase in clinical disease severity, while HC-gingivae were negative or had hardly detectable *Td*-dentilisin immunoexpression (score 0–0.5) (Figure 3, Table 1).

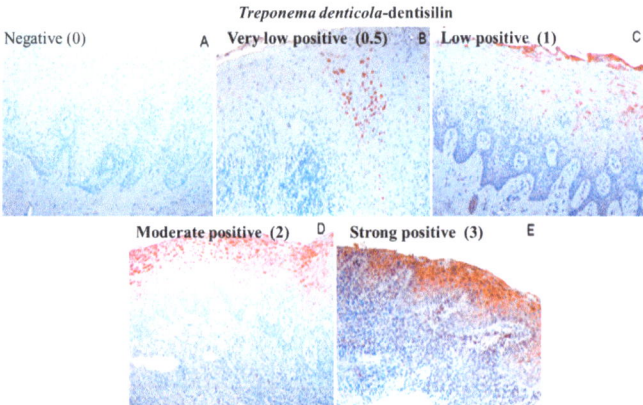

Figure 2. Immunoexpression of *Td*-dentilisin. Gingival tissue specimens were graded and scored as (**A**) negative (0), (**B**) very low-positive (0.5), (**C**) low-positive (1), (**D**) moderate-positive (2), and (**E**) strong-positive (3). The gingival tissue specimens (**A**,**B**) represent periodontitis classification stage I/grade A, specimens (**B**,**C**) stages I–II grade B, and specimens (**D**) stages III–IV/grade C, respectively. The chromogen (red) was 3-amino-9-ethylcarbazole (AEC), and the counterstain was hematoxylin. *Td*-dentilisin was detected in all red-stained regions on each tissue segment. Magnification 200×.

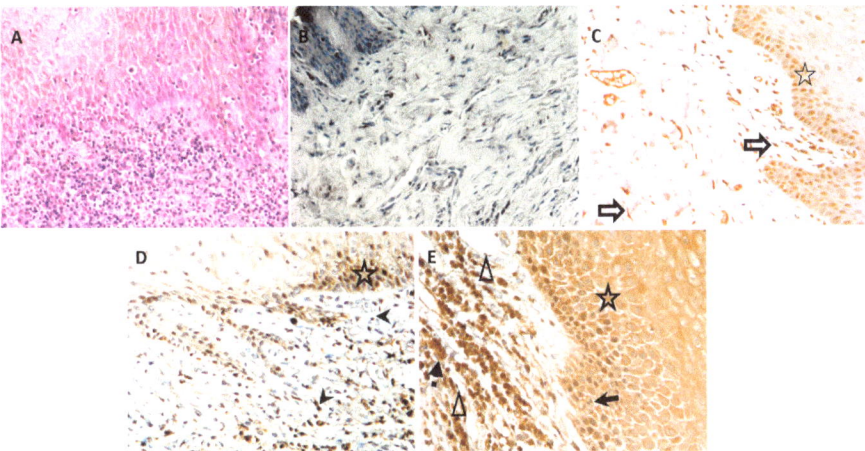

Figure 3. Immunoexpression of MMP-8. (**A**) Hematoxyline eosin staining of the periodontitis gingival tissue. (**B**) Immunohistochemical staining of the gingival tissues is scored as negative (0). (**C**) Low-positive (scored 1). (**D**) Moderate-positive (scored 2). (**E**) Strong-positive (scored 3). The gingival tissue specimen (**C**) represents periodontitis classification stages O–I/grade A; specimen (**D**) represents stages II–III grade B; specimen (**E**) represents stages III–IV grade C. The cells show MMP-8 expression, including epithelial cells (star), neutrophils (black arrow), lymphocytes (arrowhead), macrophage (black arrow with dash), endothelial cells (blank arrowhead/triangle), and fibroblasts (blank arrow) of periodontitis gingival tissues. DAB is used as a chromogen (brown) and hematoxyline as a counterstain. All brown-stained areas on each tissue section indicate specific detection of MMP-8. Magnification 200×.

Table 1. Immunoexpression of *Td*-dentilisin, MMP-8, and RNA expressions of MMP-8 and its regulators MMP-7, MMP-2, TIMP-1, and IL-1β in CP-stages III/IV grades B/C gingivae vs. HC gingivae. In IHC, n = 10 for HC, and n = 9 for CP, and in RNA sequencing/transcriptomics, n = 20 for HC, and n = 18 for CP.

Parameters	Healthy (HC)	Periodontitis (CP)	Significance (p-Value)
Immunohistochemical staining of gingival tissue			
Td-dentilisin	1.00 ± 0.21	2.44 ± 0.06	*, p = 0.0038
MMP-8	1.00 ± 0.20	4.33 ± 0.41	*, p = 0.0001
RNA sequencing/transcriptomics			
MMP-8	0.35 ± 0.62	0.46 ± 0.84	-
MMP-7	1.78 ± 4.17	49.92 ± 106.16	*, p = 0.0280
MMP-2	191.27 ± 138.23	147.05 ± 138.66	-
TIMP-1	47.28 ± 16.62	66.01 ± 49.47	-
IL-1β	14.73 ± 16.78	71.47 ± 61.32	*, p = 0.0001
GAPDH	2491.42 ± 630.29	2596.36 ± 840.13	

* = significantly different, p < 0.05, *t*-test. Abbreviations: MMP-8 = matrix metalloproteinase 8; MMP-7 = matrix metalloproteinase 7; MMP-2 = matrix metalloproteinase 2; TIMP-1 = tissue inhibitor matrix metalloproteinase 1; IL-1β = interleukin 1 beta; GAPDH = glyceraldehyde 3-phosphate-dehydrogenase; HC = healthy control; CP = chronic periodontitis.

In CP, MMP-8 immunoexpression was significantly higher in lamina propria compared to epithelium (p < 0.05). Lamina propria expression of MMP-8 was higher in CP compared with HC-gingivae (p < 0.05). Immunoexpression of MMP-8 in CP-gingivae increased according to the increase in periodontal disease severity (stages and grades). There are no detectable differences in MMP-8 expressions observed between epithelium and lamina propria in HC-gingivae.

The normalized counts for the genes MMP-8, MMP-7, MMP-2, TIMP-1, and IL-1β in CP and HC are demonstrated in Table 1. In CP-gingivae (stages III/IV, grades B/C), the translations of IL-1β and MMP-7 were significantly increased. The elevation of TIMP-1 transcription was noticed without reaching statistical significance (Table 1). MMP-2 translation was reduced in CP-gingivae vs. HC-gingivae without statistical significance. MMP-8 translation was low and similar, barely detectable in either CP-gingivae or HC-gingivae (Table 1). The expression of the housekeeping gene GAPDH was similar in CP- and HC-gingivae (Table 1).

The treatment effects of anti-infective treatment (scaling and root planing) in 12 patients with stages III/IV grades B/C CP-patients were monitored by four different MMP-8 assays (aMMP-8 IFMA, aMMP-8 Oralyzer, rate of MMP-8 activity [RFU per minute] and total MMP-8 ELISA) (Figure 4). Clinical periodontal parameters were also measured (Figure 5). Furthermore, these two figures present the successful treatment's effect assessed by both clinical parameters and by MMP-8 assays' levels of CP-patients vs. HCs. aMMP-8 assays (IFMA, Oralyzer, aMMP-8 activity/RFU assay) more precisely than total MMP-8 assay demonstrated and reflected the clinically beneficial reducing effects of the anti-infective treatment. Furthermore, when comparing MMP-8 assay levels of 12 CP-patients to 25 HCs revealed that only total MMP-8 levels could reach healthy control levels, while aMMP-8 IFMA, aMMP-8 Oralyzer, and aMMP-8 activity (RFU per minute) assays all decrease significantly but did not reach those observed in healthy subjects (Figures 4 and 5).

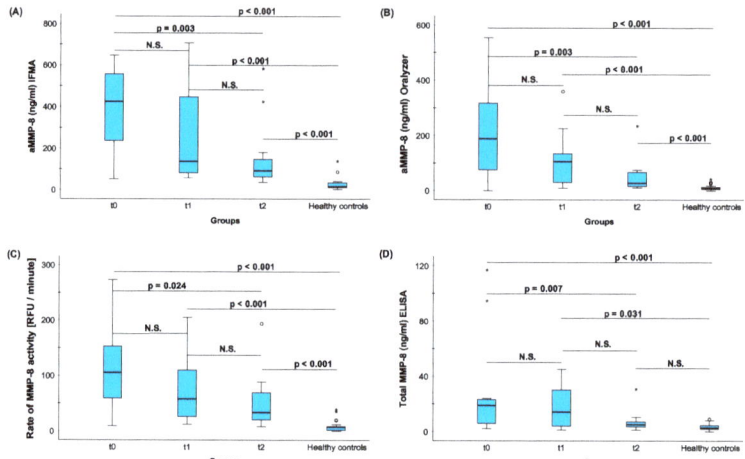

Figure 4. The treatment effects of anti-infective treatment in 12 CP-patients to the aMMP-8 and total MMP-8 levels assessed by four different a/tMMP-8 assays. (**A**) Active matrix metalloproteinase-8 (aMMP-8) (ng/mL) IFMA; (**B**) aMMP-8 (ng/mL) Oralyzer; (**C**) MMP-8 activity assay (RFU per minute); and (**D**) total MMP-8 (ng/mL) ELISA vs. levels in HC. Patients were examined based on baseline level at t0, 1st recall visit t1 (5 weeks), and 2nd recall visit t2 (10 weeks). The differences in a/t MMP-8 assay levels between t0, t1, and t2 were tested with Friedman's test (asymptotic, 2-sided) (**A**) $p = 0.005$, (**B**) $p = 0.005$, (**C**) $p = 0.017$, and (**D**) $p = 0.009$; and pairwise post hoc comparisons by Dunn–Bonferroni test are marked in the plots. The differences between 25 HCs (healthy controls) and 12 CP-patients in t0, t1, and t2 in the four different MMP-8 assay levels calculated by Bonferroni-corrected Kruskal–Wallis test are marked in the plots. Asterisk (*) and circle (o) represent outliers of more than 3 times the interquartile range and between 1.5 and 3 times the interquartile range, respectively.

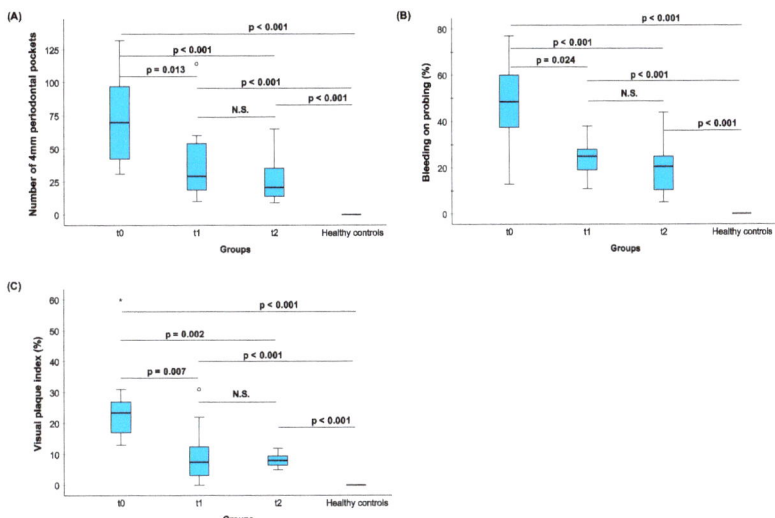

Figure 5. The treatment effects of anti-infective treatment in 12 CP patients to the recorded clinical periodontal parameters. (**A**) The number of at least 4mm periodontal pockets; (**B**) bleeding on probing (%), and (**C**) visual plaque index (%) in relation to HCs. Patients were examined at base level t0, 1st recall visit t1 (5 weeks), and 2nd recall visit t2 (10 weeks). The differences in the clinical parameters between t0, t1, and t2 were tested with Friedman's test (asymptotic, 2-sided) (**A**) $p < 0.001$, (**B**) $p < 0.001$, and (**C**) $p < 0.001$; and pairwise post hoc comparisons by Dunn–Bonferroni test are marked in the plots. The differences between 25 HCs (healthy controls) and 12 CP-patients at t0, t1, and t2 in the recorded clinical indices calculated by Bonferroni-corrected Kruskal–Wallis test are marked in the plots. Asterisk (*) and circle (o) represent outliers of more than 3 times the interquartile range and between 1.5 and 3 times the interquartile range, respectively.

4. Discussion

In the present study, we addressed the regulation of MMP-8 expression in vivo in chronic adult periodontitis gingiva vs. healthy gingiva by immunohistochemical and transcriptomic (TRNSCRMS) analysis. In addition, we compared various aMMP-8 and total MMP-8 assays as adjunctive diagnostic tools to monitor their levels in mouth rinse in periodontal treatment vs. systemically and periodontally healthy controls. MMP-8, also known as neutrophil collagenase (collagenase-2), has been regarded to be solely released by human neutrophilic leukocytes [19–21], but the protease and its RNA have also been identified in the non neutrophil-lineage cells, such as human articular chondrocytes, synovial and gingival fibroblasts, endothelial cells, odontoblasts and T-cell line as well as malignant cells [8,19,22]. Differing from MMP-1 and -2, which are constitutively de novo-transcribed and expressed by various non-malignant and malignant mesenchymal-type cells, MMP-8, after maturation in the bone marrow in latent proform, is prepacked and stored in subcellular specific granules in mature circulating neutrophils (PMNs) [4,7,8,19–21]. MMP-8 regulation at the sites of inflammation is thus regarded to occur mainly through the selective PMN degranulation and activation of the released latent proMMP-8 to active MMP-8 (aMMP-8) [18–21]. In periodontitis, periodontal pathobionts and their proteolytic virulence factors can effectively induce the selective PMN-degranulation and related proteolytic activation of latent proMMP-8 to aMMP-8 in vitro [19–21].

Immunohistochemical results of the present study revealed that the presence of *Td*-dentilisin in CP-gingival tissues was increasingly associated with the increase in MMP-8 immunoexpression along with an increase in clinical stage and grade disease severity of periodontitis. Our present results, thus, further support and extend the concept that the *Td*-dentilisin can eventually invade from the dysbiotic dental plaque biofilm into the diseased periodontitis-affected gingival tissue and up-regulate the degranulation of neutrophils and related activation of the released latent proMMP-8 to aMMP-8 [2,20]. The increased MMP-8 immunoexpression was found not only in epithelium but also in lamina propria. This showed that the inflammation occurred both in epithelium and lamina propria. The inflammatory immune response is triggered by the interaction of resident cells with the bacterial biofilm attached to the tooth surface, including *Td*. The epithelium, especially junctional epithelium, is the first periodontal structure to face the *Td* invasion. Dentilisin produced by *Td* facilitates this spirochaeta to invade and penetrate the deeper epithelium layer [28], stimulating the gingival epithelial cells and the underlying cell in lamina propria to trigger the initial inflammatory responses. The inflammatory response will activate host cells to produce MMP-8 as one of the inflammatory mediators. The MMP-8 secretory cells, being mainly infiltrating neutrophils and also other reported potential non-PMN-lineage cellular sources of MMP-8 in the diseased human inflamed gingiva, including epithelial cells, resident fibroblasts, endothelial cells, and mononuclear inflammatory cells, as shown in this study.

In degranulating mature circulating neutrophils, the de novo expression of MMP-8 cannot be induced as the gene expression is carried out during the neutrophil's maturation in the bone marrow and the latent/inactive MMP-8 is stored in its granules [17–19,21], but in non-PMN-lineage cells, such fibroblasts, endothelial cells, chondrocytes and epithelial cells, de novo expression of MMP-8 and its mRNA is inducible at the sites of inflammations. Our present transcriptomic data of MMP-8 mRNA and its potential regulators (IL-1β, MMP-7, and TIMP-1) mRNAs revealed that MMP-8 RNA was not transcriptionally up-regulated in CP-gingivae vs. HC-gingivae. On the other hand, it is known that the MMP-8's up-regulator's IL-1β mRNA [19,22] and activator MMP-7 mRNA [29] and potential endogenous inhibitor TIMP-1 mRNA can be de novo transcriptionally up-regulated in the diseased periodontitis gingivae [4,7,8,30,31]. Enhanced transcriptional and inductive IL-1β and MMP-7 expressions [4,7,8,30,31] in periodontitis-affected gingiva can eventually potentiate and complement the *Td*-dentilisin-mediated microbial-dependent activation of the degranulated latent proMMP-8 to aMMP-8 [20]. TIMP-1 mRNA up-regulation in the diseased gingiva eventually reflects the host's endogenous defense, attempting to inhibit the elevated MMP-8 and -7 [31].

Previous in vitro studies have shown that IL-1β and other proinflammatory cytokines can up-regulate MMP-8 and its RNA [19,22]. The de novo transcriptomic in vitro expression of MMP-8 and its RNA in articular chondrocytes, gingival, and synovial fibroblast, as well as endothelial cells, has been demonstrated [19,22]. MMP-7 and its RNA can transcriptionally be up-regulated by proinflammatory mediators, including IL-1β and TNF-α previously detected in increasing amounts in diseased and inflamed tissues, including gingiva and synovium [30,31]. Nonetheless, previous in vivo studies have also revealed rather low or barely detectable de novo transcriptional expression of MMP-8 RNA in the diseased periodontitis-affected gingiva and peri-apical periodontitis-affected lesions [31–33]. Our present ex vivo MMP-8 mRNA transcriptomic findings support and further extend those previous in vivo [32–34] rather than the in vitro studies [17,19,22] revealing rather low de novo transcriptional expression of MMP-8 RNA in the periodontitis-affected gingiva vs. healthy gingiva [32–34]. Our present data support the conjuncture that cytokine (IL-1β) induced neutrophil extravasation and selective degranulation together with periodontopathogenic-dependent (*Td*-dentilisin) activation of the released proMMP-8 to aMMP-8 contributes to periodontal tissue destruction [19,20].

The potential benefit and usefulness of utilizing aMMP-8 POCT as the biomarker in the new periodontitis staging and grading categorization have been demonstrated by Sorsa et al. [9], Keskin et al. [10], Deng et al. [15,16], and Sahni [35], as well independently confirmed by Deng et al. [31,32]. The implementation of aMMP-8 as the selected biomarker in the new periodontitis classification was successfully confirmed and further extended in the current study [7,9,10,15,16]. Furthermore, we showed that aMMP-8 levels in HC mouth rinses were significantly lower (i.e., below 20 ng/mL) than aMMP-8 levels in CP patients. These systemically and periodontally healthy adults (HCs) were 23–25-year-old dental students with very good oral health habits who had never experienced periodontal disease [10], and their low aMMP-8 levels indicated no/low risk of collagenolytic disease activity in the near future. Noteworthy, in HCs, the low MMP-8 levels do not represent active MMP-8 but instead represent mainly total latent proMMP-8. In that regard, Ganghar et al. [36], Overall et al. [37], Lee et al. [38], Mancini et al. [39], and Romanelli et al. [40] have shown that in oral fluid of periodontally healthy patients, the MMP-8 is latent proMMP-8 rather than aMMP-8.

In the present study, it was observed that only total MMP-8 decreased back to a healthy control level due to the treatment effect. However, aMMP-8 levels, despite being reduced significantly due to the non-antibiotic anti-infective scaling and root planing treatment affecting and reflecting clinical indices, were not reduced back to healthy control levels (Figure 4). It is possible that when periodontitis develops to stages III/IV grade B/C periodontitis, it is difficult, or almost impossible thereafter, for active collagenolytic activity to reduce back to healthy levels again. Doxycycline, an aMMP-8 inhibitor, can aid in reducing MMP-8 activation but not completely [41]. Furthermore, Romanelli et al. [40], Mancini et al. [39], Gellibolian [42], and Overall et al. [37] have demonstrated by using different and independent collagenase activity assay and immunoassays that the major type of MMP-8 in progressive periodontitis lesions is aMMP-8 and not latent total proMMP-8. MMP-8 is not activated and fragmented in gingivitis, but it is activated and fragmented in periodontitis [40]. In this regard, many studies using total MMP-8 as the oral fluid periodontitis and periimplantitis biomarker have failed. Noteworthy, aMMP-8 is collagenolytic and proteolytic, whereas total latent proMMP-8 is neither collagenolytic nor proteolytic [19,21]. Therefore, it is an aMMP-8 and not a total MMP-8 [43–45], which reflects clinically active and progressive periodontitis in oral fluids [9,10,38–40]. And hence, moving ahead, aMMP-8 should not be regarded as synonymous with total MMP-8 in periodontitis diagnosis [35].

These findings strongly suggest that low aMMP-8 levels (<20 ng/mL), as detected by aMMP-8 POCT, may be regarded as a biomarker of periodontal health [9,10], as determined by independent aMMP-8 catalytic activity assay [27], as well as by aMMP-8 IFMA immunoassay utilizing the same aMMP-8 selective monoclonal antibody [10], as in the aMMP-8 POC test [9,10,35]. All three independent aMMP-8 assays were found to correlate with each other well, and all also reflect clinical indices of periodontal disease before, during, and after successful anti-infective periodontal treatment.

5. Conclusions

Consistent with similar independent tests for aMMP-8, such as the catalytic aMMP-8-RFU activity assay [27] and aMMP-8 IFMA [10], the use of aMMP-8 POCT in chair-side applications lasting only 5 min has been shown to be convenient [9,15,16]. It serves as a reliable method for real-time quantitative diagnostics and ongoing monitoring during periodontal treatment with scaling and root planing, supplementing its effectiveness. Analysis of aMMP-8 levels following successful scaling and root planing treatment indicates a significant reduction, approaching levels observed in healthy individuals. This contrasts with total MMP-8, which lacks precision as a biomarker for periodontitis. Levels of aMMP-8 can be influenced by microbial proteases, such as those released by *Td*, which trigger specific release of neutrophils in the gingiva affected by chronic periodontitis (CP), as well as by the direct action of *Td*-dentilisin, activating MMP-8 to aMMP-8. This mechanism, rather than de novo expression of neutrophil MMP-8 in the gingiva, is a key contributor to tissue damage in CP. The use of aMMP-8 POCT is, thus, advantageous as a supplementary diagnostic, point-of-care, treatment-monitoring, and preventive tool in adult chronic periodontitis.

Author Contributions: N.R.A.S.A., T.Y.-L., I.T.R., H.K., F.T.L., D.L., S.G. and T.S. contributed to the conception and design of this study; N.R.A.S.A., T.Y.-L., H.K., M.T.C.M.C., D.L., A.L. and F.T.L. were involved in data collection; N.R.A.S.A., I.T.R., T.Y.-L., M.T.N., D.L., F.T.L. and T.S. were involved in data analysis and/or interpretation; N.R.A.S.A., T.S. and I.T.R. verified the underlying data. The original draft was written and was critically reviewed and edited by N.R.A.S.A., T.Y.-L., I.T.R., H.K.,

M.T.N., M.T.C.M.C., F.T.L., D.L., A.L., S.G. and T.S. All authors have read and agreed to the published version of the manuscript.

Funding: This research was funded by the Helsinki and Uusimaa Hospital District (HUS), Finland, grant number Y1014SULE1, Y1014SL018, Y1014SL017, TYH2019319, TYH2018229, TYH2017251, TYH2016251, TYH2020337, TYH2022225, Y2519SU010 (T.S.), the Finnish Dental Association Apollonia, Finland (T.S.), and Karolinska Institutet, Sweden (T.S.); the Swedish Research Council (T.Y.-L.); the Patent Revenue Fund for Research in Preventive Odontology (T.Y.-L.); the steering group KI/Region Stockholm for dental research—SOF (T.Y.-L.). Additionally, N.R.A.S.A. received the Indonesian Education Scholarship from PUSLAPDIK and LPDP Republic of Indonesia with a Grant number: 202231103652 for his dissertation work. The funders had no role in the design of this study, in the collection, analyses, or interpretation of data, in the writing of this manuscript, or in the decision to publish the results. Open access funding provided by University of Helsinki.

Institutional Review Board Statement: This study was conducted in accordance with the Declaration of Helsinki and approved by the Regional Ethics Board in Stockholm (Regionala etikprövingsnämnden i Stockholm, EPN) (numbers 2008/1935-31/3 and 2016-08-24/2016/1:8 and 2016-1-24; Dnr 2016/1410-31/1) and the local ethical committee of the Helsinki University Hospital, Finland (106§/26.06.2019; dnro HUS/1271/2019).

Informed Consent Statement: Written informed consent was obtained from all subjects involved in this study.

Data Availability Statement: Data supporting reported that the results can be obtained from the authors on request.

Acknowledgments: Open access funding provided by University of Helsinki.

Conflicts of Interest: Professor Timo Sorsa is the inventor of US patents 5652223, 5736341, 5866432, 6143476, 20170023571A1 (granted 6.6.2019), WO2018/060553A1 (granted 31.5.2018), 10488415B2, a Japanese patent 2016-554676, and South Korean Patent No. 10-2016-7025378. Other authors report no conflicts of interest related to this study. The funders had no role in the design of this study, in the collection, analyses, or interpretation of data, in the writing of this manuscript, or in the decision to publish the results.

References

1. Papapanou, P.N.; Sanz, M.; Buduneli, N.; Dietrich, T.; Feres, M.; Fine, D.H.; Flemmig, T.F.; Garcia, R.; Giannobile, W.V.; Graziani, F.; et al. Periodontitis: Consensus report of workgroup 2 of the 2017 World Workshop on the Classification of Periodontal and Peri-Implant Diseases and Conditions. *J. Periodontol.* **2018**, *89* (Suppl. 1), S173–S182. [CrossRef] [PubMed]
2. Cogoni, V.; Morgan-Smith, A.; Fenno, J.C.; Jenkinson, H.F.; Dymock, D. Treponema denticola chymotrypsin-like proteinase (CTLP) integrates spirochaetes within oral microbial communities. *Microbiology* **2012**, *158 Pt 3*, 759–770. [CrossRef] [PubMed] [PubMed Central]
3. Silva, N.; Abusleme, L.; Bravo, D.; Dutzan, N.; Garcia-Sesnich, J.; Vernal, R.; Hernández, M.; Gamonal, J. Host response mechanisms in periodontal diseases. *J. Appl. Oral Sci.* **2015**, *23*, 329–355. [CrossRef] [PubMed] [PubMed Central]
4. Khuda, F.; Anuar, N.N.; Baharin, B.; Nasruddin, N.S. A Mini Review on the Associations of Matrix Metalloproteinases (MMPs) -1, -8, -13 with Periodontal Disease. *AIMS Mol. Sci.* **2021**, *8*, 13–31, Gale Academic OneFile. Available online: https://go.gale.com/ps/i.do?p=AONE&u=anon~ebca9381&id=GALE%7CA684120359&v=2.1&it=r&sid=googleScholar&asid=f2e29a65 (accessed on 28 February 2024). [CrossRef]
5. Hajishengallis, G.; Chavakis, T.; Lambris, J.D. Current understanding of periodontal disease pathogenesis and targets for host-modulation therapy. *Periodontology 2000* **2020**, *84*, 14–34. [CrossRef] [PubMed]
6. Kinane, D.F.; Stathopoulou, P.G.; Papapanou, P.N. Periodontal diseases. *Nat. Rev. Dis. Primers.* **2017**, *3*, 17038. [CrossRef] [PubMed]
7. Cui, N.; Hu, M.; Khalil, R.A. Biochemical and Biological Attributes of Matrix Metalloproteinases. *Prog. Mol. Biol. Transl. Sci.* **2017**, *147*, 1–73. [CrossRef] [PubMed] [PubMed Central]
8. Chakraborti, S.; Mandal, M.; Das, S.; Mandal, A.; Chakraborti, T. Regulation of matrix metalloproteinases: An overview. *Mol. Cell. Biochem.* **2003**, *253*, 269–285. [CrossRef] [PubMed]
9. Sorsa, T.; Alassiri, S.; Grigoriadis, A.; Räisänen, I.T.; Pärnänen, P.; Nwhator, S.O.; Gieselmann, D.-R.; Sakellari, D. Active MMP-8 (aMMP-8) as a Grading and Staging Biomarker in the Periodontitis Classification. *Diagnostics* **2020**, *10*, 61. [CrossRef]
10. Keskin, M.; Rintamarttunen, J.; Gülçiçek, E.; Räisänen, I.T.; Gupta, S.; Tervahartiala, T.; Pätilä, T.; Sorsa, T. A Comparative Analysis of Treatment-Related Changes in the Diagnostic Biomarker Active Metalloproteinase-8 Levels in Patients with Periodontitis. *Diagnostics* **2023**, *13*, 903. [CrossRef]

11. Arias-Bujanda, N.; Regueira-Iglesias, A.; Balsa-Castro, C.; Nibali, L.; Donos, N.; Tomás, I. Accuracy of single molecular biomarkers in gingival crevicular fluid for the diagnosis of periodontitis: A systematic review and metaanalysis. *J. Clin. Periodontol.* **2019**, *46*, 1166–1182. [CrossRef] [PubMed]
12. Atanasova, T.; Stankova, T.; Bivolarska, A.; Vlaykova, T. Matrix Metalloproteinases in Oral Health—Special Attention on MMP-8. *Biomedicines* **2023**, *11*, 1514. [CrossRef] [PubMed]
13. Arias-Bujanda, N.; Regueira-Iglesias, A.; Balsa-Castro, C.; Nibali, L.; Donos, N.; Tomás, I. Accuracy of single molecular biomarkers in saliva for the diagnosis of periodontitis: A systematic review and meta-analysis. *J. Clin. Periodontol.* **2020**, *47*, 2–18. [CrossRef] [PubMed]
14. Alassy, H.; Parachuru, P.; Wolff, L. Peri-Implantitis Diagnosis and Prognosis Using Biomarkers in Peri-Implant Crevicular Fluid: A Narrative Review. *Diagnostics* **2019**, *9*, 214. [CrossRef] [PubMed]
15. Deng, K.; Pelekos, G.; Jin, L.; Tonetti, M.S. Diagnostic accuracy of a point-of-care aMMP-8 test in the discrimination of periodontal health and disease. *J. Clin. Periodontol.* **2021**, *48*, 1051–1065. [CrossRef] [PubMed]
16. Deng, K.; Wei, S.; Xu, M.; Shi, J.; Lai, H.; Tonetti, M.S. Diagnostic accuracy of active matrix metalloproteinase-8 point-of-care test for the discrimination of periodontal health status: Comparison of saliva and oral rinse samples. *J. Periodontal Res.* **2022**, *57*, 768–779. [CrossRef] [PubMed]
17. A Hasty, K.; Pourmotabbed, T.F.; I Goldberg, G.; Thompson, J.P.; Spinella, D.G.; Stevens, R.M.; Mainardi, C.L. Human neutrophil collagenase. A distinct gene product with homology to other matrix metalloproteinases. *J. Biol. Chem.* **1990**, *265*, 11421–11424. [CrossRef] [PubMed]
18. Devarajan, P.; Mookhtiar, K.; Van Wart, H.; Berliner, N. Structure and expression of the cDNA encoding human neutrophil colla-genase. *Blood* **1991**, *77*, 2731–2738. [CrossRef] [PubMed]
19. Tschesche, H.; Wenzel, H. Chapter 153—Neutrophil Collagenase. In *Handbook of Proteolytic Enzymes*, 3rd ed.; Rawlings, N.D., Salvesen, G., Eds.; Academic Press: Cambridge, MA, USA, 2013; pp. 725–734, ISBN 9780123822192. Available online: https://www.sciencedirect.com/science/article/pii/B9780123822192001538 (accessed on 28 February 2024). [CrossRef]
20. Ding, Y.; Uitto, V.-J.; Haapasalo, M.; Lounatmaa, K.; Konttinen, Y.; Salo, T.; Grenier, D.; Sorsa, T. Membrane Components of Treponema denticola Trigger Proteinase Release from Human Polymorphonuclear Leukocytes. *J. Dent. Res.* **1996**, *75*, 1986–1993. [CrossRef]
21. Weiss, S.J. Tissue destruction by neutrophils. *N. Engl. J. Med.* **1989**, *320*, 365–376. [CrossRef]
22. Cole, A.A.; Chubinskaya, S.; Schumacher, B.; Huch, K.; Cs-Szabo, G.; Yao, J.; Mikecz, K.; Hasty, K.A.; Kuettner, K.E. Chondrocyte Matrix Metalloproteinase-8: HUMAN ARTICULAR CHONDROCYTES EXPRESS NEUTROPHIL COLLAGENASE. *J. Biol. Chem.* **1996**, *271*, 11023–11026. [CrossRef] [PubMed]
23. Deng, K.; Zonta, F.; Yang, H.; Pelekos, G.; Tonetti, M.S. Development of a machine learning multiclass screening tool for per-iodontal health status based on non-clinical parameters and salivary biomarkers. *J. Clin. Periodontol.* **2023**. [CrossRef] [PubMed]
24. Al-Samadi, A.; Kouri, V.; Salem, A.; Ainola, M.; Kaivosoja, E.; Barreto, G.; Konttinen, Y.T.; Hietanen, J.; Häyrinen-Immonen, R. IL-17C and its receptor IL-17RA/IL-17RE identify human oral epithelial cell as an inflammatory cell in recurrent aphthous ulcer. *J. Oral Pathol. Med.* **2014**, *43*, 117–124. [CrossRef] [PubMed]
25. Verhulst, M.J.L.; Teeuw, W.J.; Bizzarro, S.; Muris, J.; Su, N.; Nicu, E.A.; Nazmi, K.; Bikker, F.J.; Loos, B.G. A rapid, non-invasive tool for periodontitis screening in a medical care setting. *BMC Oral Health* **2019**, *19*, 87. [CrossRef] [PubMed]
26. Lundmark, A.; Davanian, H.; Båge, T.; Johannsen, G.; Koro, C.; Lundeberg, J.; Yucel-Lindberg, T. Transcriptome analysis reveals mucin 4 to be highly associated with periodontitis and identifies pleckstrin as a link to systemic diseases. *Sci. Rep.* **2015**, *5*, 18475. [CrossRef] [PubMed]
27. Mc Crudden, M.T.C.; Irwin, C.R.; El Karim, I.; Linden, G.J.; Lundy, F.T. Matrix metalloproteinase-8 activity in gingival crevicular fluid: Development of a novel assay. *J. Periodontal Res.* **2016**, *52*, 556–561. [CrossRef] [PubMed]
28. Listyarifah, D.; Nieminen, M.T.; Mäkinen, L.K.; Haglund, C.; Grenier, D.; Häyry, V.; Nordström, D.; Hernandez, M.; Yucel-Lindberg, T.; Tervahartiala, T.; et al. Treponema denticola chymotrypsin-like proteinase is present in early-stage mobile tongue squamous cell carcinoma and related to the clinicopathological features. *J. Oral Pathol. Med.* **2018**, *47*, 764–772. [CrossRef] [PubMed]
29. Balbín, M.; Fueyo, A.; Knäuper, V.; Pendás, A.M.; López, J.M.; Jiménez, M.G.; Murphy, G.; López-Otín, C. Collagenase 2 (MMP-8) expression in murine tissue-remodeling processes. Analysis of its potential role in postpartum involution of the uterus. *J. Biol. Chem.* **1998**, *273*, 23959–23968. [CrossRef] [PubMed]
30. Tervahartiala, T.; Pirilä, E.; Ceponis, A.; Maisi, P.; Salo, T.; Tuter, G.; Kallio, P.; Törnwall, J.; Srinivas, R.; Konttinen, Y.; et al. The in vivo expression of the collagenolytic matrix metalloproteinases (MMP-2, -8, -13, and -14) and matrilysin (MMP-7) in adult and localized juvenile periodontitis. *J. Dent. Res.* **2000**, *79*, 1969–1977. [CrossRef] [PubMed]
31. Nomura, T.; Takahashi, T.; Hara, K. Expression of TIMP-1, TIMP-2 and collagenase mRNA in periodontitis-affected human gingival tissue. *J. Periodontal Res.* **1993**, *28*, 354–362. [CrossRef]
32. Tonetti, M.S.; Freiburghaus, K.; Lang, N.P.; Bickel, M. Detection of interleukin-8 and matrix metalloproteinases transcripts in healthy and diseased gingival biopsies by RNA/PCR. *J. Periodontal Res.* **1993**, *28*, 511–513. [CrossRef] [PubMed]
33. Aiba, T.; Akeno, N.; Kawane, T.; Okamoto, H.; Horiuchi, N. Matrix metalloproteinases-1 and -8 and TIMP-1 mRNA levels in normal and diseased human gingivae. *Eur. J. Oral Sci.* **1996**, *104*, 562–569. [CrossRef] [PubMed]

34. Fernández, A.; Cárdenas, A.M.; Astorga, J.; Veloso, P.; Alvarado, A.; Merino, P.; Pino, D.; Reyes-Court, D.; Hernández, M. Expression of Toll-like receptors 2 and 4 and its association with matrix metalloproteinases in symptomatic and asymptomatic apical periodontitis. *Clin. Oral Investig.* **2019**, *23*, 4205–4212. [CrossRef] [PubMed]
35. Sahni, V. Point of care technology for screening and referrals. *Br. Dent. J.* **2024**, *236*, 230. [CrossRef] [PubMed]
36. Gangbar, S.; Overall, C.M.; McCulloch, C.A.G.; Sodek, J. Identification of polymorphonuclear leukocyte collagenase and gelatinase activities in mouthrinse samples: Correlation with periodontal disease activity in adult and juvenile periodontitis. *J. Periodontal Res.* **1990**, *25*, 257–267. [CrossRef]
37. Overall, C.M.; Sodek, J.; A McCulloch, C.; Birek, P. Evidence for polymorphonuclear leukocyte collagenase and 92-kilodalton gelatinase in gingival crevicular fluid. *Infect. Immun.* **1991**, *59*, 4687–4692. [CrossRef] [PubMed]
38. Lee, W.; Aitken, S.; Sodek, J.; McCulloch, C.A.G. Evidence of a direct relationship between neutrophil collagenase activity and periodontal tissue destruction *in vivo*: Role of active enzyme in human periodontitis. *J. Periodontal Res.* **1995**, *30*, 23–33. [CrossRef] [PubMed]
39. Mancini, S.; Romanelli, R.; Laschinger, C.A.; Overall, C.M.; Sodek, J.; McCulloch, C.A. Assessment of a novel screening test for neutrophil collagenase activity in the diagnosis of periodontal diseases. *J. Periodontol.* **1999**, *70*, 1292–1302. [CrossRef] [PubMed]
40. Romanelli, R.; Mancini, S.; Laschinger, C.; Overall, C.M.; Sodek, J.; McCulloch, C.A. Activation of neutrophil collagenase in periodontitis. *Infect. Immun.* **1999**, *67*, 2319–2326. [CrossRef]
41. Golub, L.M.; Lee, H.-M. Periodontal therapeutics: Current host-modulation agents and future directions. *Periodontology 2000* **2020**, *82*, 186–204. [CrossRef]
42. Gellibolian, R.; Miller, C.S.; Markaryan, A.N.; Weltman, R.L.; Van Dyke, T.E.; Ebersole, J.L. Precision periodontics: Quantitative measures of disease progression. *J. Am. Dent. Assoc.* **2022**, *153*, 826–828. Available online: https://www.sciencedirect.com/science/article/pii/S0002817722001532 (accessed on 28 February 2024). [CrossRef] [PubMed]
43. Wohlfahrt, J.C.; Aass, A.M.; Granfeldt, F.; Lyngstadaas, S.P.; Reseland, J.E. Sulcus fluid bone marker levels and the outcome of surgical treatment of peri-implantitis. *J. Clin. Periodontol.* **2014**, *41*, 424–431. [CrossRef] [PubMed]
44. Wang, H.; Garaicoa-Pazmino, C.; Collins, A.; Ong, H.; Chudri, R.; Giannobile, W.V. Protein biomarkers and microbial profiles in peri-implantitis. *Clin. Oral Implant. Res.* **2016**, *27*, 1129–1136. [CrossRef] [PubMed]
45. Romero-Castro, N.S.; Vázquez-Villamar, M.; Muñoz-Valle, J.F.; Reyes-Fernández, S.; Serna-Radilla, V.O.; García-Arellano, S.; Castro-Alarcón, N. Relationship between TNF-α, MMP-8, and MMP-9 levels in gingival crevicular fluid and the subgingival microbiota in periodontal disease. *Odontology* **2020**, *108*, 25–33. [CrossRef] [PubMed]

Disclaimer/Publisher's Note: The statements, opinions and data contained in all publications are solely those of the individual author(s) and contributor(s) and not of MDPI and/or the editor(s). MDPI and/or the editor(s) disclaim responsibility for any injury to people or property resulting from any ideas, methods, instructions or products referred to in the content.

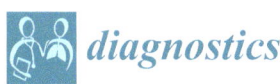

Systematic Review

Exploring the Applications of Artificial Intelligence in Dental Image Detection: A Systematic Review

Shuaa S. Alharbi *[ ] and Haifa F. Alhasson [ ]

Department of Information Technology, College of Computer, Qassim University, Buraydah 52571, Saudi Arabia; hhson@qu.edu.sa
* Correspondence: shuaa.s.alharbi@qu.edu.sa

Abstract: Background: Dental care has been transformed by neural networks, introducing advanced methods for improving patient outcomes. By leveraging technological innovation, dental informatics aims to enhance treatment and diagnostic processes. Early diagnosis of dental problems is crucial, as it can substantially reduce dental disease incidence by ensuring timely and appropriate treatment. The use of artificial intelligence (AI) within dental informatics is a pivotal tool that has applications across all dental specialties. This systematic literature review aims to comprehensively summarize existing research on AI implementation in dentistry. It explores various techniques used for detecting oral features such as teeth, fillings, caries, prostheses, crowns, implants, and endodontic treatments. AI plays a vital role in the diagnosis of dental diseases by enabling precise and quick identification of issues that may be difficult to detect through traditional methods. Its ability to analyze large volumes of data enhances diagnostic accuracy and efficiency, leading to better patient outcomes. Methods: An extensive search was conducted across a number of databases, including Science Direct, PubMed (MEDLINE), arXiv.org, MDPI, Nature, Web of Science, Google Scholar, Scopus, and Wiley Online Library. Results: The studies included in this review employed a wide range of neural networks, showcasing their versatility in detecting the dental categories mentioned above. Additionally, the use of diverse datasets underscores the adaptability of these AI models to different clinical scenarios. This study highlights the compatibility, robustness, and heterogeneity among the reviewed studies. This indicates that AI technologies can be effectively integrated into current dental practices. The review also discusses potential challenges and future directions for AI in dentistry. It emphasizes the need for further research to optimize these technologies for broader clinical applications. Conclusions: By providing a detailed overview of AI's role in dentistry, this review aims to inform practitioners and researchers about the current capabilities and future potential of AI-driven dental care, ultimately contributing to improved patient outcomes and more efficient dental practices.

Keywords: artificial intelligent; diagnostic imaging; diagnosis; deep learning; deep neural networks; machine learning; medical image processing; systematic review

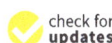

Citation: Alharbi, S.S.; Alhasson, H.F. Exploring the Applications of Artificial Intelligence in Dental Image Detection: A Systematic Review. *Diagnostics* **2024**, *14*, 2442. https://doi.org/10.3390/diagnostics14212442

Academic Editor: Luis Eduardo Almeida

Received: 22 August 2024
Revised: 10 October 2024
Accepted: 12 October 2024
Published: 31 October 2024

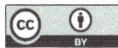

Copyright: © 2024 by the authors. Licensee MDPI, Basel, Switzerland. This article is an open access article distributed under the terms and conditions of the Creative Commons Attribution (CC BY) license (https://creativecommons.org/licenses/by/4.0/).

1. Introduction

Over the last few decades, medical imaging methods such as Computerized Tomography (CT) and X-rays have been used to identify, detect, and treat many illnesses. Moreover, there are various methods for developing rapid diagnosis equipment for dental caries, such as assessing commonly used machine learning approaches on the impacts of annual parenteral examinations, and the use of classification techniques employing two distinct phases: digital image processing and characterization.

From the 1970s to the 1990s, clinical image recognition was initially performed by sequential-based low-level raster production (edge and line spectrometer filters, morphological operation) and numerical methods (appropriate lines, groups, and elliptical) to begin building rule-based mechanisms that solved specific tasks [1,2]. Dental informatics is a new and developing topic in dentistry with the potential to enhance treatment and diagnostics, save time, and lessen stress and exhaustion in daily practice [3,4]. In general, and in dentistry in particular, a variety of types of data are generated, including high-resolution radiography, continuously monitoring biosensors, and electronic records [5]. Computer applications can assist dental professionals in making decisions regarding, among other things, protection, diagnostics, and treatment planning [6].

In a prior Korean survey, only 21% of individuals visited dental centers and hospitals for dental care and examinations [7]. Therefore, the frequency may be much lower in low- and intermediate-income societies where dental inspections are costly and not reimbursed by insurance. Therefore, advanced screening systems that most of the public can conveniently use will help boost the number of dental caries assessments.

Artificial Intelligence (AI) has profoundly advanced the field of dentistry, integrating seamlessly into clinical workflows. It has transformed dentistry by enhancing diagnostic imaging, treatment planning, patient management, and workflow optimization. It improves image analysis, automates charting, and predicts treatment outcomes. It enhances diagnostic imaging through sophisticated algorithms that improve the accuracy of radiographic and CT scan analysis, identifying pathologies such as caries and bone resorption with precision. In treatment planning, AI employs predictive analytics for personalized therapeutic strategies and optimizes orthodontic device fabrication, such as aligners. Furthermore, AI provides real-time clinical decision support and comprehensive risk assessments, improving patient outcomes. It also contributes to professional education through advanced simulation training. Also robotic surgery could used to assist in precise surgical procedures, enhancing accuracy and reducing recovery time. Despite challenges like integration and data privacy, AI significantly boosts efficiency and accuracy in dental practices. Deep learning (DL) has been demonstrated to work well in image-based diagnostics across various disciplines [8]. Convolutional neural networks (CNNs) are a popular option for interpreting medical images in DL applications, which have progressed incredibly quickly over the past decade [9]. In medicine, CNNs have been successfully used to detect skin cancer during skin screenings, diabetic retinopathy during eye examinations, and breast cancer during mammograms [10].

CNNs have lately been used in dentistry to identify apical lesions, caries on bitewing radiographs, and periodontal bone loss, as well as to classify medical images [11,12]. These types of Artificial Neural Networks (ANNs) can be used to segment and classify structures, such as teeth or cavities, as well as to detect them [13]. An image database is required for the training and optimization of ANNs.

This study rationally focused on reviewing the current state of Artificial Intelligence (AI) in dentistry and state-of-the-art applications, including the recognition of teeth cavities, filled teeth, crown predictions, oral surgery, and endodontic therapy.

The purpose of this systematic review is to understand and compare the current applications of machine learning in the care of dental patients. This will enable us to assess their diagnostic and prognostic accuracy. As part of the study, we will identify areas of development for ML applications in the dental care field. In addition, we will suggest improvements to research methodology that will facilitate the implementation of ML technologies in services and improve clinical treatment guidelines based on the results of future studies.

2. Materials and Methods

This review was conducted in accordance with PRISMA guidelines [14] for preferred reporting items for systematic reviews and meta-analyses of diagnostic test accuracy studies.

2.1. Research Questions

1. How\Which the ML\DL Technique can be used to built an efficient dentistry diagnostic support system?

2. What are the possible optimizition techniques used by different methods to improve their performance?
3. What are each optimal methods for each teeth target?
4. What is the future of clinical applications in dentistry filed?

2.2. Data Source

To ensure a comprehensive and relevant collection of data for this systematic review, an extensive search of electronic databases was performed. The selection criteria were carefully designed to capture the forefront of research in artificial intelligence applications within dentistry. This search targeted major databases recognized for their rich accumulation of peer-reviewed articles, including Science Direct, PubMed (MEDLINE), arXiv.org, MDPI, Nature, Google Scholar, Scopus, and Wiley Online Library. The period from January 2013 to February 2024 was covered to include the most recent advances. Keywords were meticulously chosen to reflect critical areas in dental AI research, such as 'teeth segmentation', 'detection of dental caries', and 'computer-aided diagnosis', among others. This strategy was aimed not only at harnessing the most pertinent studies but also at ensuring that the scope of findings remained tightly aligned with the evolving landscape of AI in dental practice. Table 1 below summarizes the databases, time range, and specific keywords that framed our research strategy.

Table 1. Overview of Databases and Keywords Used in Systematic Review of Diagnostic AI Applications in Dentistry (2013–2024).

Database	Search Strategy	Search Data	# of Identify Records
IEEE Xplore			195
Science Direct	"Dental OR Oral OR Dental Diseases OR Periodontal		608
PubMed (MIDLINE)	Disease OR Tooth Decay & Cavities OR Oral Cancer		3000
arXiv.org	OR Gums Disease OR Age Estimation OR Bone	2 August 2024	17
MDPI	Loos" AND "Machine learning OR Deep Learning		70
Nature	OR Artificial intelligence" OR "Full Text OR Paper		251
Scopus	Title" OR "Survey" OR "Overview"		1002
Wiley Online Library			85

2.3. Resources Selection

Full-length articles were retrieved from the journals. As part of the screening process, the two authors organize a focus group in order to ensure that the eligibility criteria and inclusion criteria are met. A list of the titles, authors, dates of publication, places of publication, and full abstracts of the literature obtained through the above-mentioned search protocol was imported into Microsoft Excel 2023. Using the software, duplicates were removed from the list of literature and the remaining article abstracts were screened using eligibility criteria. The required articles for this review study were selected in two stages. The first stage was the selection of articles based on the title and abstracts related to our research topic. The preliminary search yielded 5228 articles that were appropriate to address the study's aim, then due to duplication, 4012 articles were removed. Hence, the two authors retrieved 1216 articles at the second stage of selection. In the next stage, they followed a criterion to include research papers. For the purposes of the review, all authors were satisfied with the exclusion and inclusion of papers. In order to avoid missing relevant literature, criteria were devised after a focus group consisting of the two authors above reviewed preliminary papers. Figure 1 shows the detailed flowchart of our study selection based on PRISMA-DTA methodology.

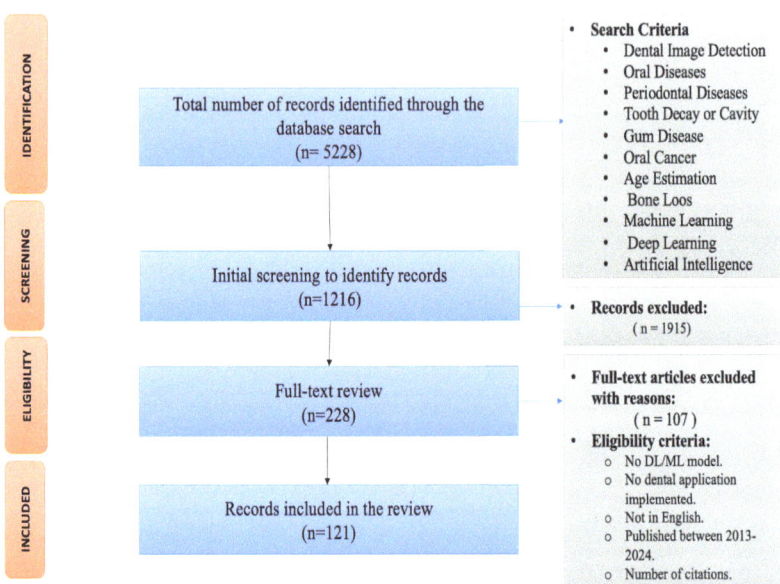

Figure 1. Detailed flowchart of study selection.

2.4. Inclusion and Exclusion Criteria

- The article must be focused on AI, and its application should be one of the related assigned dentistry applications and including the statistical analysis for the results.
- The article must include reference to or creation of datasets that are used to assess a model.

This criterion reduced the number of articles to (121). All the articles were read completely.

2.5. Performance and Accuracy Measures

Our study of the evolution of AI trends in dentistry over the years was based on the developments contained in these articles. As a general rule, the following performance evaluation metrics are most frequently used in the classification, segmentation, and detection of teeth problems: Accuracy, Precision, Sensitivity, Specificity, F1-score, Jaccard index, MAE, RMSE, R2, MRE and SDR. Table 2 summarize the statistical performance indicators used in the analyzed papers.

Table 2. Summary of statistical performance indicators used in the analyzed papers. See notes a–f for detailed definitions and additional information.

Metrics	Formula	Definition
Accuracy	$\dfrac{TP^a + TN^b}{TP + TN + FP^c + FN^d}$	The accuracy of a measurement is the degree to which it is close to the true value.
Precision	$\dfrac{TP}{TP + FP}$	Precision refers to how closely the measurements are related.

Table 2. Cont.

Metrics	Formula	Definition
Recall (Sensitivity)	$\dfrac{TP}{TP + FN}$	The recall indicates whether the model is capable of detecting positive samples.
Specificity	$\dfrac{TN}{TN + FP}$	It is defined as the proportion of true negatives that the model correctly predicts.
F1 score (Dice Coefficient)	$\dfrac{2 \cdot TP}{2 \cdot TP + FP + FN}$	In the F1 score, the precision and recall are calculated as a harmonic mean.
Jaccard index (Intersection over Union (IoU))	$\dfrac{TP}{TP + FN + FP}$	A Jaccard similarity coefficient, also known as the Jaccard index, measures the similarity and diversity of sample sets.
Mean Absolute Error (MAE)	$\dfrac{1}{n}\sum_{i=1}^{n} \lvert(\widehat{y}_i - y_i)\rvert^e$	It is a measure of the difference in error between pairs of observations expressing the same phenomenon.
Root Mean Square Error (RMSE)	$\dfrac{1}{n}\sum_{i=1}^{n} (\widehat{y}_i - y_i)^2$	Typically refers to the difference between the values predicted by a model or an estimator and the values observed.
Correlation Coefficient (R2)	$\dfrac{\frac{1}{n}\sum_{i=1}^{n}(\widehat{y}_i - \underline{y})^2 - \frac{1}{n}\sum_{i=1}^{n}(\widehat{y}_i - y_i)^2}{\frac{1}{n}\sum_{i=1}^{n}(y_i - \underline{y})^2}$	An estimation method based on statistics used to evaluate the performance of a regression model.
Mean Radial Errors (MRE)	$\dfrac{\sum_{i=1}^{n} R_i}{n}{}^f$	It is the mean Euclidian distance between the reference turning point and the predicted point.
Successful Detection Rate (SDR)	$\dfrac{\text{number of accurate samples}}{\text{number of samples}} \times 100\%$	When the error between the estimated coordinates and the correct position is less than a precision range, the estimated coordinates are considered correct.

a—TP is true positive. b—TN is true negative. c—FP is false positive. d—FN is false negative. e—The n indicates the total number of samples. y_i refers to the estimated value, while $\widehat{y}_i$ stands for actual value and $\underline{y}$ demonstrate the true mean value. f—n represents the size of the set, where radial error R is defined as the distance between the predicted coordinates and the actual coordinates based on the Euclidean distance.

Due to the inclusion of accuracy terms in the search criteria, no papers were excluded for containing accuracy measurements not specified in the search criteria.

2.6. Data Synthesis and Analysis

Main characteristics of included caries and teeth targeted studies were used to group the extracted data according to its depth. They were also grouped based on their validation metrics used and their values that allowed direct comparison of data between studies. As part of the study, all outcome measures were extracted and analyzed in a standard format, including a complete definition of accuracy regardless of the measure used by the included papers to document this. In addition, each study included was evaluated based on QUADAS-2 quality assessment [15]. More details can be found later in Section 3.1.

3. Results

In total, 5228 papers were identified in this review paper. After eliminating duplicate titles, we were left with 1216, which were then evaluated for abstracts and excluded based on exclusion criteria (i.e., ref. [16] is excluded because no DL or ML model applied). The remaining articles (n = 228) were reviewed in their full-text forms. Based on the eligibility criteria displayed in Table 1, 121 studies were selected with multiple forms of machine learning. The included papers have been conducted over the past decade (between 2013–2024) as illustrated in Figure 2.

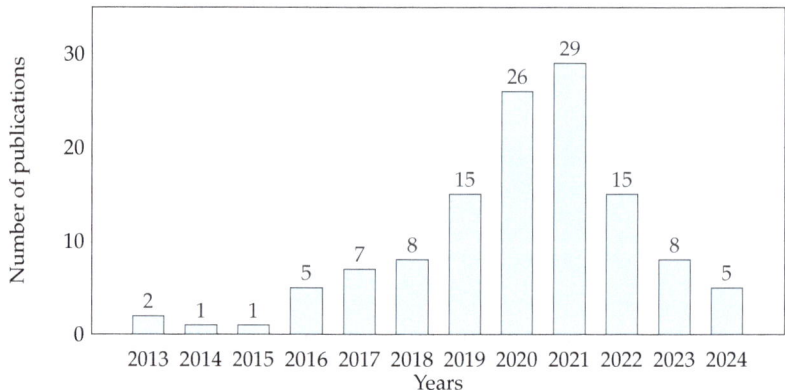

Figure 2. Artificial intelligence in dentistry research trends.

As the study contains many studies with a variety of characteristics and demographics. Tables 3 and 4 provide a comprehensive comparison of study characteristics, Section 4 provide a details description of the included studies. All the papers included in this review were published between 2013 and 2022 and used a different set of data radiography listed before in Table 5. There was a wide variation in the Machine Learning algorithms have been applied across studies. The majority of studies used convolutional neural networks (CNN), U-nets, or R-CNNs. As display in Figure 3, around 60% of the studies used CNNs, including their two extensions, U-net (n = 12) or 3D U-net (n = 3) and faster R-CNN (n = 13) or mask R-CNN (n = 9).

3.1. Risks of Bias Assessment

Throughout all of the studies, AI has been assessed for its diagnostic accuracy in a variety of specific areas of dentistry. QUADAS-2, a commonly used tool in the literature for risk of bias assessment, was used to assess the risk of bias [15]. There was a high level of risk associated with the studies conducted on humans in order to establish the reference standard. There were 7% of studies in the present analysis that reported a high risk of bias for the reference standard. Approximately 7% of the studies in the present analysis reported a high risk of bias regarding the reference standard. As AI technology relies on standardized data feeds, AI had little impact on final output flow or timeframe and was thus classified as a low-risk technology. The current systematic review reported a low risk of bias in the index test and in flow and timing (50%). However, the applicability arm of QUADAS-2 provided comparable results, as shown in Figure 4.

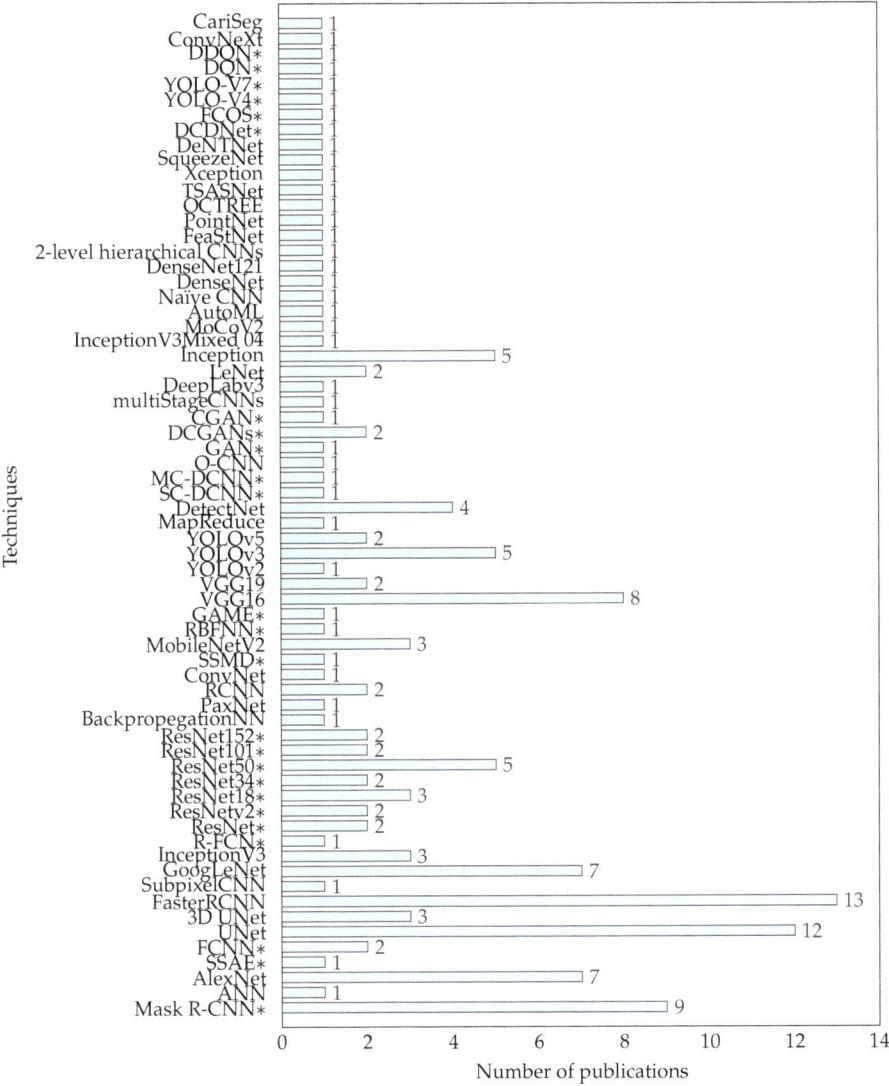

Region-based CNN (RCNN), Stacked Sparse Autoencoder Encoders (SSAE), Fully Connected Neural Networks (FCNN), Region-based Fully CNN (RFCN), Residual Networks (v2,18,34,50,101, 152), Single Shot MultiBox Detector (SSMD), Radial Basis Functions NN (RBNN), Group of Adaptive Models Evolution (GAME), Highly-Scalable Deep CNN (SCD-CNN), Multi Channel-Deep CNN (MCDCNN), Generative Adversarial Network (GAN), Deep Convolutional GAN (DCGANs), Conditional GAN (CGAN), Dental Caries Detection Network (DCDNet), Fully Convolutional One-Stage (FCOS), You Only Look Once V4 (YOLO-V4),You Only Look Once V7 (YOLO-V7), Deep Q-Networks (DQN) and Double Deep Q-Networks (DDQN). The bar chart depicts the number of publications included in this review (n=116), in which each type of machine or deep learning was referenced by an outcome measure.

Figure 3. Graphical display of machine and deep learning models in included studies, where (*) indicates the full name of the model.

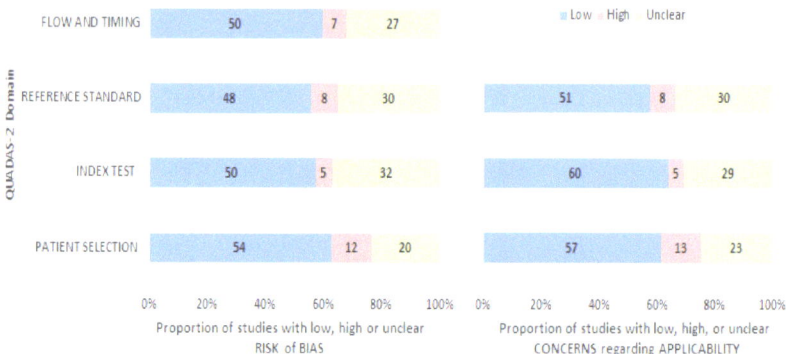

Figure 4. QUADAS-2 quality assessment graphs depict individual bias risk and concerns regarding applicability.

There is a great deal of interest in the topic of teeth caries as shown in Table 3. In some approaches, caries were detected in a large or small dataset, while in others, caries depth was used to determine treatment protocols.

The most notable growth in dental segmentation and classification, as shown in Table 4 can be summarized in two points:

1. In the segmentation domain, graph-based CNN overcomes many other segmentation methods due to the graph's ability to avoid ambiguous labeling of other teeth [17]. Some approaches yielded good accuracy in detecting the 3D dental model using the 3D CNN model based on hierarchical voxel OCTREE and conditional random field CRF model [18].
2. In the classification domain, several studies focused on classifying the teeth, such as [19–21]. Some studies used the same models to detect the problems that affect the teeth [22] or their condition [23].

The most widely used network to enhance outcomes of teeth detection and teeth numbering is faster R-CNN because of its algorithm for selectively generating search region proposals.

Assessment measurement are varieties among included studies. Summarize of these assessment measurement describe in Table 2. According to Tables 3 and 4, there were 11 out of 29 using Accuracy as assessment measurement. To this end, it is important to note that [24] and have unclear information about the value of accuracy test for their approach.

A shown in Figure 5b, panoramic X-ray images are the most popular radiographic method used in the literature [13,25]. In panoramic dental X-rays, a relatively modest dosage of ionizing radiation is used to produce an image that includes the whole mouth. Therefore, this type of image is more suitable in diagnoses of teeth diseases, in order to plan root treatment [26,27], in diagnosis of gum [28,29] and jaw bone [30] diseases. In addition, it is frequently used by dentists and oral surgeons in routine practice or for non-medical purposes such as age estimation [24] or for preprocessing tasks such as teeth numbering [4], classification [31] and segmentation [32]. The techniques of NN and AI can be applied to a variety of radiological studies, such as the periapical X-ray and the CBCT. However, there is a shortage of data availability for both periapical X-rays and CBCT. It is worth to mention missing information regarding the dataset. Some methods [33,34] have missing data such as radiography type and number of images. Others such as [21] has missing number of images used in there method.

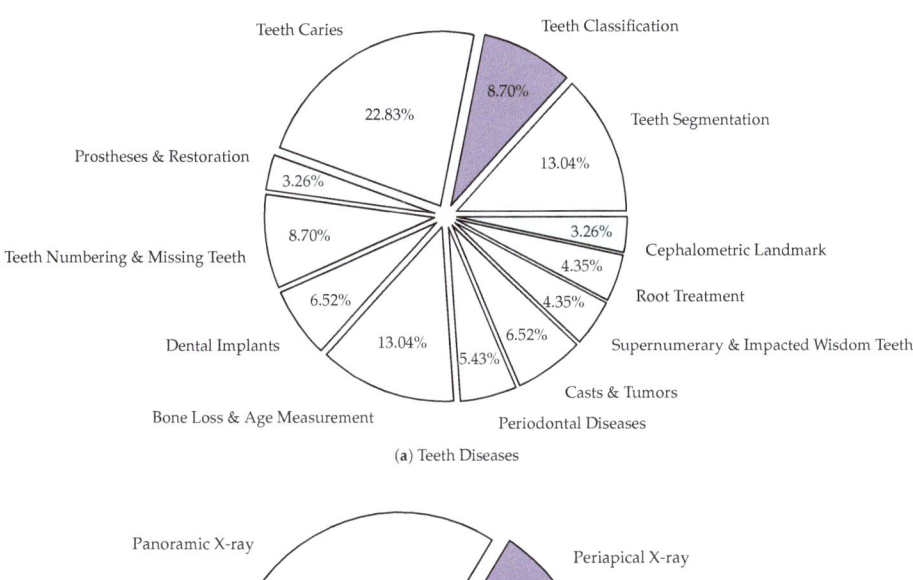

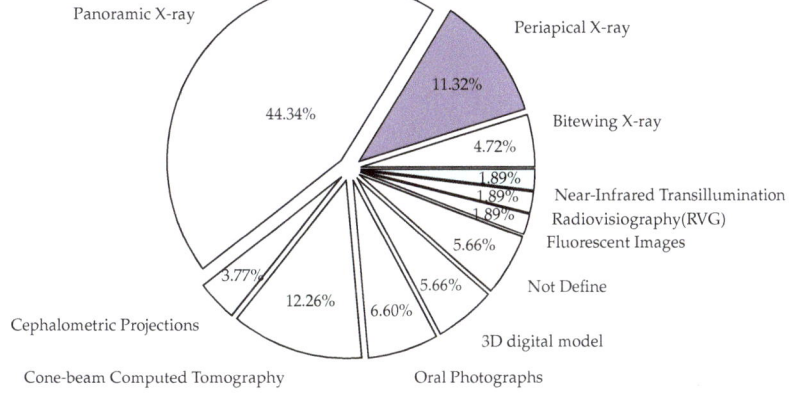

Figure 5. The focus distribution of dental detection: (**a**) Percentage of research published based on the types of teeth diseases, (**b**) Percentage of research published based on the types of radiography images.

4. Machine Learning/Deep Learning for Dental Disease Detection

Currently, there is a growing interest in applying Artificial Intelligent (AI) strategies and image processing for medical image classification, detection, segmentation, and analysis. Generally, many dental applications and different modalities are used in dental imaging [13]. Some researchers design applications for specific types of dental diseases, while others focus on distinguishing and recognizing different variables, such as distinguishing the teeth from other tissues.

4.1. Caries Targeted Studies

Early detection of dental caries (a.k.a cavity) can prevent tooth damage and save expensive healthcare costs. Thus, an effective modality for the early detection of dental caries is a crucial subject in dental research [35]. From 2015 to 2024, twenty four studies were conducted on dental caries. The details of these studies can be found in Supplementary File Section (S1.1).

Table 3 summarizes the main characteristics and outcomes that were measured of included (caries) targeted studies.

Table 3. Main characteristics of included caries targeted studies.

Author	Year	Journal Rank (SJR)/ Conference Rank (Qualis)	Radiography	# of Images	ML/DL Model	Validation Metrics	Values
Ali et al. [33]	2016	B3	—	—	Stacked Sparse Autoencoder Encoders (SSAE)	AUC ROC	97%
Prajapati et al. [36]	2017	Not Yet Assigned	Radiovisiogra-phy image	251	—	Accuracy	0.875
Srivastava et al. [37]	2017	ArXiv	Bitewing	3000	FCNN (deep fully CNN)	Recall, Precision, F1-Score	0.805, 0.615, 0.7
Hatvani et al. [38]	2018	Q1	CBCT	5680 cross-sectional and 1824 slices	U-net & Subpixel CNN	Peak Signal-to-Noise Ratio(PSNR) Similarity index	0.9101
Lee et al. [39]	2018	Q1	Periapical image	3000	GoogLeNet Inception v3	Accuracy, AUC	premolar, molar, and both premolar and molar: 0.89, 0.88, 0.82, 0.917, 0.89, 0.845
Zhang et al. [40]	2018	Q1	Periapical	700	Faster-R-CNN,region-based fully convolutional networks (R-FCN)	Precision, Recall	0.958, 0.961
Casalengo et al. [41]	2019	Q1	Near-infrared transillumination	217	U-net	AUC	0.836 (occlusal lesion) and 0.856 (proximal lesion)
Schwendicke et al. [10]	2019	Q1	Near-infrared light transillumination	226	ResNet18 ResNet50	AUC, Sensitivity, Specificity and Positive,Negative predictive Values (PPV/NPV)	0.74, 0.59, 0.76
Geetha et al. [42]	2020	Not Yet Assigned	Radiovisiography image	105	Back-propagation NN	Accuracy, Precision, Recall	0.971, 0.987
Haghanifar et al. [43]	2020	ArXiv	Panoramic X-rays	470	PaXNet	Accuracy, Recall	86.05%, 69.44%, 90.52%

Table 3. *Cont.*

Author	Year	Journal Rank (SJR)/ Conference Rank (Qualis)	Radiography	# of Images	ML/DL Model	Validation Metrics	Values
Lee et al. [44]	2020	Q2	Panoramic X-rays	846	R-CNN	F1 score, precision, Recall, mean Intersection over Union (IoU)	0.875, 0.858, 0.893, 0.877
Sonavane et al. [45]	2021	Not Yet Assigned	Oral photographs	74	Sequential model	Accuracy	71.43%
Sonavane et al. [45]	2021	Q1	Bitewing	304	U-Net	Precision, Recall, F1-score	63.29%, 65.02%, 64.14%
Bui et al. [46]	2021	Q2	Panoramic X-rays	533	Fusion feature and deep activated	Accuracy, Sensitivity, Specificity	91.70%, 90.43%, 92.67%
Ding et al. [47]	2021	Q3	Oral photographs	3990	YOLOv3	mAP, Precision, Recall, F1-score, AP	56.20%, 76.92%, 49.59%, 55.63%
Zheng et al. [48]	2021	Q3	Panoramic X-rays	844	VGG19, Inception V3, ResNet18	Accuracy, Precision, Sensitivity, Specificity	0.82, 0.81, 0.85, 0.82
Cantu et al. [49]	2020	Q1	Bitewing	3686	U-Net	Intersection-over-Union (IoU)	0.80
Zhang et al. in [50]	2022	Q1	Oral photographs	3932	ConvNet, Single Shot MultiBox Detector	AUC, Confidence interval	85.65% (95%, 82.48% to 88.71%).
kuhnisch et al. [51]	2022	Q1	Oral photographs	2417	MobileNet-V2	Sensitivity, Specificity and AUC	89.6%, 94.3%, 0.964
Day et al. [52]	2023	Q2	Panoramic X-rays	746 occlusal, 1627 proximal and 378 cervical caries	DCDNet	F-score, mIoU and Accuracy	97.79% 93.64%, 93.61%
Esmaeilyfard et al. [53]	2024	Q1	CBCT	382 (with caries) and 403 (noncarious)	Multiple-input CNN	Accuracy, Sensitivity, Specificity and F-score	95.3%, 92.1%, 96.3%, 93.2%
Chaves et al. [54]	2024	Q1	Bitewing X-ray	425	Mask-RCNN	ROC, Sensitivity, Specificity and F-score	0.806, 0.804, 0.689, 0.719

4.2. Teeth Targeted Studies

4.2.1. Teeth Segmentation

Teeth detection has been a research subject for at least the last two decades, mainly relying on threshold and region-based, and machine learning methods [55]. This paper explores the progress made through machine/deep learning methods in segmenting teeth. The segmentation of teeth from different radiography images has been investigated in sixteen studies. Supplementary File Section (S1.2.1) contains details of these studies.

4.2.2. Tooth Classification

This section contains the tooth classification methods that classify the type of teeth, the problem affecting the teeth, or the condition. Other classification studies focusing on solving other dental fields are distributed in other sections. The classification of tooth types was carried out in seven studies between 2012 and 2024. Where tow study proposed to classified different teeth problems. In addition, there are two other studies that aimed to classified the conditions of teeth. These studies are described in Section (S1.2.2) of the Supplemental File.

4.2.3. Detection of Prostheses and Restorations

Dental Prostheses are dental appliances that a dentist can use to replace or restore a missing tooth or missing parts of tooth structure, or structures that need to be removed to prevent decay. These various prostheses include fillings, crowns and bridges, all of which may cause pain in the future. There have been four studies conducted to detect different types of crowns and dental materials. The Supplemental File contains an overview of these studies in Section (S1.2.3).

4.2.4. Teeth Numbering and Missing Teeth

An important part of a dentist's diagnostic process is the evaluation of dental radiographs. The detection and numbering of teeth is part of the interpretation process carried out by a dental expert. Dental implant placement requires the detection of missing teeth regions. There have been nine studies conducted for teeth numbering and detecting missing teeth. There is a brief overview of these studies in Section (S1.2.4) of the Supplemental File.

4.2.5. Detection of Dental Implants

The application of deep learning offers promising performance in computer vision tasks, and is especially suitable for the analysis and recognition of dental images in dental implants [56]. The detection of dental implants has been the subject of eight papers in this systematic review. In the supplemental file, Section (S1.2.5) provides a brief overview of these studies.

4.2.6. Detection of Bone Loss (Osteoporosis) and Bone Age Measurement (BAM)

In clinical practice, peri-implant bone level detection relies on imaging findings. Commonly used imaging modalities include CBCT (2 studies), panoramic radiography (2 studies), and periapical radiography (6 studies). Furthermore, there are four studies available to estimate the age based on different dental images. These studies is summarized in Section (S1.2.6) of the Supplemental File.

4.2.7. Detection of Periodontal Diseases

A periodontal disease is an oral inflammation that affects the gingival tissues as well as the tissues supporting the teeth. Aside from the fact that they cause tooth loss, they are also linked to cardiovascular diseases, diabetes, and rheumatoid arthritis. There are six papers for detection of periodontal diseases included in this review. The Supplemental File contains a summary of this study in Section (S1.2.7).

4.2.8. Detection of Cysts and Tumors

There are six papers for detection of cysts and tumors are included in this review. An overview of this study can be found in Section (S1.2.8) of the Supplemental File.

4.2.9. Supernumerary and Impacted Wisdom Teeth Detection

"Supernumerary teeth" refer to teeth that are not part of the deciduous or permanent teeth series. Five papers are available for the detection of supernumerary and impacted wisdom teeth. Section (S1.2.9) of the Supplemental File provides an overview of these studies.

4.2.10. Detection of Root (Endodontic) Treatment

There are four papers available regarding the detection of root treatment. Endodontic treatment can be adversely affected by an extra root on the distal root of the mandibular (lower jaw) first molar [57]. An overview of these studies is provided in Section (S1.2.10) of the Supplemental File.

4.2.11. Detection of Cephalometric Landmark

A growing role has been played by quantitative cephalometry in clinical diagnosis, treatment, and surgery. It is essential to develop fully automated methods for these procedures in order to ensure that computerized analyses are accurate. In this systematic review, five papers discuss the detection of cephalometric landmarks. The Supplemental File provides a brief overview of these studies in Section (S1.2.11). Table 4 summarizes the main characteristics of the teeth-targeted studies and all outcomes measured in the study.

4.3. Different Dental X-Ray Images

Many types of images, especially the X-ray, have been used in the literature [25]. In the dentistry field, there are different types of X-ray detectors: Orthopantomogram (OPG) and Radiovisiography (RVG). The X-ray image produced using the OPG detector shows both the upper and lower teeth in one image. While RVG takes intraoral radiographs which are useful for diagnosing an individual tooth [36]. In general, there are different types of dental X-rays that dentist uses to evaluate the oral health of teeth:

4.3.1. Intraoral X-Rays Images

The most widely used form of dental X-ray in dental clinics. These X-rays give great information about individual teeth, allowing the dentist to track overall dental and jawbone health. In this type of X-ray image, the film is placed inside the mouth of the patient. There are several types of intraoral X-rays, each showing different aspects of teeth: Bitewing X-rays, Periapical X-rays, and Occlusal X-rays.

Table 4. Main characteristics of included teeth targeted studies.

Author	Year	Journal Rank (SJR)/ Conference Rank (Qualis)	Variable Measured	Radiography	# of Images	ML/DL Model	Validation Metrics	Values
Velemínská et al. [24]	2013	Q2	Age Estimation	Panoramic X-rays	1393	RBFNN GAME	Accuracy	-
Oktay et al. [31]	2017	Not Yet Assigned	Tooth classification	Panoramic X-rays	105	AlexNet	Accuracy, Precision recall	0.971, 0.987
Miki et al. [19]	2017	Q1	Tooth classification	CBCT	52	AlexNet	Accuracy	0.88
Raith et al. [34]	2017	Q1	Tooth classification	-	-	ANN	Performance	0.93
Jader et al. [32]	2018	B1	Tooth segmentation	Panoramic X-rays	1500	Mask R-CNN	Precision, Accuracy, Recall, F1-score, Specificity	0.98, 0.88, 0.94, 0.84, 0.99
Lee et al. [12]	2018	Q2	Periodontal diseases	Periapical images	1740	VGG-19	Accuracy	81.0%
Moriyama et al. [58]	2019	B4	Periodontal Pockets	Oral images	2625	YOLOv2, MapReduce	Accuracy, True Positive Rate (TPR), False Positive Rate (FPR), AUC	91.7%, 93.2%, 6.8%, 0.917%
Chen et al. [59]	2019	Q1	Teeth numbering/Missing teeth	Periapical images	1250	Faster R-CNN	Recall, Precision	0.728, 0.771
Ariji et al. [28]	2019	Q1	Cysts and Tumors	Panoramic X-rays	210	DetectNet	Intersection over Union (IoU)	0.88
Tuzoff et al. [4]	2019	Q1	Teeth detection/Teeth numbering	Panoramic X-rays	1352	Faster R-CNN and VGG16	Sensitivity, Precision	0.9941, 0.9945
Lee et al. [30]	2019	Q1	Bone Loss	Panoramic X-rays	1500	SC-DCNN, MC-DCNN	AUC	0.9763, 0.9991 and 0.9987, respectively

Table 4. *Cont.*

Author	Year	Journal Rank (SJR)/ Conference Rank (Qualis)	Variable Measured	Radiography	# of Images	ML/DL Model	Validation Metrics	Values
Vinayaha-lingam et al. [60]	2021	Q1	Teeth classification	Panoramic X-rays	400	MobileNet-V2	Accuracy, Sensitivity, Specificity, AUC	0.87, 0.86, 0.88, 0.90
Siva-sundaram et al. [61]	2021	Q2	Cysts and Tumors	Panoramic X-rays	–	Modified LeNet	Accuracy, Sensitivity	99.63% 98.3%
Chandr-ashekar et al. [62]	2022	Q1	Teeth segmentation	Panoramic X-rays	1500	Faster R-CNN and YOLOv5	AUC	98.77%
Oztekin et al. [63]	2022	Q2	Prostheses and Restorations	Panoramic X-rays	250	U-Net and YOLOv5	Accuracy	99.81%
Widiasri et al. [64]	2022	Q1	Bone Loss	CBCT	75	3D U-Net	Accuracy	95.3%
Seo et al. [65]	2022	Q2	Age Estimation	Cephalometric projections	900	DeepLabv3 and Inception-ResNet-v2	Accuracy, IoU, F1 scores	0.956, 0.913, 0.895
Atas et al. [66]	2022	ArXiv	Age Estimation	Panoramic X-rays	1332	InceptionV3 and InceptionV3Mixed 04	MAE, RMSE, R2	3.13, 4.77, 87%
Chen et al. [21]	2021	Q1	Teeth classification	3D dental model	–	DCGANs	Accuracy, macro precision, macro-recall, and macro-F1	91.35%, 91.49%, 91.29%, 0.9139
kim et al. [67]	2021	Q1	Cephalo-metric Landmark	CBCT	430	multi-stage CNNs	SDR, MRE	87.10% and 1.03 mm average MRE.
Yu et al. [68]	2022	Q1	Cysts and Tumors	Panoramic X-rays	10,000 healthy images and 872 lesion images	Two-branch network architecture (MoCoV2, U-Net)	Accuracy, Precision, Sensitivity, Specificity, F1 score	88.72%, 65.81%, 66.56%, 92.66%, 66.14%

Table 4. *Cont.*

Author	Year	Journal Rank (SJR)/ Conference Rank (Qualis)	Variable Measured	Radiography	# of Images	ML/DL Model	Validation Metrics	Values
Mine et al. [69]	2022	Q1	Supernumerary Teeth	Panoramic X-rays	220	AlexNet, VGG16-TL, InceptionV3-TL	Accuracy, Sensitivity, Specificity, ROC curve	84.0%, 85.0%, 83.0%
Almalki et al. [70]	2022	Q1	Teeth classification	Panoramic X-rays	1200	YOLOv3	Accuracy	99.33%
Xie et al. [71]	2023	Q1	Teeth Segmentation	CBCT	1000	FCOS	Dice index	–
Rubiu et al. [72]	2023	Q2	Teeth Segmentation	Panoramic X-rays	1000	Mask-RCNN	Accuracy, Dice index	98.4%, 0.87
Yilmaz et al. [73]	2023	Q2	Teeth Classification	Panoramic X-rays	–	RCNN	–	–
Yilmaz et al. [73]	2023	Q2	Teeth Classification	Panoramic X-rays	1200	RCNN and YOLO-V4	precision, recall, F1 score	99.90%, 99.18%, 99.54% for YOLO-V4
karaoglu et al. [74]	2023	Q1	Teeth Numbring	Panoramic X-rays	2702	Mask RCNN	precision, recall, F1 score	92.49%, 96.08%, 95.65% and 95.87%
Park et al. [75]	2023	Q1	Dental Implants	Panoramic and Periapical radiographic	156,965	customized DL model	Accuracy, Precision, Recall, F1 score	88.53%, 85.70%, 82.30%, 84.00%
Hong et al. [76]	2023	Q1	Cephalo-metric Landmark	CBCT	500	DQN and DDQN	Accuracy	67.33% and 66.04%
Ayhan et al. [77]	2024	Q1	Teeth detection /Teeth numbering	Bitewing X-ray	1170	Improved YOLOv7	Accuracy, Recall, Specificity, Precision and F1-Score	0.934, 0.834, 0.961, 0.851, 0.842
Kurtulus et al. [78]	2024	Q2	Dental Implants	Panoramic X-rays	1258	VGG16, ResNet-50, EfficientNet, ConvNeXt	Accuracy, Precision, Recall, F1-score	95.74%, 96.01%, 94.72% 95.22%
Marginean et al. [79]	2024	Q1	Teeth Segmentation	Panoramic X-rays	150	CariSeg	Accuracy, Dice coefficient	99.42%, 68.2%

4.3.2. Extraoral X-Rays Images

Extraoral X-ray images are diagnostic tools used to capture detailed views of the teeth, jaw, and facial structures from outside the mouth, aiding in comprehensive dental assessment and treatment planning. Dentists use various extraoral X-rays, such as Panoramic X-rays, Cephalometric Projections (CP), and Cone-beam Computed Tomography (CBCT). These imaging techniques provide comprehensive views of dental structures, aiding in accurate diagnosis and effective treatment planning. Panoramic X-rays offer a wide view of the jaw and teeth, while CP focuses on the skull and jaw relationships offer insights into the relationships between the jaw and skull, crucial for orthodontic planning. In addition, AI in 3D dental imaging enhances diagnostics and treatment planning by analyzing CBCT scans to accurately identify issues like cavities and fractures. CBCT stands out by providing high-resolution 3D images, allowing for precise diagnosis and treatment planning, particularly in complex cases like implants and orthodontics. These 3D images provide a detailed view of dental structures, aiding in the creation of precise treatment plans for implants and orthodontics by simulating scenarios and predicting outcomes. These advancements in 3D imaging enhance the dentist's ability to accurately identify and address dental issues, ultimately improving patient outcomes. Automated measurements and AI-generated models improve efficiency and patient communication, while predictive analytics aid in informed decision-making. CBCT provides detailed 3D images, crucial for complex procedures like implants and orthodontics, ensuring precise assessments and interventions.

4.3.3. Oral Photographs

Oral images can be captured with the help of a consumer camera in a cost-effective and simple manner. It has become increasingly common for consumers to carry cameras, including smartphones, which are easy to use and have enhanced functionality [50,80].

4.3.4. Near-Infrared Transillumination

Near-infrared transillumination (TI) is a promising and effective imaging technique for the detection of early teeth lesions (i.e., caries) in real-time without film [41,81]. Increased mineral loss (caries lesion) leads to an increase in scattering and absorption of light. Therefore, caries appears as dark regions because less light reaches the detector [81].

4.3.5. Fluorescent Imaging

Fluorescence occurs when a substance absorbs higher-energy light and then emits light (photons). It is more intense in the dentine than in the enamel in natural teeth, and it has a bluish-white color [82].

4.3.6. 3D Digital Dental Model

In addition to intraoral scanning technology, digital dental models can be obtained through advancements in digital technology. A resinic dental model can then be created using the stereolithographic data collected from the scanner [83]. Table 5 summarizes the different characteristics and usage of X-ray images.

Table 5. Main characteristics and usage of dental X-ray images in literature.

Type	Publication Used	Variable Measured	Sample Image	Features
Bitewing X-rays	[37,49,54,77,84–86]	Caries detection (posterior initial proximal caries)		Accuracy

Table 5. Cont.

Type	Publication Used	Variable Measured	Sample Image	Features
Occlusal X-ray	N.A	Detecting abnormal, extra teeth, jaw fractures, a cleft palate, cysts and abscesses		Displaying a section or entire arch of teeth in the upper or lower jaw
Periapical X-rays	[12,39,40,59,86–93]	Diagnosing invisible proximal dental caries		Display the entire tooth, from the crown to the root, where it connects to the jaw.
Radiovisiography (RVG)	[36,42]	Diagnosis of an individual tooth and classification of dental diseases.		No films placed inside the patient mouth.
Cephalometric projections	[65,94–96]	Orthodontic treatment planning. It captures a single film's anterior, posterior, and lateral image of the skull bones and soft tissues.		Typically collected from individuals who need orthodontic or orthognathic surgery.
Cone-beam Computed Tomography (CBCT)	[19,38,53,64,67,93,97–104]	Endodontics, orthodontics, implant, oral surgery, and oral medicine		High resolution 3D volumetric data.
Panoramic X-rays	[4,11,20,22–24,26,27,30–32,43,44,57,58,60–63,66,68,69,89,105–127]	Full visualization of jaw, such as tumors, teeth included, infections, post-accident fractures, temporomandibular joint disorders		Captured outside the mouth which makes them more acceptable for the patient, they cause a lower infection rate, and lower radiation exposure, they are simple to apply and require less time but they are the most challenging type due to uneven lighting, the presence of noise and low resolution.
Ora Photographs	[50,51,58,89,128–131]	Gathered by consumer cameras		They are easier and more cost-effective to capture.
Near-Infrared Transillumination	[10,41]	Early teeth lesions (i.e., caries) in real time		The near-infrared light shows as a dark region in a caries lesion because of light scattering and absorption.

Table 5. Cont.

Type	Publication Used	Variable Measured	Sample Image	Features
Fluorescent imaging	[132,133]	Identification and analysis of dental plaque to detect disease		Accuracy
3D digital dental model	[17,18,21,34,106,134]	Planning of treatment in surgery		View the dental occlusion in 3D spatial perspective

To conclude, radiographic images are very challenging for the following reasons:
- There are different levels of noise in radiographic images due to the moving imaging device that captures the patient's teeth.
- The segmentation of objects in panoramic radiographic images can be made difficult by problems such as light imbalances caused by superimposition and other positioning errors [135].

The resolution of panoramic radiographic images is usually low, which contributes to the presence of noise in the image. It is therefore necessary to distinguish between the area of interest (ROI) and the background when processing dental X-ray images [115]. It is important to note that, when compared to other radiographic images, such as intraoral images (bitewing and periapical), these images offer greater patient comfort and provide less radiation exposure to the patient. Additionally, it has ability to examine a larger area of the jaw and maxilla [108].

5. Discussion

This study aims to summarize the current state of artificial intelligence's ability to detect various dental conditions, including dental caries, fillings, endodontic treatment, dental implants, and endodontic treatments. The NN structures vary from single layer to multiple layers with a different number of interconnected nodes, showing different modes of traveling through the network. An increasing interest is being shown in the use of different NN structures, especially for the analysis of medical images. This is because these models are capable of processing large amounts of relevant data for analysis, diagnosis, and surveillance of disease [136].

There has been a general growth in the research that applies AI (specially deep learning) to dentistry fields. Figure 2 shows that the year 2020 followed by year 2021 had the most articles published in this field. This literature review includes studies utilizing a variety of NN architectures, see Figure 3. CNNs are designed to process data that consists of multiple arrays and different backbones. As the detection of dental images has emerged over time, more dense CNNs have been used for this purpose, such as Faster RCNN [137], that utilizes a faster region proposal network (RPN) and a detection network that share convolutional features based on the full-image convolutions. UNet [138] architecture is used to segment images in a fast and precise manner. So far, it has outperformed a sliding-window convolutional network among the most effective methods. Moreover, Compared to the traditional CNN, FCNN [139] improves the computational efficiency and detection accuracy. Some of the convolution layers are weighted directly by Gabor filters [37,40]. The YOLO family [140] architecture is one of the most popular model architectures for detecting objects in real time. The main reason for its popularity is that it utilizes one of the most effective neural network architectures to produce high reliability and efficient processing performance. DetectNet [28] is a deep neural network for detecting objects that provides the XY coordinates of an object detected [27,99,118]. More recent modification of

Faster R-CNN is Mask R-CNN [141], which predict segmentation masks for each region of interest (ROI) [126]. Recently, Mask R-CNN and U-net have outperformed other teeth detection and segmentation structures for further teeth diagnosis tasks.

Generally, NNs require large amounts of different types of dental images in order to ensure high levels of targeted accuracy. Overfitting occurs when neural networks learn too well from their training data. So far, NNs cannot be applied to another group of images beyond those trained. This emphasizes the importance of using a variety of data that is matched to a given population. Training on a large amount of data has resulted in very efficient deep CNN algorithms [37,39,50]. Srivastava et al. [37] collect the dataset from approximately 100 clinics across the United States provided them with over 3000 bitewing radiographs, which allowed them to achieve optimal results in finding dental professionals. Lee et al. [39] in their study utilized a total of approximately 3000 periapical radiographs, divided into training and validation sets, where [50] during the development and evaluation of the model, 3932 oral photographs were collected from 625 volunteers with consumer cameras.

In theory, performance of networks with deeper layers is expected to be better than the performance of networks with shallower layers. It appears, however, deep networks perform less well in practice than shallow networks. This is because there was an optimization problem rather than an overfitting problem. To put it simply, the deeper a network is, the more challenging it is to optimize. Therefore, Transfer Learning (TL) is another way to provide a rapid straight-forward progress or improved performance for certain problem such as oral field. Pre-trained Models (AlexNet, GoogLeNet, ResNet, VGG, Inception Networks etc. and more) are an examples of TL that enrich the dentistry diagnostic support system. AlexNet [142] is composed of eight layers, in which five convolutional layers are employed, two hidden layers are fully connected, and a single output layer is fully connected. GoogLeNet [143] has 20 layers and VGG-16 [144] has 16 layers, both trained on ImageNet [142] classifies images into 1000 object categories. Inception [143] is concerned with computation costs, whereas ResNet family [145] is concerned with computation accuracy. As an example of TL, Prajapati et al. [36] and Haghanifar et al. [43] experimented with the performance of CNN for diagnosis by employing transfer learning to classify dental caries.

Alternatively, combining different CNN architectures in one model (hybrid model) shows significant results [38,127]. Using U-net combined with subpixel CNN models resulted in improved quality metrics as well as image segmentation-based analysis compared with techniques for super-resolution reconstruction based on the state-of-the-art [38]. Where [127] utilizes three different U-Net networks with Faster R-CNN and VGG-16 for tooth detection and tooth numbering.

There have been numerous target applications employing NN in the dental field. In our study, we focus on explore the maximum number of teeth target that can be in one research (12 targets). Figure 5a,b demonstrate the emphasis of dental detection in terms of disease or type of radiography, respectively. As can be seen in Figure 5a, teeth caries is the most searched topic [146]. Some approaches focused on the detection of caries in a large [37] or small dataset [36], whereas other suggested a treatment plan based on caries depth [147]. Moreover, teeth segmentation seems to be an effective preprocessing step for further dental disease diagnosis in 2D images [32] or/and 3D teeth models [18,134]. The teeth segmentation aids in distinguishing the teeth from other tissues (i.e., gums and jaw bones). Due to the public availability of datasets, studies have been increasingly focused on measuring the bone level as preprocessing for other treatments (i.e., implant) [30,113] or in measuring the age of bone [24].

There have been variety of data types have been used in the computerized dental targets. In our study, we focus on explore the maximum number of data types that can be used in research (11 types). As can be seen in Figure 5b, Panoramic X-Rays is the most popular data type in literature (with 44.34%) as it provide full visualization of jaw, such as tumors, teeth included, infections, post-accident fractures, temporomandibular joint disorders. This is because it captures outside the mouth which makes them more acceptable for the patient with a lower infection rate, and lower radiation exposure. Also, they are simple to apply and require less time but they are the most challenging type due to uneven lighting, the presence of noise and low resolution (such as [68,69]). CBCT comes in second place (with 12.26%), where it used in endodontics, orthodontics, implant, oral surgery, and oral medicine due to the high resolution 3D volumetric data (such as [64,67]). Then, Periapical X-rays in third place (with 11.32%) for diagnosing invisible proximal dental caries because it displays the entire tooth, from the crown to the root, where it connects to the jaw (such as [40,59]). Recently, the use of Oral Photographs (such as [50,51]) rapidly evolved in recent research from (2019–2022) enabling end-users cameras to capture using mobile applications because it is easier and more cost-effective to capture. A further barrier to setting up training data is the requirement for annotation by medical experts.

Many researcher optimized the performance of their architecture by different techniques such as: augmentation. For example, Miki et al. [19] augmented the data by image rotation and intensity transformation, and Sivasundaram et al. [61] enhanced the number of input samples and performed a threefold cross-validation in order to evaluate the accuracy of the results by using data augmentation and threefold cross-validation. Also, Almalki et al. [70] used it to increase the dataset size, several augmentation functions were used to increase the number of images, including rotation, shear, zooming, and horizontal and vertical flipping. In the other hand, Other diagnoses focus on integrating image analysis tools with dental radiography as pre-processing or post-processing such as [88,148]. Sabharwal et al. [148] reviewed different methods that combine DL with image analysis for implant and periodontal diseases to understand their impact and how this can lead to improved treatment results. Also, Choi et al. in [88] used a preprocessing step (i.e., horizontal alignment of pictured teeth) followed by a fully convolutional network model with Naïve classifier [149]. For post-processsing, Chen et al. [59] proposed three post-processing techniques to improve detection precision of faster R-CNN.

To this end, there are a variety of alternatives available to researchers in dental-care problems. According to our study, we found that there is little guidance in the literature on selecting appropriate methods for each target. Therefore, there is a need to collaborate between dentists and DL developers to clarify the optimal model for each teeth target.

In future clinical applications, hybrid models will be taken into account in order to increase accuracy for each target. It is likely that more TL-based techniques will be applied in the future, especially for more successful techniques (U-net [38,49,101], Mask R-CNN [23,125] and Faster R-CNN [23,125]). Additionally, prediction target networks will probably be seen more in the future, such as [12,147].

6. Conclusions

The recognition of dental images has progressively advanced with the introduction of more complex convolutional neural networks (CNNs), achieving significant enhancements in accuracy. As the acquisition of big data grows, the demand for the efficient processing capabilities of deep CNN technologies becomes increasingly critical. Given the substantial diversity in image databases, as well as the variability in types, outcomes, and frameworks of neural networks (NNs), a standardized approach is essential to enhance comparability and robustness across studies. To further advance standardization, generalizability, and reproducibility in dental imaging, future research should focus on identifying the most effective imaging modality for each specific dental application. Additionally, the potential of transfer learning and hybrid models has shown promising results in terms of performance improvement. However, more experimental studies are required to verify their effectiveness across various dental target studies. Future research in dental imaging should focus on developing standardized protocols for image acquisition and processing to enhance comparability across studies. Identifying the most effective imaging modalities for specific dental applications is crucial to improve diagnostic accuracy. Additionally, exploring the potential of transfer learning and hybrid models through experimental studies can ensure their applicability across diverse datasets. Efficient management of big data is essential, emphasizing advanced storage, retrieval, and processing techniques. Robust frameworks that accommodate variability in neural network architectures are needed to ensure consistent performance. Enhancing the generalizability and reproducibility of CNN models should be prioritized, possibly through cross-validation with diverse datasets. Interdisciplinary collaboration between dental researchers, data scientists, and software developers is vital for innovating and refining AI applications in dentistry. AI in dentistry faces challenges such as insufficient data quality and quantity, lack of standardization, and difficulties in model interpretability. Models often struggle with generalizability across diverse datasets and integrating into clinical workflows. There are also ethical and legal concerns, including patient privacy and liability issues. Additionally, high costs and the need for specialized expertise can limit accessibility, while resistance from dental professionals may hinder adoption. Addressing these issues is essential for effective AI integration in dental practices.

Limitation of Included Research

In systematic review methodology, the use of filters is generally discouraged due to the potential risk of omitting relevant studies. However, in this review, the filters applied did not significantly impact the retrieval of pertinent articles. The limitations were carefully chosen to minimize the inclusion of irrelevant articles without compromising the scope of relevant findings. Specifically, the review was restricted to human studies, and only papers published between 2013 and 2022 were considered. These criteria were deemed appropriate given the focus of the review and are unlikely to have biased the results significantly.

The temporal restriction was particularly considered to reflect recent advancements and current practices, thereby enhancing the review's relevance to contemporary research and practice in the field. This approach ensured that the most up-to-date and applicable findings were included, providing a modern perspective on the use of neural networks in dental imaging. However, it is acknowledged that this may also limit the historical perspective and exclude seminal works published prior to 2013 that could still be relevant to understanding the full landscape of the field.

Supplementary Materials: The following supporting information can be downloaded at: https://www.mdpi.com/article/10.3390/diagnostics14212442/s1.

Author Contributions: S.S.A. developed the theoretical formalism, performed the analytic calculations and performed the numerical simulations. Both S.S.A. and H.F.A. authors contributed to the final version of the manuscript. S.S.A. supervised the project. All authors have read and agreed to the published version of the manuscript.

Funding: The Researchers would like to thank the Deanship of Graduate Studies and Scientific Research at Qassim University for financial support (QU-APC-2024-9/1).

Institutional Review Board Statement: Not applicable.

Informed Consent Statement: Not applicable.

Data Availability Statement: The data used in this study has been provided in the references of this paper and Supplementary File. PRISMA 2020 Checklist available at: https://shorturl.at/rV8BC (accessed on 22 August 2024).

Conflicts of Interest: The authors declare no conflicts of interest.

References

1. Thanh, M.T.G.; Van Toan, N.; Ngoc, V.T.N.; Tra, N.T.; Giap, C.N.; Nguyen, D.M. Deep Learning Application in Dental Caries Detection Using Intraoral Photos Taken by Smartphones. *Appl. Sci.* **2022**, *12*, 5504. [CrossRef]
2. Lakshmi, M.M.; Chitra, P. Classification of Dental Cavities from X-ray images using Deep CNN algorithm. In Proceedings of the 2020 4th International Conference on Trends in Electronics and Informatics (ICOEI)(48184), Tirunelveli, India, 15–17 June 2020; IEEE: Piscataway, NJ, USA, 2020; pp. 774–779. [CrossRef]

3. Ehtesham, H.; Safdari, R.; Mansourian, A.; Tahmasebian, S.; Mohammadzadeh, N.; Pourshahidi, S. Developing a new intelligent system for the diagnosis of oral medicine with case-based reasoning approach. *Oral Dis.* **2019**, *25*, 1555–1563. [CrossRef] [PubMed]
4. Tuzoff, D.V.; Tuzova, L.N.; Bornstein, M.M.; Krasnov, A.S.; Kharchenko, M.A.; Nikolenko, S.I.; Sveshnikov, M.M.; Bednenko, G.B. Tooth detection and numbering in panoramic radiographs using convolutional neural networks. *Dentomaxillofac. Radiol.* **2019**, *48*, 20180051. [CrossRef] [PubMed]
5. Topol, E.J. High-performance medicine: The convergence of human and artificial intelligence. *Nat. Med.* **2019**, *25*, 44–56. [CrossRef]
6. Mendonça, E.A. Clinical decision support systems: Perspectives in dentistry. *J. Dent. Educ.* **2004**, *68*, 589–597. [CrossRef]
7. Tarvonen, P.L.; Suominen, A.; Yang, G.; Ri, Y.; Sipilä, K. Association between oral health habits and dental caries among children in Pyongyang, Democratic People's Republic of Korea. *Int. J. Dent. Hyg.* **2017**, *15*, e136–e142. [CrossRef]
8. Xue, Y.; Zhang, R.; Deng, Y.; Chen, K.; Jiang, T. A preliminary examination of the diagnostic value of deep learning in hip osteoarthritis. *PLoS ONE* **2017**, *12*, e0178992. [CrossRef] [PubMed]
9. Sklan, J.E.; Plassard, A.J.; Fabbri, D.; Landman, B.A. Toward content-based image retrieval with deep convolutional neural networks. In Proceedings of the Medical Imaging 2015: Biomedical Applications in Molecular, Structural, and Functional Imaging, Orlando, FL, USA, 21–26 February 2015; Volume 9417, p. 94172C. [CrossRef]
10. Schwendicke, F.; Elhennawy, K.; Paris, S.; Friebertshäuser, P.; Krois, J. Deep learning for caries lesion detection in near-infrared light transillumination images: A pilot study. *J. Dent.* **2020**, *92*, 103260. [CrossRef]
11. Krois, J.; Ekert, T.; Meinhold, L.; Golla, T.; Kharbot, B.; Wittemeier, A.; Dörfer, C.; Schwendicke, F. Deep learning for the radiographic detection of periodontal bone loss. *Sci. Rep.* **2019**, *9*, 8495. [CrossRef]
12. Lee, J.H.; Kim, D.h.; Jeong, S.N.; Choi, S.H. Diagnosis and prediction of periodontally compromised teeth using a deep learning-based convolutional neural network algorithm. *J. Periodontal Implant. Sci.* **2018**, *48*, 114–123. [CrossRef]
13. Schwendicke, F.; Golla, T.; Dreher, M.; Krois, J. Convolutional neural networks for dental image diagnostics: A scoping review. *J. Dent.* **2019**, *91*, 103226. [CrossRef] [PubMed]
14. Page, M.J.; McKenzie, J.E.; Bossuyt, P.M.; Boutron, I.; Hoffmann, T.C.; Mulrow, C.D.; Shamseer, L.; Tetzlaff, J.M.; Akl, E.A.; Brennan, S.E.; et al. The PRISMA 2020 statement: An updated guideline for reporting systematic reviews. *Syst. Rev.* **2021**, *10*, 1–11. [CrossRef] [PubMed]
15. Whiting, P.F.; Rutjes, A.W.; Westwood, M.E.; Mallett, S.; Deeks, J.J.; Reitsma, J.B.; Leeflang, M.M.; Sterne, J.A.; Bossuyt, P.M.; QUADAS-2 Group. QUADAS-2: A revised tool for the quality assessment of diagnostic accuracy studies. *Ann. Intern. Med.* **2011**, *155*, 529–536. [CrossRef]
16. Kidd, E.; Fejerskov, O. Detection, diagnosis, and recording in the clinic. In *Essentials of Dental Caries*; Oxford Academic: Oxford, UK, 2016; Volume 49, p. 1. [CrossRef]
17. Sun, D.; Pei, Y.; Song, G.; Guo, Y.; Ma, G.; Xu, T.; Zha, H. Tooth segmentation and labeling from digital dental casts. In Proceedings of the 2020 IEEE 17th International Symposium on Biomedical Imaging (ISBI), Iowa City, IA, USA, 3–7 April 2020; pp. 669–673. [CrossRef]
18. Tian, S.; Dai, N.; Zhang, B.; Yuan, F.; Yu, Q.; Cheng, X. Automatic classification and segmentation of teeth on 3D dental model using hierarchical deep learning networks. *IEEE Access* **2019**, *7*, 84817–84828. [CrossRef]
19. Miki, Y.; Muramatsu, C.; Hayashi, T.; Zhou, X.; Hara, T.; Katsumata, A.; Fujita, H. Classification of teeth in cone-beam CT using deep convolutional neural network. *Comput. Biol. Med.* **2017**, *80*, 24–29. [CrossRef]
20. Muramatsu, C.; Morishita, T.; Takahashi, R.; Hayashi, T.; Nishiyama, W.; Ariji, Y.; Zhou, X.; Hara, T.; Katsumata, A.; Ariji, E.; et al. Tooth detection and classification on panoramic radiographs for automatic dental chart filing: Improved classification by multi-sized input data. *Oral Radiol.* **2021**, *37*, 13–19. [CrossRef]
21. Chen, Q.; Huang, J.; Salehi, H.S.; Zhu, H.; Lian, L.; Lai, X.; Wei, K. Hierarchical CNN-based occlusal surface morphology analysis for classifying posterior tooth type using augmented images from 3D dental surface models. *Comput. Methods Programs Biomed.* **2021**, *208*, 106295. [CrossRef]
22. Muresan, M.P.; Barbura, A.R.; Nedevschi, S. Teeth Detection and Dental Problem Classification in Panoramic X-Ray Images using Deep Learning and Image Processing Techniques. In Proceedings of the 2020 IEEE 16th International Conference on Intelligent Computer Communication and Processing (ICCP), Cluj-Napoca, Romania, 3–5 September 2020; pp. 457–463. [CrossRef]
23. Başaran, M.; Çelik, Ö.; Bayrakdar, I.S.; Bilgir, E.; Orhan, K.; Odabaş, A.; Aslan, A.F.; Jagtap, R. Diagnostic charting of panoramic radiography using deep-learning artificial intelligence system. *Oral Radiol.* **2021**, *38*, 363–369. [CrossRef]
24. Velemínská, J.; Pilný, A.; Cepek, M.; Koťová, M.; Kubelková, R. Dental age estimation and different predictive ability of various tooth types in the Czech population: Data mining methods. *Anthropol. Anzeiger; Ber. Uber Die Biol.-Anthropol. Lit.* **2013**, *70*, 331–345. [CrossRef]
25. Kumar, A.; Bhadauria, H.S.; Singh, A. Descriptive analysis of dental X-ray images using various practical methods: A review. *PeerJ Comput. Sci.* **2021**, *7*, e620. [CrossRef]
26. Ekert, T.; Krois, J.; Meinhold, L.; Elhennawy, K.; Emara, R.; Golla, T.; Schwendicke, F. Deep learning for the radiographic detection of apical lesions. *J. Endod.* **2019**, *45*, 917–922. [CrossRef] [PubMed]
27. Fukuda, M.; Inamoto, K.; Shibata, N.; Ariji, Y.; Yanashita, Y.; Kutsuna, S.; Nakata, K.; Katsumata, A.; Fujita, H.; Ariji, E. Evaluation of an artificial intelligence system for detecting vertical root fracture on panoramic radiography. *Oral Radiol.* **2020**, *36*, 337–343. [CrossRef] [PubMed]

28. Ariji, Y.; Yanashita, Y.; Kutsuna, S.; Muramatsu, C.; Fukuda, M.; Kise, Y.; Nozawa, M.; Kuwada, C.; Fujita, H.; Katsumata, A.; et al. Automatic detection and classification of radiolucent lesions in the mandible on panoramic radiographs using a deep learning object detection technique. *Oral Surg. Oral Med. Oral Pathol. Oral Radiol.* **2019**, *128*, 424–430. [CrossRef]
29. Lee, J.H.; Kim, D.H.; Jeong, S.N. Diagnosis of cystic lesions using panoramic and cone beam computed tomographic images based on deep learning neural network. *Oral Dis.* **2020**, *26*, 152–158. [CrossRef]
30. Lee, J.S.; Adhikari, S.; Liu, L.; Jeong, H.G.; Kim, H.; Yoon, S.J. Osteoporosis detection in panoramic radiographs using a deep convolutional neural network-based computer-assisted diagnosis system: A preliminary study. *Dentomaxillofacial Radiol.* **2019**, *48*, 20170344. [CrossRef]
31. Oktay, A.B. Tooth detection with convolutional neural networks. In Proceedings of the 2017 Medical Technologies National Congress (TIPTEKNO), Trabzon, Turkey, 12–14 October 2017; pp. 1–4. [CrossRef]
32. Jader, G.; Fontineli, J.; Ruiz, M.; Abdalla, K.; Pithon, M.; Oliveira, L. Deep instance segmentation of teeth in panoramic X-ray images. In Proceedings of the Conference on Graphics, Patterns and Images (SIBGRAPI), Parana, Brazil, 29 October–1 November 2018; pp. 400–407. [CrossRef]
33. Ali, R.B.; Ejbali, R.; Zaied, M. Detection and classification of dental caries in X-ray images using deep neural networks. In Proceedings of the ICSEA 2016: The Eleventh International Conference on Software Engineering Advances, Rome, Italy, 21–25 August 2016. [CrossRef]
34. Raith, S.; Vogel, E.P.; Anees, N.; Keul, C.; Güth, J.F.; Edelhoff, D.; Fischer, H. Artificial Neural Networks as a powerful numerical tool to classify specific features of a tooth based on 3D scan data. *Comput. Biol. Med.* **2017**, *80*, 65–76. [CrossRef] [PubMed]
35. Forouzeshfar, P.; Safaei, A.A.; Ghaderi, F.; Hashemi Kamangar, S.; Kaviani, H.; Haghi, S. Dental caries diagnosis using neural networks and deep learning: A systematic review. *Multimed. Tools Appl.* **2024**, *83*, 30423–30466. [CrossRef]
36. Prajapati, S.A.; Nagaraj, R.; Mitra, S. Classification of dental diseases using CNN and transfer learning. In Proceedings of the International Symposium on Computational and Business Intelligence (ISCBI), Dubai, United Arab Emirates, 11–14 August 2017; pp. 70–74. [CrossRef]
37. Srivastava, M.M.; Kumar, P.; Pradhan, L.; Varadarajan, S. Detection of tooth caries in bitewing radiographs using deep learning. *arXiv* **2017**, arXiv:1711.07312. [CrossRef]
38. Hatvani, J.; Horváth, A.; Michetti, J.; Basarab, A.; Kouamé, D.; Gyöngy, M. Deep learning-based super-resolution applied to dental computed tomography. *IEEE Trans. Radiat. Plasma Med. Sci.* **2018**, *3*, 120–128. [CrossRef]
39. Lee, J.H.; Kim, D.H.; Jeong, S.N.; Choi, S.H. Detection and diagnosis of dental caries using a deep learning-based convolutional neural network algorithm. *J. Dent.* **2018**, *77*, 106–111. [CrossRef]
40. Zhang, K.; Wu, J.; Chen, H.; Lyu, P. An effective teeth recognition method using label tree with cascade network structure. *Comput. Med. Imaging Graph.* **2018**, *68*, 61–70. [CrossRef] [PubMed]
41. Casalegno, F.; Newton, T.; Daher, R.; Abdelaziz, M.; Lodi-Rizzini, A.; Schürmann, F.; Krejci, I.; Markram, H. Caries detection with near-infrared transillumination using deep learning. *J. Dent. Res.* **2019**, *98*, 1227–1233. [CrossRef]
42. Geetha, V.; Aprameya, K.; Hinduja, D.M. Dental caries diagnosis in digital radiographs using back-propagation neural network. *Health Inf. Sci. Syst.* **2020**, *8*, 8. [CrossRef] [PubMed]
43. Haghanifar, A.; Majdabadi, M.M.; Ko, S.B. Paxnet: Dental caries detection in panoramic X-ray using ensemble transfer learning and capsule classifier. *arXiv* **2020**, arXiv:2012.13666. [CrossRef]
44. Lee, J.H.; Han, S.S.; Kim, Y.H.; Lee, C.; Kim, I. Application of a fully deep convolutional neural network to the automation of tooth segmentation on panoramic radiographs. *Oral Surg. Oral Med. Oral Pathol. Oral Radiol.* **2020**, *129*, 635–642. [CrossRef] [PubMed]
45. Sonavane, A.; Yadav, R.; Khamparia, A. Dental cavity classification of using convolutional neural network. *IOP Conf. Ser. Mater. Sci. Eng.* **2021**, *1022*, 012116. [CrossRef]
46. Bui, T.H.; Hamamoto, K.; Paing, M.P. Deep fusion feature extraction for caries detection on dental panoramic radiographs. *Appl. Sci.* **2021**, *11*, 2005. [CrossRef]
47. Ding, B.; Zhang, Z.; Liang, Y.; Wang, W.; Hao, S.; Meng, Z.; Guan, L.; Hu, Y.; Guo, B.; Zhao, R.; et al. Detection of dental caries in oral photographs taken by mobile phones based on the YOLOv3 algorithm. *Ann. Transl. Med.* **2021**, *9*, 1–11. [CrossRef]
48. Zheng, L.; Wang, H.; Mei, L.; Chen, Q.; Zhang, Y.; Zhang, H. Artificial intelligence in digital cariology: A new tool for the diagnosis of deep caries and pulpitis using convolutional neural networks. *Ann. Transl. Med.* **2021**, *9*. [CrossRef]
49. Cantu, A.G.; Gehrung, S.; Krois, J.; Chaurasia, A.; Rossi, J.G.; Gaudin, R.; Elhennawy, K.; Schwendicke, F. Detecting caries lesions of different radiographic extension on bitewings using deep learning. *J. Dent.* **2020**, *100*, 103425. [CrossRef]
50. Zhang, X.; Liang, Y.; Li, W.; Liu, C.; Gu, D.; Sun, W.; Miao, L. Development and evaluation of deep learning for screening dental caries from oral photographs. *Oral Dis.* **2022**, *28*, 173–181. [CrossRef] [PubMed]
51. Kühnisch, J.; Meyer, O.; Hesenius, M.; Hickel, R.; Gruhn, V. Caries detection on intraoral images using artificial intelligence. *J. Dent. Res.* **2022**, *101*, 158–165. [CrossRef] [PubMed]
52. Dayı, B.; Üzen, H.; Çiçek, İ.B.; Duman, Ş.B. A Novel Deep Learning-Based Approach for Segmentation of Different Type Caries Lesions on Panoramic Radiographs. *Diagnostics* **2023**, *13*, 202. [CrossRef] [PubMed]
53. Esmaeilyfard, R.; Bonyadifard, H.; Paknahad, M. Dental Caries Detection and Classification in CBCT Images Using Deep Learning. *Int. Dent. J.* **2024**, *74*, 328–334. [CrossRef] [PubMed]
54. Chaves, E.T.; Vinayahalingam, S.; van Nistelrooij, N.; Xi, T.; Romero, V.H.D.; Flügge, T.; Saker, H.; Kim, A.; da Silveira Lima, G.; Loomans, B.; et al. Detection of caries around restorations on bitewings using deep learning. *J. Dent.* **2024**, 104886. [CrossRef]

55. Chen, X.; Ma, N.; Xu, T.; Xu, C. Deep learning-based tooth segmentation methods in medical imaging: A review. *PRoceedings Inst. Mech. Eng. Part H J. Eng. Med.* **2024**, 09544119231217603. [CrossRef]
56. Chaurasia, A.; Namachivayam, A.; Koca-Ünsal, R.B.; Lee, J.H. Deep-learning performance in identifying and classifying dental implant systems from dental imaging: A systematic review and meta-analysis. *J. Periodontal Implant. Sci.* **2024**, *54*, 3–12. [CrossRef]
57. Hiraiwa, T.; Ariji, Y.; Fukuda, M.; Kise, Y.; Nakata, K.; Katsumata, A.; Fujita, H.; Ariji, E. A deep-learning artificial intelligence system for assessment of root morphology of the mandibular first molar on panoramic radiography. *Dentomaxillofac. Radiol.* **2019**, *48*, 20180218. [CrossRef]
58. Moriyama, Y.; Lee, C.; Date, S.; Kashiwagi, Y.; Narukawa, Y.; Nozaki, K.; Murakami, S. A MapReduce-like Deep Learning Model for the Depth Estimation of Periodontal Pockets. In Proceedings of the HEALTHINF, Prague, Czech Republic, 22–24 February 2019; pp. 388–395. [CrossRef]
59. Chen, H.; Zhang, K.; Lyu, P.; Li, H.; Zhang, L.; Wu, J.; Lee, C.H. A deep learning approach to automatic teeth detection and numbering based on object detection in dental periapical films. *Sci. Rep.* **2019**, *9*, 3840. [CrossRef]
60. Vinayahalingam, S.; Kempers, S.; Limon, L.; Deibel, D.; Maal, T.; Hanisch, M.; Bergé, S.; Xi, T. Classification of caries in third molars on panoramic radiographs using deep learning. *Sci. Rep.* **2021**, *11*, 12609. [CrossRef]
61. Sivasundaram, S.; Pandian, C. Performance analysis of classification and segmentation of cysts in panoramic dental images using convolutional neural network architecture. *Int. J. Imaging Syst. Technol.* **2021**, *31*, 2214–2225. [CrossRef]
62. Chandrashekar, G.; AlQarni, S.; Bumann, E.E.; Lee, Y. Collaborative deep learning model for tooth segmentation and identification using panoramic radiographs. *Comput. Biol. Med.* **2022**, *148*, 105829. [CrossRef]
63. Oztekin, F.; Katar, O.; Sadak, F.; Aydogan, M.; Yildirim, T.T.; Plawiak, P.; Yildirim, O.; Talo, M.; Karabatak, M. Automatic semantic segmentation for dental restorations in panoramic radiography images using U-Net model. *Int. J. Imaging Syst. Technol.* **2022**, *32*, 1990–2001. [CrossRef]
64. Widiasri, M.; Arifin, A.Z.; Suciati, N.; Fatichah, C.; Astuti, E.R.; Indraswari, R.; Putra, R.H.; Za'in, C. Dental-YOL: Alveolar Bone and Mandibular Canal Detection on Cone Beam Computed Tomography Images for Dental Implant Planning. *IEEE Access* **2022**, *10*, 101483–101494. [CrossRef]
65. Seo, H.; Hwang, J.; Jung, Y.H.; Lee, E.; Nam, O.H.; Shin, J. Deep focus approach for accurate bone age estimation from lateral cephalogram. *J. Dent. Sci.* **2023**, *18*, 34–43. [CrossRef]
66. Atas, I.; Ozdemir, C.; Atas, M.; Dogan, Y. Forensic Dental Age Estimation Using Modified Deep Learning Neural Network. *arXiv* **2022**, arXiv:2208.09799. [CrossRef]
67. Kim, M.J.; Liu, Y.; Oh, S.H.; Ahn, H.W.; Kim, S.H.; Nelson, G. Automatic cephalometric landmark identification system based on the multi-stage convolutional neural networks with CBCT combination images. *Sensors* **2021**, *21*, 505. [CrossRef]
68. Yu, D.; Hu, J.; Feng, Z.; Song, M.; Zhu, H. Deep learning based diagnosis for cysts and tumors of jaw with massive healthy samples. *Sci. Rep.* **2022**, *12*, 1855. [CrossRef]
69. Mine, Y.; Iwamoto, Y.; Okazaki, S.; Nakamura, K.; Takeda, S.; Peng, T.Y.; Mitsuhata, C.; Kakimoto, N.; Kozai, K.; Murayama, T. Detecting the presence of supernumerary teeth during the early mixed dentition stage using deep learning algorithms: A pilot study. *Int. J. Paediatr. Dent.* **2022**, *32*, 678–685. [CrossRef]
70. Almalki, Y.E.; Din, A.I.; Ramzan, M.; Irfan, M.; Aamir, K.M.; Almalki, A.; Alotaibi, S.; Alaglan, G.; Alshamrani, H.A.; Rahman, S. Deep Learning Models for Classification of Dental Diseases Using Orthopantomography X-ray OPG Images. *Sensors* **2022**, *22*, 7370. [CrossRef]
71. Xie, R.; Yang, Y.; Chen, Z. WITS: Weakly-supervised individual tooth segmentation model trained on box-level labels. *Pattern Recognit.* **2023**, *133*, 108974. [CrossRef]
72. Rubiu, G.; Bologna, M.; Cellina, M.; Cè, M.; Sala, D.; Pagani, R.; Mattavelli, E.; Fazzini, D.; Ibba, S.; Papa, S.; et al. Teeth Segmentation in Panoramic Dental X-ray Using Mask Regional Convolutional Neural Network. *Appl. Sci.* **2023**, *13*, 7947. [CrossRef]
73. Yilmaz, S.; Tasyurek, M.; Amuk, M.; Celik, M.; Canger, E.M. Developing deep learning methods for classification of teeth in dental panoramic radiography. *Oral Surg. Oral Med. Oral Pathol. Oral Radiol.* **2024**, *138*, 118–127. [CrossRef] [PubMed]
74. Karaoglu, A.; Ozcan, C.; Pekince, A.; Yasa, Y. Numbering teeth in panoramic images: A novel method based on deep learning and heuristic algorithm. *Eng. Sci. Technol. Int. J.* **2023**, *37*, 101316. [CrossRef]
75. Park, W.; Huh, J.K.; Lee, J.H. Automated deep learning for classification of dental implant radiographs using a large multi-center dataset. *Sci. Rep.* **2023**, *13*, 4862. [CrossRef]
76. Hong, W.; Kim, S.M.; Choi, J.; Ahn, J.; Paeng, J.Y.; Kim, H. Automated Cephalometric Landmark Detection Using Deep Reinforcement Learning. *J. Craniofacial Surg.* **2023**, *34*, 2336–2342. [CrossRef]
77. Ayhan, B.; Ayan, E.; Bayraktar, Y. A novel deep learning-based perspective for tooth numbering and caries detection. *Clin. Oral Investig.* **2024**, *28*, 178. [CrossRef]
78. Kurtulus, I.L.; Lubbad, M.; Yilmaz, O.M.D.; Kilic, K.; Karaboga, D.; Basturk, A.; Akay, B.; Nalbantoglu, U.; Yilmaz, S.; Ayata, M.; et al. A robust deep learning model for the classification of dental implant brands. *J. Stomatol. Oral Maxillofac. Surg.* **2024**, *125*, 101818. [CrossRef]
79. Marginean, A.C.; Mureşan, S.; Hedeşiu, M.; Dioşan, L. Teeth Segmentation and Carious Lesions Segmentation in Panoramic X-Ray Images using CariSeg, a Networks' Ensemble. *Heliyon* **2024**, *10*, e30826. [CrossRef]
80. Lee, J.H. Future of the smartphone for patients and healthcare providers. *Healthc. Inform. Res.* **2016**, *22*, 1–2. [CrossRef]

81. Karlsson, L.; Maia, A.M.A.; Kyotoku, B.B.; Tranaeus, S.; Gomes, A.S.L.; Margulis, W. Near-infrared transillumination of teeth: Measurement of a system performance. *J. Biomed. Opt.* **2010**, *15*, 036001. [CrossRef]
82. Volpato, C.A.M.; Pereira, M.R.C.; Silva, F.S. Fluorescence of natural teeth and restorative materials, methods for analysis and quantification: A literature review. *J. Esthet. Restor. Dent.* **2018**, *30*, 397–407. [CrossRef] [PubMed]
83. Morris, R.S.; Hoye, L.N.; Elnagar, M.H.; Atsawasuwan, P.; Galang-Boquiren, M.T.; Caplin, J.; Viana, G.C.; Obrez, A.; Kusnoto, B. Accuracy of Dental Monitoring 3D digital dental models using photograph and video mode. *Am. J. Orthod. Dentofac. Orthop.* **2019**, *156*, 420–428. [CrossRef] [PubMed]
84. Lee, S.; Oh, S.i.; Jo, J.; Kang, S.; Shin, Y.; Park, J.w. Deep Learning for Early Dental Caries Detection in Bitewing Radiographs. *Sci. Rep.* **2021**, *11*, 16807. [CrossRef]
85. Moran, M.; Faria, M.; Giraldi, G.; Bastos, L.; Oliveira, L.; Conci, A. Classification of Approximal Caries in Bitewing Radiographs Using Convolutional Neural Networks. *Sensors* **2021**, *21*, 5192. [CrossRef]
86. Karatas, O.; Cakir, N.N.; Ozsariyildiz, S.S.; Kis, H.C.; Demirbuga, S.; Gurgan, C.A. A deep learning approach to dental restoration classification from bitewing and periapical radiographs. *Quintessence Int.* **2021**, *52*, 568–574. [CrossRef]
87. Huang, P.W.; Huang, P.Y.; Lin, P.L.; Hsu, H.C. Alveolar bone-loss area detection in periodontitis radiographs using hybrid of intensity and texture analyzed based on FBM model. In Proceedings of the 2014 International Conference on Machine Learning and Cybernetics, Lanzhou, China, 13–16 July 2014; Volume 2, pp. 487–492. [CrossRef]
88. Choi, J.; Eun, H.; Kim, C. Boosting proximal dental caries detection via combination of variational methods and convolutional neural network. *J. Signal Process. Syst.* **2018**, *90*, 87–97. [CrossRef]
89. Lee, J.H.; Kim, Y.T.; Lee, J.B.; Jeong, S.N. A performance comparison between automated deep learning and dental professionals in classification of dental implant systems from dental imaging: A multi-center study. *Diagnostics* **2020**, *10*, 910. [CrossRef]
90. Cha, J.Y.; Yoon, H.I.; Yeo, I.S.; Huh, K.H.; Han, J.S. Peri-implant bone loss measurement using a region-based convolutional neural network on dental periapical radiographs. *J. Clin. Med.* **2021**, *10*, 1009. [CrossRef]
91. Moran, M.; Faria, M.; Giraldi, G.; Bastos, L.; Conci, A. Do Radiographic Assessments of Periodontal Bone Loss Improve with Deep Learning Methods for Enhanced Image Resolution? *Sensors* **2021**, *21*, 2013. [CrossRef]
92. Liu, M.; Wang, S.; Chen, H.; Liu, Y. A pilot study of a deep learning approach to detect marginal bone loss around implants. *BMC Oral Health* **2022**, *22*, 11. [CrossRef] [PubMed]
93. Mori, M.; Ariji, Y.; Fukuda, M.; Kitano, T.; Funakoshi, T.; Nishiyama, W.; Kohinata, K.; Iida, Y.; Ariji, E.; Katsumata, A. Performance of deep learning technology for evaluation of positioning quality in periapical radiography of the maxillary canine. *Oral Radiol.* **2022**, *38*, 147–154. [CrossRef]
94. Arik, S.Ö.; Ibragimov, B.; Xing, L. Fully automated quantitative cephalometry using convolutional neural networks. *J. Med. Imaging* **2017**, *4*, 014501. [CrossRef]
95. Qian, J.; Cheng, M.; Tao, Y.; Lin, J.; Lin, H. CephaNet: An improved faster R-CNN for cephalometric landmark detection. In Proceedings of the 2019 IEEE 16th International Symposium on Biomedical Imaging (ISBI 2019), Venice, Italy, 8–11 April 2019; pp. 868–871. [CrossRef]
96. Song, Y.; Qiao, X.; Iwamoto, Y.; Chen, Y.w. Automatic cephalometric landmark detection on X-ray images using a deep-learning method. *Appl. Sci.* **2020**, *10*, 2547. [CrossRef]
97. Okada, K.; Rysavy, S.; Flores, A.; Linguraru, M.G. Noninvasive differential diagnosis of dental periapical lesions in cone-beam CT scans. *Med. Phys.* **2015**, *42*, 1653–1665. [CrossRef]
98. Dutra, K.L.; Haas, L.; Porporatti, A.L.; Flores-Mir, C.; Santos, J.N.; Mezzomo, L.A.; Correa, M.; Canto, G.D.L. Diagnostic accuracy of cone-beam computed tomography and conventional radiography on apical periodontitis: A systematic review and meta-analysis. *J. Endod.* **2016**, *42*, 356–364. [CrossRef]
99. Ariji, Y.; Fukuda, M.; Kise, Y.; Nozawa, M.; Yanashita, Y.; Fujita, H.; Katsumata, A.; Ariji, E. Contrast-enhanced computed tomography image assessment of cervical lymph node metastasis in patients with oral cancer by using a deep learning system of artificial intelligence. *Oral Surg. Oral Med. Oral Pathol. Oral Radiol.* **2019**, *127*, 458–463. [CrossRef]
100. Chung, M.; Lee, M.; Hong, J.; Park, S.; Lee, J.; Lee, J.; Yang, I.H.; Lee, J.; Shin, Y.G. Pose-aware instance segmentation framework from cone beam CT images for tooth segmentation. *Comput. Biol. Med.* **2020**, *120*, 103720. [CrossRef]
101. Zheng, Z.; Yan, H.; Setzer, F.C.; Shi, K.J.; Mupparapu, M.; Li, J. Anatomically constrained deep learning for automating dental cbct segmentation and lesion detection. *IEEE Trans. Autom. Sci. Eng.* **2020**, *18*, 603–614. [CrossRef]
102. Yang, Y.; Xie, R.; Jia, W.; Chen, Z.; Yang, Y.; Xie, L.; Jiang, B. Accurate and automatic tooth image segmentation model with deep convolutional neural networks and level set method. *Neurocomputing* **2021**, *419*, 108–125. [CrossRef]
103. Kurt Bayrakdar, S.; Orhan, K.; Bayrakdar, I.S.; Bilgir, E.; Ezhov, M.; Gusarev, M.; Shumilov, E. A deep learning approach for dental implant planning in cone-beam computed tomography images. *BMC Med. Imaging* **2021**, *21*, 86. [CrossRef] [PubMed]
104. Orhan, K.; Bilgir, E.; Bayrakdar, I.S.; Ezhov, M.; Gusarev, M.; Shumilov, E. Evaluation of artificial intelligence for detecting impacted third molars on cone-beam computed tomography scans. *J. Stomatol. Oral Maxillofac. Surg.* **2021**, *122*, 333–337. [CrossRef] [PubMed]
105. ALbahbah, A.A.; El-Bakry, H.M.; Abd-Elgahany, S. Detection of caries in panoramic dental X-ray images using back-propagation neural network. *Int. J. Electron. Commun. Comput. Eng.* **2016**, *7*, 250. [CrossRef]
106. Naam, J.; Harlan, J.; Madenda, S.; Wibowo, E.P. The algorithm of image edge detection on panoramic dental X-ray using multiple morphological gradient (mmg) method. *Int. J. Adv. Sci. Eng. Inf. Technol.* **2016**, *6*, 1012–1018. [CrossRef]

107. Avuçlu, E.; Başçiftçi, F. Novel approaches to determine age and gender from dental X-ray images by using multiplayer perceptron neural networks and image processing techniques. *Chaos Solitons Fractals* **2019**, *120*, 127–138. [CrossRef]
108. Kim, J.; Lee, H.S.; Song, I.S.; Jung, K.H. DeNTNet: Deep Neural Transfer Network for the detection of periodontal bone loss using panoramic dental radiographs. *Sci. Rep.* **2019**, *9*, 17615. [CrossRef] [PubMed]
109. Vinayahalingam, S.; Xi, T.; Bergé, S.; Maal, T.; de Jong, G. Automated detection of third molars and mandibular nerve by deep learning. *Sci. Rep.* **2019**, *9*, 9007. [CrossRef]
110. Zhao, Y.; Li, P.; Gao, C.; Liu, Y.; Chen, Q.; Yang, F.; Meng, D. TSASNet: Tooth segmentation on dental panoramic X-ray images by Two-Stage Attention Segmentation Network. *Knowl.-Based Syst.* **2020**, *206*, 106338. [CrossRef]
111. Kim, C.; Kim, D.; Jeong, H.; Yoon, S.J.; Youm, S. Automatic tooth detection and numbering using a combination of a CNN and heuristic algorithm. *Appl. Sci.* **2020**, *10*, 5624. [CrossRef]
112. Sukegawa, S.; Yoshii, K.; Hara, T.; Yamashita, K.; Nakano, K.; Yamamoto, N.; Nagatsuka, H.; Furuki, Y. Deep neural networks for dental implant system classification. *Biomolecules* **2020**, *10*, 984. [CrossRef]
113. Chang, H.J.; Lee, S.J.; Yong, T.H.; Shin, N.Y.; Jang, B.G.; Kim, J.E.; Huh, K.H.; Lee, S.S.; Heo, M.S.; Choi, S.C.; et al. Deep learning hybrid method to automatically diagnose periodontal bone loss and stage periodontitis. *Sci. Rep.* **2020**, *10*, 7531. [CrossRef] [PubMed]
114. Sharifonnasabi, F.; Jhanjhi, N.; John, J.; Alaboudi, A.; Nambiar, P. A Review on Automated Bone Age Measurement Based on Dental OPG Images. *Int. J. Eng. Res. Technol.* **2020**, *13*, 5408–5422. [CrossRef]
115. Kahaki, S.M.; Nordin, M.; Ahmad, N.S.; Arzoky, M.; Ismail, W. Deep convolutional neural network designed for age assessment based on orthopantomography data. *Neural Comput. Appl.* **2020**, *32*, 9357–9368. [CrossRef]
116. Thanathornwong, B.; Suebnukarn, S. Automatic detection of periodontal compromised teeth in digital panoramic radiographs using faster regional convolutional neural networks. *Imaging Sci. Dent.* **2020**, *50*, 169. [CrossRef]
117. Kwon, O.; Yong, T.H.; Kang, S.R.; Kim, J.E.; Huh, K.H.; Heo, M.S.; Lee, S.S.; Choi, S.C.; Yi, W.J. Automatic diagnosis for cysts and tumors of both jaws on panoramic radiographs using a deep convolution neural network. *Dentomaxillofac. Radiol.* **2020**, *49*, 20200185. [CrossRef]
118. Kuwada, C.; Ariji, Y.; Fukuda, M.; Kise, Y.; Fujita, H.; Katsumata, A.; Ariji, E. Deep learning systems for detecting and classifying the presence of impacted supernumerary teeth in the maxillary incisor region on panoramic radiographs. *Oral Surg. Oral Med. Oral Pathol. Oral Radiol.* **2020**, *130*, 464–469. [CrossRef] [PubMed]
119. Lian, L.; Zhu, T.; Zhu, F.; Zhu, H. Deep Learning for Caries Detection and Classification. *Diagnostics* **2021**, *11*, 1672. [CrossRef]
120. Cui, W.; Zeng, L.; Chong, B.; Zhang, Q. Toothpix: Pixel-Level Tooth Segmentation in Panoramic X-Ray Images based on Generative Adversarial Networks. In Proceedings of the 2021 IEEE 18th International Symposium on Biomedical Imaging (ISBI), Nice, France, 13–16 April 2021; pp. 1346–1350. [CrossRef]
121. Leite, A.F.; Gerven, A.V.; Willems, H.; Beznik, T.; Lahoud, P.; Gaêta-Araujo, H.; Vranckx, M.; Jacobs, R. Artificial intelligence-driven novel tool for tooth detection and segmentation on panoramic radiographs. *Clin. Oral Investig.* **2021**, *25*, 2257–2267. [CrossRef]
122. Kılıc, M.C.; Bayrakdar, I.S.; Çelik, Ö.; Bilgir, E.; Orhan, K.; Aydın, O.B.; Kaplan, F.A.; Sağlam, H.; Odabaş, A.; Aslan, A.F.; et al. Artificial intelligence system for automatic deciduous tooth detection and numbering in panoramic radiographs. *Dentomaxillofac. Radiol.* **2021**, *50*, 20200172. [CrossRef]
123. Lin, S.Y.; Chang, H.Y. Tooth Numbering and Condition Recognition on Dental Panoramic Radiograph Images Using CNNs. *IEEE Access* **2021**, *9*, 166008–166026. [CrossRef]
124. Sukegawa, S.; Yoshii, K.; Hara, T.; Matsuyama, T.; Yamashita, K.; Nakano, K.; Takabatake, K.; Kawai, H.; Nagatsuka, H.; Furuki, Y. Multi-task deep learning model for classification of dental implant brand and treatment stage using dental panoramic radiograph images. *Biomolecules* **2021**, *11*, 815. [CrossRef] [PubMed]
125. Imak, A.; Çelebi, A.; Türkoğlu, M.; Şengür, A. Dental Material Detection based on Faster Regional Convolutional Neural Networks and Shape Features. *Neural Process. Lett.* **2022**, *54*, 2107–2126. [CrossRef]
126. Park, J.; Lee, J.; Moon, S.; Lee, K. Deep Learning Based Detection of Missing Tooth Regions for Dental Implant Planning in Panoramic Radiographic Images. *Applied Sciences* **2022**, *12*, 1595. [CrossRef]
127. Estai, M.; Tennant, M.; Gebauer, D.; Brostek, A.; Vignarajan, J.; Mehdizadeh, M.; Saha, S. Deep learning for automated detection and numbering of permanent teeth on panoramic images. *Dentomaxillofacial Radiol.* **2022**, *51*, 20210296. [CrossRef]
128. Lerner, H.; Mouhyi, J.; Admakin, O.; Mangano, F. Artificial intelligence in fixed implant prosthodontics: A retrospective study of 106 implant-supported monolithic zirconia crowns inserted in the posterior jaws of 90 patients. *BMC Oral Health* **2020**, *20*, 80. [CrossRef]
129. Alalharith, D.M.; Alharthi, H.M.; Alghamdi, W.M.; Alsenbel, Y.M.; Aslam, N.; Khan, I.U.; Shahin, S.Y.; Dianišková, S.; Alhareky, M.S.; Barouch, K.K. A deep learning-based approach for the detection of early signs of gingivitis in orthodontic patients using faster region-based convolutional neural networks. *Int. J. Environ. Res. Public Health* **2020**, *17*, 8447. [CrossRef]
130. Takahashi, T.; Nozaki, K.; Gonda, T.; Mameno, T.; Ikebe, K. Deep learning-based detection of dental prostheses and restorations. *Sci. Rep.* **2021**, *11*, 1960. [CrossRef]
131. Warin, K.; Limprasert, W.; Suebnukarn, S.; Jinaporntham, S.; Jantana, P. Automatic classification and detection of oral cancer in photographic images using deep learning algorithms. *J. Oral Pathol. Med.* **2021**, *50*, 911–918. [CrossRef]

132. Imangaliyev, S.; Veen, M.H.; Volgenant, C.; Keijser, B.J.; Crielaard, W.; Levin, E. Deep learning for classification of dental plaque images. In Proceedings of the International Workshop on Machine Learning, Optimization, and Big Data, Volterra, Italy, 26–29 August 2016; pp. 407–410. [CrossRef]
133. Yauney, G.; Angelino, K.; Edlund, D.; Shah, P. Convolutional neural network for combined classification of fluorescent biomarkers and expert annotations using white light images. In Proceedings of the 2017 IEEE 17th International Conference on Bioinformatics and Bioengineering (BIBE), Washington, DC, USA, 23–25 October 2017; pp. 303–309. [CrossRef]
134. Xu, X.; Liu, C.; Zheng, Y. 3D tooth segmentation and labeling using deep convolutional neural networks. *IEEE Trans. Vis. Comput. Graph.* **2018**, *25*, 2336–2348. [CrossRef]
135. Akarslan, Z.Z.; Erten, H.; Güngör, K.; Celik, I. Common errors on panoramic radiographs taken in a dental school. *J. Contemp. Dent. Pract.* **2003**, *4*, 24–34. [CrossRef]
136. Prados-Privado, M.; Villalón, J.G.; Martínez-Martínez, C.H.; Ivorra, C. Dental images recognition technology and applications: A literature review. *Appl. Sci.* **2020**, *10*, 2856. [CrossRef]
137. Ren, S.; He, K.; Girshick, R.; Sun, J. Faster r-cnn: Towards real-time object detection with region proposal networks. *IEEE Trans. Pattern Anal. Mach. Intell.* **2015**, *39*, 1137–1149. [CrossRef] [PubMed]
138. Ronneberger, O.; Fischer, P.; Brox, T. U-net: Convolutional networks for biomedical image segmentation. In Proceedings of the International Conference on Medical Image Computing and Computer-Assisted Intervention, Munich, Germany, 5–9 October 2015; Springer: Berlin/Heidelberg, Germany, 2015; pp. 234–241. [CrossRef]
139. Long, J.; Shelhamer, E.; Darrell, T. Fully convolutional networks for semantic segmentation. In Proceedings of the IEEE Conference on Computer Vision and Pattern Recognition, Boston, MA, USA, 7–12 June 2015; pp. 3431–3440. [CrossRef]
140. Redmon, J.; Divvala, S.; Girshick, R.; Farhadi, A. You only look once: Unified, real-time object detection. In Proceedings of the IEEE Conference on Computer Vision and Pattern Recognition, Las Vegas, NV, USA, 27–30 June 2016; pp. 779–788. [CrossRef]
141. He, K.; Gkioxari, G.; Dollár, P.; Girshick, R. Mask r-cnn. In Proceedings of the IEEE International Conference on Computer Vision, Venice, Italy, 22–29 October 2017; pp. 2961–2969. [CrossRef]
142. Krizhevsky, A.; Sutskever, I.; Hinton, G.E. Imagenet classification with deep convolutional neural networks. *Commun. ACM* **2017**, *60*, 84–90. [CrossRef]
143. Szegedy, C.; Liu, W.; Jia, Y.; Sermanet, P.; Reed, S.; Anguelov, D.; Erhan, D.; Vanhoucke, V.; Rabinovich, A. Going deeper with convolutions. In Proceedings of the IEEE Conference on Computer Vision and Pattern Recognition, Boston, MA, USA, 7–12 June 2015; pp. 1–9. [CrossRef]
144. Simonyan, K.; Zisserman, A. Very deep convolutional networks for large-scale image recognition. *arXiv* **2014**, arXiv:1409.1556. [CrossRef]
145. He, K.; Zhang, X.; Ren, S.; Sun, J. Deep residual learning for image recognition. In Proceedings of the IEEE Conference on Computer Vision and Pattern Recognition, Las Vegas, NV, USA, 27–30 June 2016; pp. 770–778.
146. Selwitz, R.H.; Ismail, A.I.; Pitts, N.B. Dental caries. *Lancet* **2007**, *369*, 51–59. [CrossRef]
147. Bouchahma, M.; Hammouda, S.B.; Kouki, S.; Alshemaili, M.; Samara, K. An automatic dental decay treatment prediction using a deep convolutional neural network on X-ray images. In Proceedings of the 2019 IEEE/ACS 16th International Conference on Computer Systems and Applications (AICCSA), Abu Dhabi, United Arab Emirates, 3–7 November 2019; pp. 1–4. [CrossRef]
148. Sabharwal, A.; Kavthekar, N.; Miecznikowski, J.; Glogauer, M.; Maddi, A.; Sarder, P. Integrating Image Analysis and Dental Radiography for Periodontal and Peri-Implant Diagnosis. *Front. Dent. Med.* **2022**, *3*, 840963. [CrossRef]
149. Rish, I. An empirical study of the naive Bayes classifier. In Proceedings of the IJCAI 2001 Workshop on Empirical Methods in Artificial Intelligence, Seattle, WA, USA, 4–10 August 2001; Volume 3, pp. 41–46. [CrossRef]

Disclaimer/Publisher's Note: The statements, opinions and data contained in all publications are solely those of the individual author(s) and contributor(s) and not of MDPI and/or the editor(s). MDPI and/or the editor(s) disclaim responsibility for any injury to people or property resulting from any ideas, methods, instructions or products referred to in the content.

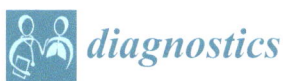

Systematic Review

Performance of Artificial Intelligence Models Designed for Automated Estimation of Age Using Dento-Maxillofacial Radiographs—A Systematic Review

Sanjeev B. Khanagar [1,2,*], Farraj Albalawi [1,2], Aram Alshehri [2,3], Mohammed Awawdeh [1,2], Kiran Iyer [1,2], Barrak Alsomaie [2,4], Ali Aldhebaib [2,4], Oinam Gokulchandra Singh [2,4] and Abdulmohsen Alfadley [2,3]

1. Preventive Dental Science Department, College of Dentistry, King Saud Bin Abdulaziz University for Health Sciences, Riyadh 11426, Saudi Arabia
2. King Abdullah International Medical Research Center, Ministry of National Guard Health Affairs, Riyadh 11481, Saudi Arabia
3. Restorative and Prosthetic Dental Sciences Department, College of Dentistry, King Saud bin Abdulaziz University for Health Sciences, Riyadh 11426, Saudi Arabia
4. Radiological Sciences Program, College of Applied Medical Sciences, King Saud bin Abdulaziz University for Health Sciences, Riyadh 11426, Saudi Arabia
* Correspondence: sanjeev.khanagar76@gmail.com

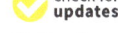

Citation: Khanagar, S.B.; Albalawi, F.; Alshehri, A.; Awawdeh, M.; Iyer, K.; Alsomaie, B.; Aldhebaib, A.; Singh, O.G.; Alfadley, A. Performance of Artificial Intelligence Models Designed for Automated Estimation of Age Using Dento-Maxillofacial Radiographs—A Systematic Review. *Diagnostics* **2024**, *14*, 1079. https://doi.org/10.3390/diagnostics14111079

Academic Editor: Jae-Ho Han

Received: 7 April 2024
Revised: 15 May 2024
Accepted: 21 May 2024
Published: 22 May 2024

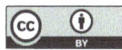

Copyright: © 2024 by the authors. Licensee MDPI, Basel, Switzerland. This article is an open access article distributed under the terms and conditions of the Creative Commons Attribution (CC BY) license (https://creativecommons.org/licenses/by/4.0/).

Abstract: Automatic age estimation has garnered significant interest among researchers because of its potential practical uses. The current systematic review was undertaken to critically appraise developments and performance of AI models designed for automated estimation using dento-maxillofacial radiographic images. In order to ensure consistency in their approach, the researchers followed the diagnostic test accuracy guidelines outlined in PRISMA-DTA for this systematic review. They conducted an electronic search across various databases such as PubMed, Scopus, Embase, Cochrane, Web of Science, Google Scholar, and the Saudi Digital Library to identify relevant articles published between the years 2000 and 2024. A total of 26 articles that satisfied the inclusion criteria were subjected to a risk of bias assessment using QUADAS-2, which revealed a flawless risk of bias in both arms for the patient-selection domain. Additionally, the certainty of evidence was evaluated using the GRADE approach. AI technology has primarily been utilized for automated age estimation through tooth development stages, tooth and bone parameters, bone age measurements, and pulp–tooth ratio. The AI models employed in the studies achieved a remarkably high precision of 99.05% and accuracy of 99.98% in the age estimation for models using tooth development stages and bone age measurements, respectively. The application of AI as an additional diagnostic tool within the realm of age estimation demonstrates significant promise.

Keywords: artificial intelligence; age estimation; deep learning; forensics; machine learning; panoramic radiographs

1. Introduction

Age plays a crucial role in defining a person's identity [1]. The pursuit of accurate age estimation methods has persisted throughout time. Whether for living or deceased individuals, the need for reliable age estimation remains significant in various scenarios. There are different approaches to determining someone's age, which include considering their chronological age, skeletal age, and dental age [2]. Chronological age refers to the length of time that has passed since birth and is the primary way of defining age [3].

Chronological age, alongside biological sex and ethnicity, is a crucial factor in anthropological and forensic studies [4]. Estimating chronological age has been successfully performed by assessing the development of bones. Various skeletal parts, such as the pubic symphysis, auricular surface, and sternal ribs, have been utilized for this purpose. It should be noted that there is not one specific method based on bone development that consistently outperforms others, as the effectiveness of each method depends on numerous factors [5].

Dental maturity is a highly dependable approach for estimating chronological age in criminal, forensic, and anthropological contexts and has the ability to serve as a reliable indicator of age [6–8]. Teeth are frequently utilized in age estimation due to their less susceptible nature to external influences, such as genetics or environment [9]. Due to their highly mineralized structure, teeth are resistant to decomposition after death and can withstand flames, alkalis, and acids [10]. While bones may degrade over time, teeth can be preserved for extended periods and are therefore a dependable method of identification in emergency scenarios [11,12].

A blend of techniques—visual, radiographic, chemical, and histological—are utilized for determining dental age. Visual assessment relies on tracking the succession of tooth emergence and functional transitions that accompany aging, like wear and alterations in tooth hue. Radiographic scans offer insight into the developmental stage of teeth, from the inception of mineralization to crown shaping and root tip maturation. Biochemical techniques help to identify changes in ion levels as an individual ages. Histological methods involve preparing tissues for thorough microscopic analysis [8,13,14]. Morphological and radiographic techniques such as Schour and Massler's method, Demirjian's method, and Kvaal's method prove to be effective in determining age in living individuals who are in their teenage and adult years. When it comes to deceased individuals, histological and biochemical techniques like Gustafson's and Johanson's method, the Bang and Ramm method, aspartic acid racemization, and the cemental annulation technique come into play for accurately determining age [1,15].

Dental age estimation relies on two distinct methods: assessing the timing of tooth eruption and analyzing the progression of dental maturity stages. The latter, dental maturity, is deemed more dependable due to its high heritability, low coefficient variation, and autonomy from external factors such as nutrition, hormones, and environmental influences [7,16]. Dental radiographic records can help determine a person's age by assessing different characteristics. These include jaw bone development, tooth germ appearance, stage of tooth crown completion and eruption, extent of deciduous teeth resorption, measurement of open apices in teeth, size of pulp chamber and root canals, formation of secondary dentin, tooth-to-pulp ratio, and development and structure of the third molar [17,18].

Estimating dental age is a complicated task, as teeth come in all shapes and sizes, making it a unique challenge. The complexities and variations within and among individuals further complicate the process [19]. As people become older, they experience changes like reduced alveolar bone levels and altered pulp-to-tooth ratios. However, using only direct measurements of the first molar may result in a significant margin of error of 8.84 years [19]. Moreover, previous methods of age estimation in dentistry have been limited, focusing only on specific aspects of teeth and often resulting in large error margins. Since existing age estimation methods are prone to errors and bias, we hypothesized that an improvement in accuracy could be achieved by removing subjective elements and automating the process. There have been continuous efforts to enhance the precision of AI-powered age estimations, such as utilizing deep learning algorithms, over the past ten years [5].

Dental radiographs have been utilized to demonstrate the dependability of convolutional neural networks (CNNs) for a range of dental ailments like dental caries [20], periodontal disease [21], odontogenic cysts and tumors [22], and conditions affecting the maxillary sinus and temporomandibular joints [23,24]. CNNs have an advantage over traditional individual feature-based techniques as they can conduct end-to-end learning and automatically extract relevant features from raw data without human intervention. They do not need human-engineered techniques, so an AI system could greatly reduce the work of human interpreters or observers in predicting dental age [25]. Additionally, since CNNs generate a comprehensive feature set from data on their own, they perform well with large datasets. Therefore, this systematic review was carried out to assess and report on the performance of AI models developed for automated age estimation from dento-maxillofacial radiographs.

2. Materials and Methods

To ensure the quality of the methodology, the authors adhered to the diagnostic test accuracy criteria specified in the Preferred Reporting Items for Systematic Reviews and Meta-Analyses Extension (PRISMA-DTA) [26]. This systematic review protocol is registered in PROSPERO with registration number CRD42024528182. The search for literature was guided by the PICO (Problem/Patient, Intervention/Indicator, Comparison, and Outcome) criteria detailed in Table 1.

Table 1. Description of the PICO (P = Population, I = Intervention, C = Comparison, O = Outcome) elements.

Research question	What are the developments and performance of the artificial intelligence models that have been used in age estimation using dento-maxillofacial radiographs?
Population	Patients who underwent dento-maxillofacial radiographs
Intervention	AI-based models developed for age estimation
Comparison	Traditional methods of age estimation, expert opinion, other AI models
Outcome	Accuracy, sensitivity, specificity, precision, recall, receiver, area under the curve (AUC), F measure, mean absolute error (MAE), root mean squared error (RMSE), R squared (R^2), root mean squared percentage error (RMSPE).

2.1. Search Strategy

We utilized an array of reputable databases, such as PubMed, Scopus, Embase, Cochrane, Web of Science, Google Scholar, and the Saudi Digital Library, to conduct a digital search for data. Our comprehensive search encompassed the years 2000 to 2024. To search for articles in electronic databases several key terms were used: artificial intelligence, age, age estimation, chronological age, precise age, age prediction, age detection, age evaluation, age assessment, dental age, age classification, tooth staging, tooth parameter, bone parameters, tooth development, convolutional neural network, automated, machine learning, deep learning, X-rays, dental radiographs, panoramic radiographs, and forensics. Further to that, we used Boolean operators (AND, OR) and applied English language filters. To supplement our electronic search, we also manually scrutinized applicable research publications and their citations. This process included inspecting the reference lists of previously gathered articles in the college library. The search was carried out by two separate authors who were specifically trained to carry out the same task.

2.2. Study Selection

Article selection was based on how relevant articles were to the field of study, alongside the allure of their titles and abstracts. Two researchers (S.B.K. and F.B.) conducted the search process independently, resulting in a bounty of 580 articles initially considered, with 578 discovered through the electronic search and 2 found through manual exploration. To safeguard against duplicity, two additional team members conducted a thorough inspection, purging 387 replicates. The remaining trove of 193 manuscripts underwent a meticulous assessment to ascertain their eligibility.

2.3. Eligibility Criteria

The papers selected for this comprehensive review had to adhere to specific guidelines: (a) original works exploring AI; (b) inclusion of quantitative data for examination and analysis; and (c) clear references to the data enabling evaluation of AI-based models. For the study design to be included in this review, no limitations were imposed. Articles not delving into AI innovation, conference papers never published or that were only available online, unpublished works, articles lacking full-text availability, pilot studies, and those not in English were excluded.

2.4. Data Extraction

After evaluating the selected papers based on their titles and abstracts and removing duplicates, the authors thoroughly examined the full texts. Following this evaluation, the count of articles meeting the criteria for inclusion in the systematic review dwindled to 28. To uphold impartiality, the publications' journal names and author details were expunged, allowing two impartial reviewers (M.A. and A.S.), unconnected to the initial search, to appraise them. Pertinent data from the chosen papers were meticulously extracted and inputted into a Microsoft Excel document, encapsulating particulars on writers, publication dates, research goals, AI algorithm varieties employed, and the data for model training, validation, and testing. Results, findings, and recommendations from the research were also recorded. Disagreements regarding the inclusion of four articles arose due to insufficient evidence supporting their results and conclusions. After consultation with another qualified author (A.F.), these four articles were excluded. As a result, a total of 26 articles were carefully curated and meticulously examined in this systematic review, as shown in Figure 1. These 26 articles were deemed worthy of consideration for inclusion and were subjected to a rigorous evaluation.

The papers were scrutinized for quality using QUADAS-2 [27], which delved into various aspects of research design and reporting, including patient selection, index test, reference standard, flow, and timing. This evaluation sought to gauge the applicability of the data across diverse clinical settings and patient cohorts, while pinpointing possible sources of bias. Two reviewers showed substantial agreement, with an 82% level of agreement measured by Cohen's kappa.

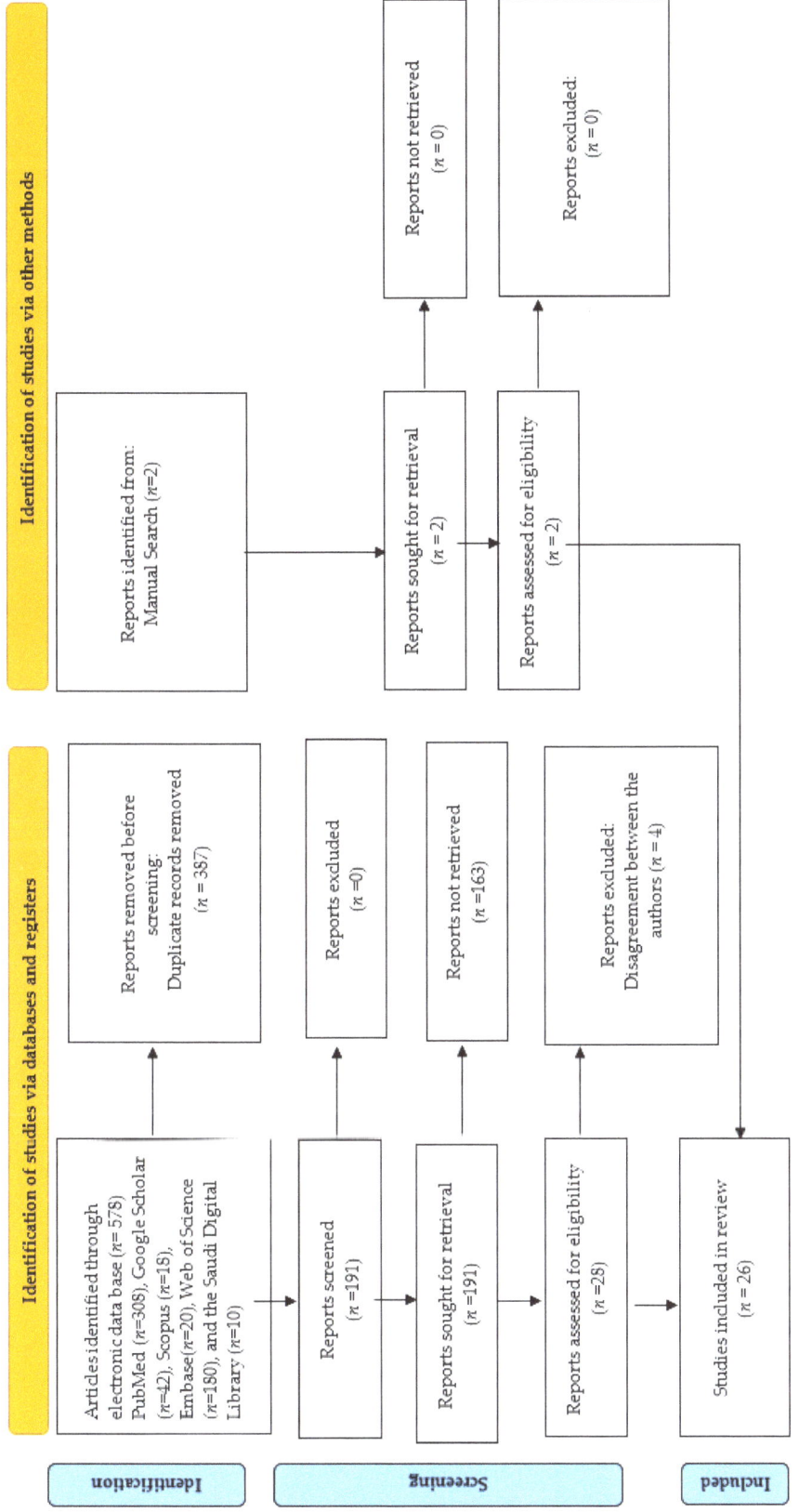

Figure 1. PRISMA 2020 flow diagram for new systematic reviews including searches of databases, registers and other sources.

3. Results

After an in-depth analysis of 26 articles, qualitative data were extracted. Most of the articles were published in the last four years, indicating a rising trend in articles focusing on the implementation of AI models for tooth numbering and detection.

3.1. Qualitative Data of the Studies

AI has primarily been used for automated age estimation by analyzing tooth development stages [28–47], tooth and bone parameters [48–50], bone age measurements [51], and pulp–tooth ratio [52,53]. We gathered data from the studies included, but due to the varied data samples used to assess AI model performance, a meta-analysis could not be conducted. The heterogeneity in the extracted data stemmed from the diverse types of data samples utilized in evaluating the AI models' performance. Therefore, this systematic review only provides descriptive data from the studies included, as shown in Table 2.

3.2. Study Characteristics

The study characteristics decoded comprised details regarding the authors; year of publication; research goals; AI model development algorithms employed; training, validation, and testing data sources; model accuracy assessment; research findings; and any guidance offered by the authors.

3.3. Outcome Measures

Efficiency in task execution was evaluated by employing different metrics, such as measurable or predictive outcomes including receiver operating characteristic (ROC), area under the curve (AUC), accuracy, sensitivity, specificity, precision, recall, F-measure, mean absolute error (MAE), root mean squared error (RMSE), R squared (R^2), and root mean squared percentage error (RMSPE).

3.4. Risk of Bias Assessment and Applicability Concern

The evaluation of study quality and risk of bias was conducted using the QUADAS-2 assessment tool (Table S1). All studies employed patient-derived secondary information in the form of dento-maxillofacial radiographs as the input for the CNNs, presuming randomization and non-randomization to be equally dispersed in primary studies. The patient-selection domain was considered to have no risk of bias. The standardized methods for entering data into AI technology helped mitigate bias in the flow and timing domain. Nevertheless, two of the studies (15.38%) [37,46] failed to clearly delineate the reference standard employed, giving rise to inherent bias concerns in the index test, reference standard, flow, and timing domains. Another (7.69%) study [46] relied on notations from solitary observations as a gold standard, culminating in a high risk of bias with respect to index tests. Despite the above-mentioned issues, both research arms exhibited minimal risk of bias in all the studies considered. The risk of bias evaluation and applicability concerns in the studies analyzed are presented in Table S1 and Figure 2.

Table 2. Details of the studies that have used automation-based models for age estimation.

Sl No.	Authors	Year of Publication	Study Design	Algorithm Architecture	Objective of the Study	No. of Patients/Images/Photographs for Testing [Datasets]	Study Factor	Modality	Comparison If Any	Evaluation Accuracy/Average Accuracy/Statistical Significance	Results (+) Effective, (−) Non-Effective (N) Neutral	Outcomes	Authors Suggestions/ Conclusions
1.	Bunyarit SS et al. [28]	2018	Retrospective cross-sectional study	ANN	To investigate the applicability of Chaillet and Demirjian's scores for the age estimation of Malaysian Chinese children and adolescents	1228 DPRs	Tooth development stages (permanent teeth from central incisor to third molar-left mandible).	DPRs	Chaillet and Demirjian's method	Accurate estimation of age and the difference between CA and DA was −0.05 ± 0.92 years for boys and −0.06 ± 1.11 years for girls using ANN–MLP networking model.	Effective (+)	Chaillet and Demirjian's method underestimated the DA. Population-specific prediction model was developed using the ANN–MLP networking model.	These ethnic-specific data can be used to estimate the DA of Malaysian Chinese children and adolescents in both clinical and forensic applications.
2.	Mualla N et al. [29]	2020	Observational study	CNN	To implement automated dental age estimation using transfer learning	1429 X-ray images	Tooth development stages	X-rays	ResNet	AlexNet (KNN classifier) Accuracy 98.8% Specificity 99.18 Precision 99.005 Recall 99.98 F-measure 98.99 ResNet Accuracy 98.8% Specificity 99.818 Precision 99.062 Recall 99.104 F-measure 99.149	Effective (+)	AlexNet-based features were better than the ResNet-based features.	Transfer learning has proved its effectiveness in many machine learning and object recognition problems. This method needs to be evaluated more using a larger dataset and other classification models.
3.	Galibourg A et al. [30]	2021	Comparative study	ML	To compare the predictive performance of ten machine learning algorithms for dental age estimation in children and young adults using left permanent mandibular teeth and third molars	3570 OPGs	Tooth development stages (seven permanent mandibular teeth and four third molars)	OPG	Age estimation methods by Demirjian et al. and Willems et al.	AI method had a mean absolute error (MAE) under 0.811 years. With Demirjian's and Willems' methods, the MAE was 1.107 and 0.927 years,	Effective (+)	WILL method was significantly more accurate than DEM, and all ML methods were more accurate than the best reference method.	This study supported the use of ML algorithms instead of using standard population tables.

Table 2. Cont.

Sl No.	Authors	Year of Publication	Study Design	Algorithm Architecture	Objective of the Study	No. of Patients/Images/Photographs for Testing [Datasets]	Study Factor	Modality	Comparison If Any	Evaluation Accuracy/Average Accuracy/Statistical Significance	Results (+) Effective, (−) Non-Effective (N) Neutral	Outcomes	Authors Suggestions/ Conclusions
4.	Isa AT al. [31]	2021	Comparative study	DL models	To estimate the forensic ages of individuals using an automated approach	1332 DPRs Training 962 (85%) testing 170 (15%), and validating 200 (15%)	Tooth development stages (teeth, gingival tissue, and upper jaw)	DPR Images	InceptionV3 DenseNet201 EfficientNetB4 MobileNetV2 VGG16, and ResNet50V2	MAE = 3.13, RMSE =4.77, and correlation coefficient R^2 was 87%.	Effective (+)	Modified InceptionV3 model delivered results faster and estimated ages more precisely compared to others.	This method proved to be potentially dependable and practical ancillary equipment in forensic sciences and dental medicine.
5.	Wallraff S et al. [32]	2021	Comparative study	CNN	To automate age estimation of adolescents using a supervised regression-based deep learning method	14000 DPRs 10,000 for training, 2500 for validation, and 244 for testing	Tooth development stages	DPR	Senior physician for oral and maxillofacial surgery and three dental students specially trained in age estimation	MAE of 1.08 years and error rate (ER) of 17.52%.	Effective (+)	This method achieved better results than manual estimation methods used by clinical experts.	This method will be useful in age estimation compared to manual methods.
6.	Kim S et al. [33]	2021	Comparative study	CNN	To estimate age group by incorporating a CNN using dental X-ray image patches of the first molars extracted via panoramic radiography	DPRs of 1586 individuals Training: 1078 Validation: 190 Test: 318	Tooth development stages (permanent first molars of both arches)	Panoramic radiographs	Subgroup comparison	The accuracy of the tooth-wise estimation was 89.05 to 90.27%. AUC scores ranged from 0.94 to 0.98 for all age groups.	Effective (+)	Study demonstrated the suitability of CNNs for accurately estimating the age groups of both the maxillary and mandibular first molars.	The prediction accuracy and heat map analyses support that this AI-based age-group determination model is plausible and useful.
7.	Shen S et al. [34]	2021	Retrospective study	ML	To utilize seven lower left permanent teeth alongside three models (RF, SVM, and LR) based on the Cameriere method for predicting children's dental age and assess their performance against Cameriere age estimation	748 OPGs Training: 598 (80%) Test: 150 (20%)	Tooth development stages (7 lower left permanent teeth)	OPG	Traditional Cameriere formula	ME, MAE, MSE, and RMSE values of the SVM model (0.004, 0.489, 0.392, and 0.625, respectively) and the RF model (−0.004, 0.495, 0.389, and 0.623, respectively) had the highest accuracy.	Effective (+)	The research showed that the ML models have better accuracy than the traditional Cameriere formula.	All tested machine learning methods were significantly more accurate than the two Cameriere formulas for all metrics.

Table 2. Cont.

Sl No.	Authors	Year of Publication	Study Design	Algorithm Architecture	Objective of the Study	No. of Patients/Images/Photographs for Testing [Datasets]	Study Factor	Modality	Comparison If Any	Evaluation Accuracy/Average Accuracy/Statistical Significance	Results (+) Effective, (−) Non-Effective (N) Neutral	Outcomes	Authors Suggestions/ Conclusions
8.	Milošević D et al. [35]	2022	Comparative study	CNN	To explore the applicability of deep learning in chronological age estimation using panoramic dental X-rays	4035 DPRs training/validation/test size is 80%/10%/10%	Tooth development stages	DPR	State of art methods	Mean absolute error of 3.96 years, a median absolute error of 2.95 years, and an R^2 of 0.8439.	(+) Effective	This research showcases the effectiveness of automated deep learning in dental imaging for precise age estimation.	The proposed approach attains the lowest estimation error in the literature for adult and senior subjects.
9.	Hann et al. [36]	2022	Cross-sectional, descriptive, analytical study.	CNN	To assess the accuracy of a machine learning model for precise age estimation with or without relying on human interference	10,257 OPGs Training set (80%), validation set (10%), and test set (10%).	Tooth development stages (8 permanent teeth of left mandible)	OPG	ADSE model based on specified manually defined features	MAE of the ADAE model is 0.83 years, being reduced by half that of the MDAE model. ADSE model for stage classification is 0.17 stages; its accuracy in dental age estimation is unsatisfactory.	(+) Effective	The ADSE model slightly improves accuracy with manually defined features and enhances evaluation efficiency. In contrast, the ADAE model, utilizing CNN, significantly boosts accuracy and efficiency without human intervention.	Fully automated feature extraction in a deep learning model without human interference performs better in dental age estimation, prominently increasing the accuracy and objectivity.
10.	Baydoğan MP et al. [37]	2022	Observational study	CNN	To estimate age by deep learning using dental panoramic radiographs	627 OPGs Training (70%) Test (30%)	Tooth development stages	OPG	Dentist	84% accuracy, 85% F-score, and 76% sensitivity values were reached using the Alexnet architecture and k-nearest neighbor (k-NN) algorithm.	(+) Effective	The proposed system will ensure age determination in less time and abate the cost compared to the traditional age determination method.	The study will support dentists in the clinical environment and can be used in education

Table 2. Cont.

Sl No.	Authors	Year of Publication	Study Design	Algorithm Architecture	Objective of the Study	No. of Patients/Images/Photographs for Testing [Datasets]	Study Factor	Modality	Comparison If Any	Evaluation Accuracy/Average Accuracy/Statistical Significance	Results (+) Effective (−) Non-Effective (N) Neutral	Outcomes	Authors Suggestions/ Conclusions
11.	Pintana P et al. [38]	2022	Observational study	CNN	To develop and implement a fully automated system for estimating dental age utilizing the ACF detector and deep learning methodologies	1000 OPGs Training: 800 Testing: 200	Tooth development stages (lower left third molars)	OPG	Demirjian's method	Localized the lower left mandibular third molar automatically with 99.5% accuracy and achieved 83.25% classification accuracy using the transfer learning strategy with the Resnet50 network.	(+) Effective	ACF detector and CNN model successfully localized third molars and identified the developmental stages automatically in order to estimate the age of the subjects.	The proposed method can be applied in clinical practice as a tool that helps clinicians reduce the time and subjectivity for dental age estimation.
12.	Saric et al. [39]	2022	Observational study	ANN	To decide on the most desirable machine learning for dental age estimation based on buccal bone level	150 CBCTs	Tooth development stages (lower seven mandibular teeth)	CBCT	Conventional ML models	Random forest classifier provided the greatest result with a correlation coefficient of 0.803 and a mean absolute error of 6.022.	(+) Effective	RF proved to be the best algorithm in our study, providing the most acceptable result for age estimation, using the three most important attributes.	We have also shown that considering sinus-related features can be a significant addition to the databases.
13.	Shen et al. [40]	2022	Comparative study	ML	To compare of the accuracy of the Cameriere and Demirjian methods of dental age estimation using ML simultaneously	748 OPGs Training: 80% Testing: 20%	Tooth development stages (seven mandibular teeth)	OPG	Demirjian method or Cameriere European formula	KNN model based on the Cameriere method had the highest accuracy (ME = 0.015, MAE = 0.473, MSE = 0.340, RMSE = 0.583, R^2 = 0.94).	(+) Effective	KNN model based on the Cameriere method was able to infer dental age more accurately in a clinical setting.	ML can be used for dental age estimation in a larger geographical area and over a larger age range.
14.	Wang et al. [41]	2022	Comparative study	CNN	To estimate chronological ages by using DENSEN for different age groups	1903 OPGs	Tooth development stages	OPG	Bayesian CNN Net and DANet	DENSEN produced MAEs of 0.6885, 0.7615, 1.3502, and 2.8770 for children, teens, young adults, and adults, respectively.	(+) Effective	DENSEN has lower errors for the adult group. The proposed model is memory-compact, consuming about 1.0 MB of memory overhead.	This approach required less laboratory work compared with existing methods.

Table 2. *Cont.*

Sl No.	Authors	Year of Publication	Study Design	Algorithm Architecture	Objective of the Study	No. of Patients/Images/Photographs for Testing [Datasets]	Study Factor	Modality	Comparison If Any	Evaluation Accuracy/Average Accuracy/Statistical Significance	Results (+) Effective, (−) Non-Effective (N) Neutral	Outcomes	Authors Suggestions/ Conclusions
15.	Kumagai A et al. [42]	2023	Comparative study	ML	To validate data-mining-based dental age estimation by comparing its accuracy and classification performance at 18-year thresholds against conventional methods	2657 DPRs Training: 900 Test sets: 857	Tooth development stages (second and third molars of both jaws)	DPRs	Conventional method	The accuracy of the conventional method with the internal test set was slightly higher than that of the data mining models, with a slight difference (mean absolute error< 0.21 years, root mean square error< 0.24 years).	Neutral (N)	The threshold was also similar between the conventional method and the data mining models.	This method proved that conventional methods can be replaced by data mining models in forensic age estimation using second and third molar maturity of Korean juveniles and young adults.
16.	Yeom HG et al. [43]	2023	Comparative study	CNN	To estimate chronological age using a hybrid method based on ResNet 50 and ViT	9663 DPRs Training: 5861 Validation: 1916 Test data: 1886	Tooth development stages	DPRs	ResNet50 or ViT.	Significant improvements were observed in both MAE and RMSE values across all network models (ResNet50, ViT, and Hybrid	(+) Effective	The age estimation model designed using the hybrid method performed better than those using only ResNet50 or ViT.	This model can perform better and be used effectively in the clinical field.
17.	Kahm SH et al. [44]	2023	Comparative study	DL	To evaluate the efficiency of an AI model by applying the entire panoramic image for age estimation	27,877 DPRs Training: 13,220 Validation: 1653 Test data: 1653	Tooth development stages	DPRs	Two experienced dentists	Incorporating ± 3years of deviation, the accuracy of type 1 and 2 was 0.2716, 0.7323, respectively; and the F1 score was 0.1709 and 0.6437, respectively.	(+) Effective	The study showed significant accurate diagnosis in type 2 grouping with ±3years of deviation in both DN and WRN models.	In the future, the application of AI is expected to assist humans in clinical and dento-maxillofacial radiology fields.
18.	Aljameel S et al. [47]	2023	Comparative study	CNN	To predict dental age using AI model	529 DPRs 423 (80% for training) 106 (20% for testing)	Tooth development stages (7 left permanent teeth and 3 molars)	DPRs	Three dentists	Xception model had the best performance, with an error rate of 1.417 for the 6–11 age group.	(+) Effective	Xception model had the best performance, with an error rate of 1.417 for the 6–11 age group.	The proposed model can assist dentists in determining the appropriate treatment for patients based on their DA rather than their chronological age.

Table 2. Cont.

Sl No.	Authors	Year of Publication	Study Design	Algorithm Architecture	Objective of the Study	No. of Patients/Images/ Photographs for Testing [Datasets]	Study Factor	Modality	Comparison If Any	Evaluation Accuracy/Average Accuracy/Statistical Significance	Results (+) Effective, (−) Non-Effective (N) Neutral	Outcomes	Authors Suggestions/ Conclusions
19.	Rin Kim et al. [46]	2023	Observational study	CNN	To classify the age group using deep neural network when precise age information is not given	10023 DPRs	Tooth development stages	DPRs	NM	The accuracies were 53.846% with a tolerance of ±5 years, 95.121% with ±15 years, and 99.581% with ±25 years, which means the probability of the estimation error being larger than one age group is 0.419%.	(+) Effective	This study confirmed the potential possibility of age estimation using AI in terms of clinical aspects of oral care, as well as forensic medicine, by determining the difference between the actual age and predicted age using panoramic radiographic images, which can be used to evaluate the overall oral conditions.	This study has the potential to be used as oral health education material using the difference between the actual age and the predicted age through AI in dental clinics.
20.	Murray J et al. [47]	2024	Observational study	CNN	To apply AI in determination of legal age	4003 DPRs. Training: 80% Testing: 20%	Tooth development stages (third molars)	DPRs	Experts	Of the subjects over 18 years of age, 88% were correctly identified, and 87.0% of subjects under the age of majority were similarly predicted.	(+) Effective	AI-based methods could improve courtroom efficiency, stand as automated assessment methods, and contribute to our understanding of biological aging.	The present model may be used as an automated assessment tool for identifying legal age. The weightings generated by this architecture can also help researchers identify which patterns are most significant for understanding this challenging age group.

Table 2. Cont.

Sl No.	Authors	Year of Publication	Study Design	Algorithm Architecture	Objective of the Study	No. of Patients/Images/Photographs for Testing [Datasets]	Study Factor	Modality	Comparison If Any	Evaluation Accuracy/Average Accuracy/Statistical Significance	Results (+) Effective, (−) Non-Effective (N) Neutral	Outcomes	Authors Suggestions/Conclusions
21.	Zaborowicz M et al. [48]	2022	Observational study	EL	To utilize deep learning neural models for accurate assessment of chronological age in children and adolescents based on tooth and bone parameters	619 OPGs	Tooth and bone parameters	OPG	Radial basis function networks	The MAE error of the produced models, depending on the learning set used, is between 2.34 and 4.61 months, while the RMSE error is between 5.58 and 7.49 months. The correlation coefficient R^2 ranges from 0.92 to 0.96.	(+) Effective	The conducted research indicates that neural modeling methods are an appropriate tool for determining the metric age based on the developed proprietary tooth and bone indices.	The initial iteration of learning the network with all developed metrics already yields high-quality deep neural models. It is advisable to construct deep neural networks using the indicators from the initial research stage.
22.	MU CC et al. [49]	2022	Comparative study	DL	To assess the accuracy of transfer learning models for age estimation from panoramic radiographs of permanent dentitions of patients	3000 DPRs Training: 2400 Validating: 300 Test set: 300	Tooth and bone parameters (teeth, maxillary sinus, and mandibular angle)	DPRs	ResNet VggNet DenseNet	MAE and RMSE of EfficientNet-B5 were 2.83 and 4.49, respectively	(+) Effective	This method of transfer learning proves to be applicable for age estimation utilizing panoramic radiographs.	This model can be used for age estimation with panoramic radiographs.
23.	Wang J et al. [50]	2023	Comparative study	CNN	To investigate the possibility of using AI-based methods for age estimation in an eastern Chinese population	9586 OPGs Training: 70% Testing: 30%	Tooth and bone parameters (molars, maxillary sinus, and nasal septum)	OPGs	ResNet101	Accuracy of VGG16 model = 93.63%. Accuracy of ResNet101 network = 88.73%.	(+) Effective	VGG16 outperformed ResNet101 in terms of DA prediction performance.	CNNs such as VGG16 hold great promise for future use in clinical practice and forensic sciences.
24.	Sharifonnasabi F et al. [51]	2022	Comparative study	CNN	To evaluate the accuracy of a hybrid HCNN-KNN model in age estimation	1922 DPRs Training: 80% Testing: 20%	Bone age measurement	OPG	ResNet, CNN, GoogLeNet Inception	Successfully estimated the age in classified studies of -year-old, 6 months, 3 months, and 1-month-old cases with accuracies of 99.98, 99.96, 99.87, and 98.78 respectively.	(+) Effective	The evaluation of our model on a diverse dataset confirms its superior performance.	The benchmarking with current existing models also showed that the HCNN-KNN model is the best model for bone age measurement.

Table 2. Cont.

Sl No.	Authors	Year of Publication	Study Design	Algorithm Architecture	Objective of the Study	No. of Patients/Images/Photographs for Testing [Datasets]	Study Factor	Modality	Comparison If Any	Evaluation Accuracy/Average Accuracy/Statistical Significance	Results (+) Effective, (−) Non-Effective (N) Neutral	Outcomes	Authors Suggestions/ Conclusions
25.	Pereira de Sousa et al. [52]	2023	Comparative study	ML	To assess and compare age estimation on panoramic radiography using the Kvaal method and machine learning	554 DPRs Training: 85% Testing: 5%	Pulp–tooth ratio	DPRs	Kvaal method	ML (MAE: 4.77) presented higher age estimation precision than the Kvaal method (MAE: 5.68).	(+) Effective	ML classifiers can improve age estimation when assessing panoramic radiography using the Kvaal method.	The use of ML on panoramic radiographs can improve age estimation.
26.	Dogan B et al. [53]	2024	Observational study	ML	To use ML algorithms to evaluate the efficacy of pulp/tooth area ratio (PTR) in cone-beam CT (CBCT) images to predict dental age classification in adults	236 CBCT Training: 70% Testing: 30%	Pulp/tooth area ratio	CBCT	CART SVM	The models' highest accuracy and confidence intervals were found to belong to the RF algorithm.	Neutral (N)	The models' performances were found to be low.	The models were found to be low in performance but were considered as a different approach.

Notes: ML = machine learning; DL = deep learning; ANN = artificial neural networks; CNN = convolutional neural networks; DPRs—digital panoramic radiographs; OPGs—orthopantomographs; CT—computed tomography; CBCT—cone-beam computed tomography; MAE—mean absolute error; RMSE—Root Mean Squared Error; R^2—R squared.

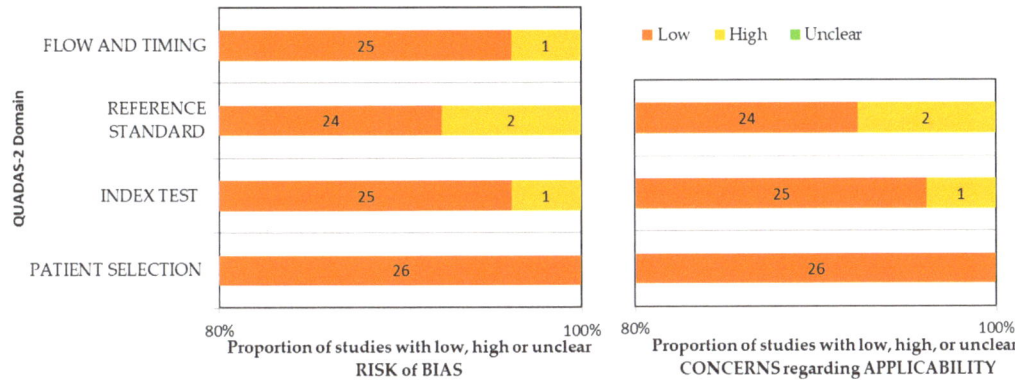

Figure 2. QUADAS-2 assessment of the individual risk of bias domains and applicability concerns.

3.5. Assessment of Strength of Evidence

The certainty of evidence was evaluated using the Grading of Recommendations Assessment Development and Evaluation (GRADE) technique [54]. There are four levels of certainty: very low, low, moderate, and high. This is determined by assessing five factors: risk of bias, inconsistency, indirectness, imprecision, and publication bias. According to the assessment, the included papers demonstrated a high level of certainty of evidence, as shown in Table 3.

Table 3. Assessment of strength of evidence.

Outcome	Inconsistency	Indirectness	Imprecision	Risk of Bias	Publication Bias	Strength of Evidence
Application of AI in automated age estimation using tooth development stages [28–47]	Not Present	Not Present	Not Present	Present	Not Present	⊕⊕⊕○
Application of AI in automated age estimation using tooth and bone parameters [48–50]	Not Present	Not Present	Not Present	Not Present	Not Present	⊕⊕⊕⊕
Application of AI in automated age estimation using bone age measurements [51]	Not Present	Not Present	Not Present	Not Present	Not Present	⊕⊕⊕⊕
Application of AI in automated age estimation using pulp–tooth ratio [52,53]	Not Present	Not Present	Not Present	Not Present	Not Present	⊕⊕⊕⊕

⊕⊕⊕⊕—high evidence; ⊕⊕⊕○—moderate evidence.

The certainty of the studies included in this systematic review was evaluated using the Grading of Recommendations Assessment Development and Evaluation (GRADE) approach. Inconsistency, indirectness, imprecision, risk of bias, and publication bias were the five domains that determine the certainty of evidence and can be categorized as very low, low, moderate, or high evidence. The overall certainty of evidence from the included studies in this review was found to be high.

4. Discussion

Determining age is crucial in various areas, like in forensic science for identifying individuals in various situations like mass casualties and criminal cases [55]. It also helps to verify the ages of athletes and immigrants to uphold equal rights and fairness [56]. Additionally, it aids in planning orthodontic and pediatric treatments by predicting jaw growth spurts [57]. To accurately estimate age, it is essential to assess sexual characteristics, bone development, and tooth development [12].

Chronological age can be estimated using three main categories: laboratory-guided molecular biology studies, dental indicators, and bone markers [50]. Dental age assessment involves comparing the developmental stages of both temporary and permanent teeth with dental development charts created by various researchers [50]. Researchers have established different scales based on the developmental stages of both permanent and temporary teeth observed in radiographs. The age of 14, when the permanent second molars erupt, marks the conclusion of the childhood and mixed dentition phase and serves as a reliable method in age estimation [37]. Two conventional methods that are commonly used for age determination are the 'Atlas method' and 'Demirjian's method'. The former compares radiographic dental development (mineralization) with published standards, and the latter is a scoring method that involves scoring the development of seven left lower mandibular teeth in eight categories (A–H) [58].

Even though these manual methods have been correctly utilized in various groups, there are still specific drawbacks in clinical settings, such as the subjectivity of the technique and potential bias in measurement. Additionally, these procedures can be tedious and time-consuming [31]. The conventional approach to dental age estimation using image processing involves a series of manual procedures, including segmentation, feature extraction, image pre-processing, classification, and regression. Each of these steps carries a risk of errors and can introduce variability in the final result. For instance, bone images obtained from radiography scans may differ between dry and wet conditions, even within the same age group [51].

Deep learning methods are known as end-to-end learning-based approaches, where deep neural networks like convolutional neural networks can directly process input images and generate the desired output without the need for intermediate steps like segmentation and feature extraction [29]. Thus, automated dental age estimation is very much essential in order to improve the accuracy and repeatability of age estimation [7]. Hence, this systematic review was undertaken to assess the development and performance of AI models in automated age estimation.

4.1. Effectiveness of AI in Automated Age Estimation Using Tooth Development Stages

Dental radiological techniques for age assessment typically involve parameters like tooth development stages, tooth eruption, open apices of teeth, development of jaw bones, and pulp–tooth ratio. Tooth development is more commonly used than eruption in age assessment as the latter can be affected by external factors, whereas formation is a continuous, cumulative, and advancing process [59]. Out of the studies reviewed, a total of 20 have delved into the application of AI for estimating age based on tooth development stages. The study conducted by Mulla et al. [29] achieved the highest accuracy of 98.8% and precision of 99.05% out of all other AI models in age estimation. Their approach was assessed using various performance metrics on a dataset containing 1429 dental X-ray images and indicated that features based on AlexNet outperformed those based on ResNet. Furthermore, the k-NN classifier demonstrated superior performance across different metrics when compared to other classifiers [29].

It was observed in our review that the major drawbacks associated with traditional age estimation methods were underestimation and overestimation of age. It was found that the Chaillet and Demirjian method underestimated the dental age of Malaysian Chinese individuals in the study conducted by Bunyarit SS et al. [28]. Therefore, a population-specific predictive model was created using an artificial neural network–multilayer perceptron (ANN-MLP) to improve the accuracy of age estimation. The discrepancy between chronological age (CA) and dental age (DA) was much lesser (-0.05 ± 0.92 years for boys and -0.06 ± 1.11 years for girls) when utilizing the ANN-MLP networking model. In contrast to this, Galibourg et al. [30] reported that Demirjian's and Willems' methods, both overestimated the age, Demirjian's by a mean of 257 days and Willems' by 80 days, and affirmed that machine learning methods outperformed traditional approaches for age estimation using radiographic dental staging from childhood to early adulthood. These findings align with a meta-analysis which indicated that Demirjian's method tends to overestimate females' ages by 0.65 years and males' ages by 0.60 years on average [60].

A dental age estimation model that is fully automated, with no human involvement, outperformed one that depended on manually defining features. The automated model achieved a mean absolute error (MAE) of 0.83 years, which was half of that of the manual model. This autonomous method might reveal previously unrecognized age-related features, thereby improving the model's overall performance as reported by Han M et al. [36].

In another study conducted by Kumagai et al. [42], it was found that the accuracy of the conventional method using the internal test set was slightly better compared to the AI models. The difference in mean absolute error was less than 0.21 years, and the root mean square error was less than 0.24 years. The discrepancies between the conventional methods and AI models were around 44 to 77 days with mean absolute error and 62 to 88 days with root mean square error. While the conventional methods showed a slight edge in accuracy in this research, it is uncertain whether this small difference has significant clinical or practical relevance. These findings suggest that dental age estimation using AI models can be done with nearly the same precision as the conventional method.

Shen et al. [34] conducted a study on estimating the dental age of seven permanent teeth in the left mandible in Eastern Chinese individuals aged 5 to 13 years. They used the Cameriere method for age estimation and compared it with linear regression, support vector machine (SVM), and random forest (RF) models. Their results showed that all three AI models had higher accuracy than the conventional method. The improved accuracy could be due to including younger participants in the study sample. As age estimation becomes more precise with the increasing number of developing teeth, the presence of younger subjects in the study could lead to higher accuracy in the derived age estimation method [61].

4.2. Effectiveness of AI in Automated Age Estimation Using Tooth and Bone Parameters

The neural model created in the research conducted by Zaborowicz M et al. [48] demonstrated the lowest prediction errors of 2.34 months in determining the metric age of boys. Specific sets of 21 tooth and bone parameters that were developed as mathematical proportions by the same author were utilized here [62]. The study used panoramic radiographs of people with normal dental development and no systemic illnesses. Cases with root canal treatment or extensive fillings were excluded to improve network construction.

In a different study [49], using the optimal EfficientNet-B5 model, the group of females aged 22 to 31 had the smallest prediction error (MAE 0.96, RMSE 1.52), whereas the group of males aged 52 to 61 had the highest error (MAE 5.12, RMSE 7.03). The discrepancy between estimated and real age increased with age. The dentition, maxillary sinus, mandibular body, and mandibular angle all contributed to age estimation. The class activation mapping results indicated that different anatomical structures were relevant in age groups. Characteristics were predominantly in the teeth in younger age groups (12 to 21 and 22 to 31 years), which is in line with conventional techniques. The emphasis turned to the maxillary sinus upon movement into the middle age groups (ages 32 to 41 and 42 to 51). Mandibular body and mandibular angle were emphasized for older age groups (52–61 and 62–71 years) [49].

In comparison to the ResNet101 network, VGG16 demonstrated superior performance in estimating DA using OPGs on a large scale using teeth and bone parameters according to the study conducted by Wang J et al. [51]. The VGG16 model yielded satisfactory predictions for younger age groups, with an accuracy of up to 93.63% in the 6- to 8-year-old category [50].

4.3. Effectiveness of AI in Automated Age Estimation Using Bone Parameters

A novel automated machine learning model for bone age estimation was proposed by Sharifonnasabi F et al. [51]. The current bone age estimation models are mainly in the research phase and have not been widely adopted in the industry. The proposed model achieved high accuracy (99.98%) levels for different age ranges and outperformed existing models. Testing on diverse datasets and races confirmed the superior performance of the HCNN-KNN model, making it a promising tool for bone age measurement [51].

4.4. Effectiveness of AI in Pulp–Tooth Ratio

Dental age estimation in adults is based on quantifying age-related morphological changes of teeth, such as the deposition of secondary dentin. Even after the completion of root formation, the odontoblasts remain functional, continuing the production of secondary dentin throughout life. As a result of this physiological process, the dimensions of the pulp chamber gradually change [63]. Various age estimation methods have been developed based on this decrease. This assessment can be definitively performed through non-radiological methods like histological and biochemical approaches. Due to the need for tooth extraction in these methods, they are not suitable for living individuals or situations where tissue collection from human remains is not feasible. Therefore, radiological methods are more easily applicable for dental age estimation. Radiological methods have progressed significantly, enabling the three-dimensional imaging of hard tissues in the jaws [64].

Pulp chamber volumes are utilized in estimating dental age, and these ratios can be analyzed through deep learning. Despite the low performance of the models as reported in a study conducted by Dogan B et al. [53], they represent a different approach. The algorithms performed most accurately for the 18–25 age group compared to other age groups. Exploring different parameters derived from various measuring techniques in CBCT data could aid in developing machine learning algorithms for age classification in forensic scenarios. The measurements should be always taken from the cementum–enamel junction level on the axial section to obtain accurate three-dimensional secondary dentine deposition [53].

A study evaluated the effectiveness of Kvaal's age estimation method using various ML attribute extraction approaches and algorithms on a population from northeastern Brazil, based on pulp–tooth ratios. The findings suggested a positive outcome for the semantic–radiomic association attribute. Kvaal's method and ML yielded better results for the male dataset, with ML outperforming the Kvaal method by around 1 year across all analyzed scenarios [52].

5. Challenges and Future Considerations in AI

AI models developed for age estimation using dento-maxillofacial radiographs can be applied for various tasks like determining identities of dead people in explosions and bomb blasts, evaluating athletes in competitive sports, judging juvenile delinquencies, clinical and forensic purposes, adopting undocumented children of uncertain ages, handling international refugees, and planning treatment for patients. Despite promising results from studies evaluating the performance of AI models for automated age estimation from dento-maxillofacial radiographs, various factors need to be considered before a definitive conclusion can be reached. The limitations and challenges reported in most of the studies are mainly related to the limited number of datasets and the lack of a good number of previously reported studies for a comparison of the results. Hence, it is necessary to conduct more studies with abundant sample sizes and in diverse populations in order to improve the applicability of this approach. The requirement for abundant data can also be addressed through the application of data augmentation methods. Furthermore, the training datasets need to be precise, reliable, and free from significant errors to ensure optimal performance [65]. Some studies reviewed had used a limited number of dental radiograph datasets compared to the wealth of data utilized in medical AI research. This may lead to the development of AI models that are excessively specialized, potentially skewing results towards overly optimistic outcomes. The essence of this issue lies in the fact that AI algorithms typically require a substantial amount of data for effective generalization to diverse scenarios. Consequently, it is crucial to validate the sample size and possibly conduct statistical analyses to ensure that the findings have broader applicability. The overall findings of the studies included in the paper suggest that AI-based models which include ML and DL display high accuracy and minimal average error and outperform the classical methods applied for age estimation [34,39]. However, the mean error of deep learning techniques is claimed to be somewhat greater than that of machine learning regression approaches, despite the fact that they can save more time in object detection [34]. When applying ML models for age estimation, we should consider individual variability and use additional predictors in order to reduce the variability [66]. Deep learning techniques can perform a more detailed analysis process, where they can work directly on input images and provide the desired output without requiring the completion of intermediate processes like feature extraction and segmentation. However, designing and training a deep neural network is an expensive, time-consuming, and difficult process. Therefore, new approaches are developed that can utilize pre-trained deep neural networks and perform the necessary tasks, and these approaches are termed transfer learning methods [31]. These transformers have made a breakthrough in computer vision. Age estimation models that were developed using transfer learning were more feasible in terms of cost, time spent in developing the model, and performing the task more precisely [31,49].

6. Conclusions

This systematic review found that AI models demonstrated superior performance in automatic age estimation utilizing dento-maxillofacial radiographic images with increased accuracy and precision and decreased mean absolute errors. Given this specific situation, AI has the potential to act as a valuable partner in supporting the efforts of dental and forensic professionals by allowing them to handle numerous images simultaneously. However, it is crucial to recognize that the results of AI radiographic analyses are not inherently flawless, as their precision depends on the quality of the training data and the effectiveness of their model's selection and training procedures. Thus, it remains essential for experts to provide their ultimate interpretation as the final assessment.

Supplementary Materials: The following supporting information can be downloaded at: https://www.mdpi.com/article/10.3390/diagnostics14111079/s1, Table S1: Risk of bias and applicability concerns.

Author Contributions: Conceptualization, S.B.K. and F.A.; methodology, M.A., A.A. (Aram Alshehri), A.A. (Ali Aldhebaib) and O.G.S. software, K.I.; validation, A.A. (Abdulmohsen Alfadley), B.A. and A.A. (Aram Alshehri); formal analysis, K.I.; investigation, M.A. and B.A.; resources, F.A.; data curation, A.A. (Ali Aldhebaib); writing—original draft preparation, S.B.K.; writing—review and editing, F.A., B.A. and O.G.S. visualization, F.A.; supervision, A.A. (Abdulmohsen Alfadley); project administration, F.A. All authors have read and agreed to the published version of the manuscript.

Funding: This research received no external funding.

Institutional Review Board Statement: Not applicable.

Informed Consent Statement: Not applicable.

Data Availability Statement: Not applicable.

Conflicts of Interest: The authors declare no conflicts of interest.

References

1. Limdiwala, P.; Shah, J. Age Estimation by Using Dental Radiographs. *J. Forensic Dent. Sci.* **2013**, *5*, 118. [CrossRef] [PubMed]
2. Willems, G.; Moulin-Romsee, C.; Solheim, T. Non-Destructive Dental-Age Calculation Methods in Adults: Intra- and Inter-Observer Effects. *Forensic Sci. Int.* **2002**, *126*, 221–226. [CrossRef]
3. Maltoni, R.; Ravaioli, S.; Bronte, G.; Mazza, M.; Cerchione, C.; Massa, I.; Balzi, W.; Cortesi, M.; Zanoni, M.; Bravaccini, S. Chronological Age or Biological Age: What Drives the Choice of Adjuvant Treatment in Elderly Breast Cancer Patients? *Transl. Oncol.* **2022**, *15*, 101300. [CrossRef] [PubMed]
4. Franklin, D. Forensic Age Estimation in Human Skeletal Remains: Current Concepts and Future Directions. *Leg. Med.* **2010**, *12*, 1–7. [CrossRef]
5. Vila-Blanco, N.; Varas-Quintana, P.; Tomás, I.; Carreira, M.J. A Systematic Overview of Dental Methods for Age Assessment in Living Individuals: From Traditional to Artificial Intelligence-Based Approaches. *Int. J. Leg. Med.* **2023**, *137*, 1117–1146. [CrossRef] [PubMed]

6. Lewis, J.M.; Senn, D.R. Dental Age Estimation Utilizing Third Molar Development: A Review of Principles, Methods, and Population Studies Used in the United States. *Forensic Sci. Int.* **2010**, *201*, 79–83. [CrossRef]
7. Celik, S.; Zeren, C.; Çelikel, A.; Yengil, E.; Altan, A. Applicability of the Demirjian Method for Dental Assessment of Southern Turkish Children. *J. Forensic Leg. Med.* **2014**, *25*, 1–5. [CrossRef] [PubMed]
8. Uzuner, F.D.; Kaygısız, E.; Darendeliler, N. Defining Dental Age for Chronological Age Determination. *Post Mortem Exam. Autops.* **2017**, *6*, 77–104. [CrossRef]
9. Willems, G. A Review of the Most Commonly Used Dental Age Estimation Techniques. *J. Forensic Odonto-Stomatol.* **2001**, *19*, 9–17.
10. Reesu, G.V.; Augustine, J.; Urs, A.B. Forensic Considerations When Dealing with Incinerated Human Dental Remains. *J. Forensic Leg. Med.* **2015**, *29*, 13–17. [CrossRef]
11. Stavrianos, C.; Mastagas, D.; Stavrianou, I.; Karaiskou, O. Dental Age Estimation of Adults: A Review of Methods and Principles. *Res. J. Med. Sci.* **2008**, *2*, 258–268.
12. Panchbhai, A. Dental Radiographic Indicators, a Key to Age Estimation. *Dentomaxillofacial Radiol.* **2011**, *40*, 199–212. [CrossRef] [PubMed]
13. AlQahtani, S.J.; Hector, M.P.; Liversidge, H.M. Brief Communication: The London Atlas of Human Tooth Development and Eruption. *Am. J. Phys. Anthropol.* **2010**, *142*, 481–490. [CrossRef] [PubMed]
14. Blenkin, M.; Taylor, J. Age Estimation Charts for a Modern Australian Population. *Forensic Sci. Int.* **2012**, *221*, 106–112. [CrossRef] [PubMed]
15. Reppien, K.; Sejrsen, B.; Lynnerup, N. Evaluation of Post-Mortem Estimated Dental Age versus Real Age: A Retrospective 21-Year Survey. *Forensic Sci. Int.* **2006**, *159*, S84–S88. [CrossRef] [PubMed]
16. McKenna, C.; James, H.; Taylor, J.; Townsend, G. Tooth Development Standards for South Australia. *Aust. Dent. J.* **2002**, *47*, 223–227. [CrossRef] [PubMed]
17. Liversidge, H.M.; Smith, B.H.; Maber, M. Bias and Accuracy of Age Estimation Using Developing Teeth in 946 Children. *Am. J. Phys. Anthropol.* **2010**, *143*, 545–554. [CrossRef] [PubMed]
18. Mani, S.A.; Naing, L.; John, J.; Samsudin, A.R. Comparison of Two Methods of Dental Age Estimation in 7–15-Year-Old Malays. *Int. J. Paediatr. Dent.* **2008**, *18*, 380–388. [CrossRef] [PubMed]
19. Shah, P.; Venkatesh, R. Pulp/Tooth Ratio of Mandibular First and Second Molars on Panoramic Radiographs: An Aid for Forensic Age Estimation. *J. Forensic Dent. Sci.* **2016**, *8*, 112. [CrossRef]
20. Lee, J.-H.; Kim, D.-H.; Jeong, S.-N.; Choi, S.-H. Detection and Diagnosis of Dental Caries Using a Deep Learning-Based Convolutional Neural Network Algorithm. *J. Dent.* **2018**, *77*, 106–111. [CrossRef]
21. Chen, I.-H.; Lin, C.-H.; Lee, M.-K.; Chen, T.-E.; Lan, T.-H.; Chang, C.-M.; Tseng, T.-Y.; Wang, T.; Du, J.-K. Convolutional-Neural-Network-Based Radiographs Evaluation Assisting in Early Diagnosis of the Periodontal Bone Loss via Periapical Radiograph. *J. Dent. Sci.* **2024**, *19*, 550–559. [CrossRef]
22. Yang, H.; Jo, E.; Kim, H.J.; Cha, I.; Jung, Y.-S.; Nam, W.; Kim, J.-Y.; Kim, J.-K.; Kim, Y.H.; Oh, T.G.; et al. Deep Learning for Automated Detection of Cyst and Tumors of the Jaw in Panoramic Radiographs. *J. Clin. Med.* **2020**, *9*, 1839. [CrossRef]
23. Serindere, G.; Bilgili, E.; Yesil, C.; Ozveren, N. Evaluation of Maxillary Sinusitis from Panoramic Radiographs and Cone-Beam Computed Tomographic Images Using a Convolutional Neural Network. *Imaging Sci. Dent.* **2022**, *52*, 187. [CrossRef] [PubMed]
24. Choi, E.; Kim, D.; Lee, J.-Y.; Park, H.-K. Artificial Intelligence in Detecting Temporomandibular Joint Osteoarthritis on Orthopantomogram. *Sci. Rep.* **2021**, *11*, 10246. [CrossRef]
25. Merdietio Boedi, R.; Banar, N.; De Tobel, J.; Bertels, J.; Vandermeulen, D.; Thevissen, P.W. Effect of Lower Third Molar Segmentations on Automated Tooth Development Staging Using a Convolutional Neural Network. *J. Forensic Sci.* **2019**, *65*, 481–486. [CrossRef]
26. Page, M.J.; McKenzie, J.E.; Bossuyt, P.M.; Boutron, I.; Hoffmann, T.C.; Mulrow, C.D.; Shamseer, L.; Tetzlaff, J.M.; Akl, E.A.; Brennan, S.E.; et al. The PRISMA 2020 Statement: An Updated Guideline for Reporting Systematic Reviews. *Br. Med. J.* **2021**, *372*, n71. [CrossRef]
27. Whiting, P.F. QUADAS-2: A Revised Tool for the Quality Assessment of Diagnostic Accuracy Studies. *Ann. Intern. Med.* **2011**, *155*, 529. [CrossRef] [PubMed]
28. Bunyarit, S.S.; Nambiar, P.; Naidu, M.; Asif, M.K.; Poh, R.Y.Y. Dental Age Estimation of Malaysian Indian Children and Adolescents: Applicability of Chaillet and Demirjian's Modified Method Using Artificial Neural Network. *Ann. Hum. Biol.* **2022**, *49*, 192–199. [CrossRef] [PubMed]
29. Mualla, N.; Houssein, E.H.; Hassan, M.R. Dental Age Estimation Based on X-ray Images. *Comput. Mater. Contin.* **2020**, *62*, 591–605. [CrossRef]
30. Galibourg, A.; Cussat-Blanc, S.; Dumoncel, J.; Telmon, N.; Monsarrat, P.; Maret, D. Comparison of Different Machine Learning Approaches to Predict Dental Age Using Demirjian's Staging Approach. *Int. J. Leg. Med.* **2021**, *135*, 665–675. [CrossRef]
31. Atas, İ.; Özdemir, C.; Atas, M.; Dogan, Y. Forensic Dental Age Estimation Using Modified Deep Learning Neural Network. *Balk. J. Electr. Comput. Eng.* **2023**, *11*, 298–305. [CrossRef]
32. Wallraff, S.; Vesal, S.; Syben, C.; Lutz, R.; Maier, A. Age Estimation on Panoramic Dental X-Ray Images Using Deep Learning. In *Bildverarbeitung für die Medizin 2021*; Springer: Berlin/Heidelberg, Germany, 2021; pp. 186–191. [CrossRef]
33. Kim, S.; Lee, Y.-H.; Noh, Y.-K.; Park, F.C.; Auh, Q.-S. Age-Group Determination of Living Individuals Using First Molar Images Based on Artificial Intelligence. *Sci. Rep.* **2021**, *11*, 1073. [CrossRef]

34. Shen, S.; Liu, Z.; Wang, J.; Fan, L.; Ji, F.; Tao, J. Machine Learning Assisted Cameriere Method for Dental Age Estimation. *BMC Oral Health* **2021**, *21*, 641. [CrossRef]
35. Milošević, D.; Vodanović, M.; Galić, I.; Subašić, M. Automated Estimation of Chronological Age from Panoramic Dental X-Ray Images Using Deep Learning. *Expert Syst. Appl.* **2022**, *189*, 116038. [CrossRef]
36. Han, M.; Du, S.; Ge, Y.; Zhang, D.; Chi, Y.; Long, H.; Yang, J.; Yang, Y.; Xin, J.; Chen, T.; et al. With or without Human Interference for Precise Age Estimation Based on Machine Learning? *Int. J. Leg. Med.* **2022**, *136*, 821–831. [CrossRef]
37. Baydoğan, M.P.; Baybars, S.C.; Tuncer, S.A. Age Detection by Deep Learning from Dental Panoramic Radiographs. *Artif. Intell. Theory Appl.* **2022**, *2*, 51–58.
38. Pintana, P.; Upalananda, W.; Saekho, S.; Yarach, U.; Wantanajittikul, K. Fully Automated Method for Dental Age Estimation Using the ACF Detector and Deep Learning. *Egypt. J. Forensic Sci.* **2022**, *12*, 54. [CrossRef]
39. Saric, R.; Kevric, J.; Hadziabdic, N.; Osmanovic, A.; Kadic, M.; Saracevic, M.; Jokic, D.; Rajs, V. Dental Age Assessment Based on CBCT Images Using Machine Learning Algorithms. *Forensic Sci. Int.* **2022**, *334*, 111245. [CrossRef]
40. Shen, S.; Yuan, X.; Wang, J.; Fan, L.; Zhao, J.; Tao, J. Evaluation of a Machine Learning Algorithms for Predicting the Dental Age of Adolescent Based on Different Preprocessing Methods. *Front. Public Health* **2022**, *10*, 1068253. [CrossRef]
41. Wang, X.; Liu, Y.; Miao, X.; Chen, Y.; Cao, X.; Zhang, Y.; Li, S.; Zhou, Q. DENSEN: A Convolutional Neural Network for Estimating Chronological Ages from Panoramic Radiographs. *BMC Bioinform.* **2022**, *23*, 426. [CrossRef]
42. Kumagai, A.; Jeong, S.; Kim, D.; Kong, H.-J.; Oh, S.; Lee, S.-S. Validation of Data Mining Models by Comparing with Conventional Methods for Dental Age Estimation in Korean Juveniles and Young Adults. *Sci. Rep.* **2023**, *13*, 726. [CrossRef]
43. Yeom, H.-G.; Lee, B.-D.; Lee, W.; Lee, T.; Yun, J.P. Estimating Chronological Age through Learning Local and Global Features of Panoramic Radiographs in the Korean Population. *Sci. Rep.* **2023**, *13*, 21857. [CrossRef]
44. Kahm, S.H.; Kim, J.-Y.; Yoo, S.; Bae, S.-M.; Kang, J.-E.; Lee, S.H. Application of Entire Dental Panorama Image Data in Artificial Intelligence Model for Age Estimation. *BMC Oral Health* **2023**, *23*, 1007. [CrossRef]
45. Aljameel, S.S.; Althumairy, L.; Albassam, B.; Alsheikh, G.; Albluwi, L.; Althukair, R.; Alhareky, M.; Alamri, A.; Alabdan, A.; Shahin, S.Y. Predictive Artificial Intelligence Model for Detecting Dental Age Using Panoramic Radiograph Images. *Big Data Cogn. Comput.* **2023**, *7*, 8. [CrossRef]
46. Kim, Y.-R.; Choi, J.-H.; Ko, J.; Jung, Y.-J.; Kim, B.; Nam, S.-H.; Chang, W.-D. Age Group Classification of Dental Radiography without Precise Age Information Using Convolutional Neural Networks. *Healthcare* **2023**, *11*, 1068. [CrossRef]
47. Murray, J.; Heng, D.; Lygate, A.; Porto, L.; Abade, A.; Manica, S.; Franco, A. Applying Artificial Intelligence to Determination of Legal Age of Majority from Radiographic. *Morphol. Bull. L'association Anat.* **2023**, *108*, 100723. [CrossRef]
48. Zaborowicz, M.; Zaborowicz, K.; Biedziak, B.; Garbowski, T. Deep Learning Neural Modelling as a Precise Method in the Assessment of the Chronological Age of Children and Adolescents Using Tooth and Bone Parameters. *Sensors* **2022**, *22*, 637. [CrossRef]
49. Mu, C.C.; Li, G. Age Estimation Using Panoramic Radiographs by Transfer Learning. *Chin. J. Dent. Res.* **2022**, *25*, 119–124. [CrossRef]
50. Wang, J.; Dou, J.; Han, J.; Li, G.; Tao, J. A Population-Based Study to Assess Two Convolutional Neural Networks for Dental Age Estimation. *BMC Oral Health* **2023**, *23*, 109. [CrossRef]
51. Sharifonnasabi, F.; Jhanjhi, N.Z.; John, J.; Obeidy, P.; Band, S.S.; Alinejad-Rokny, H.; Baz, M. Hybrid HCNN-KNN Model Enhances Age Estimation Accuracy in Orthopantomography. *Front. Public Health* **2022**, *10*, 879418. [CrossRef]
52. Pereira de Sousa, D.; Diniz Lima, E.; Souza Paulino, J.A.; Dos Anjos Pontual, M.L.; Meira Bento, P.; Melo, D.P. Age Determination on Panoramic Radiographs Using the Kvaal Method with the Aid of Artificial Intelligence. *Dento Maxillo Facial Radiol.* **2023**, *52*, 20220363. [CrossRef]
53. Dogan, O.B.; Boyacioglu, H.; Goksuluk, D. Machine Learning Assessment of Dental Age Classification Based on Cone-Beam CT Images: A Different Approach. *Dento Maxillo Facial Radiol.* **2024**, *53*, 67–73. [CrossRef]
54. Granholm, A.; Alhazzani, W.; Møller, M.H. Use of the GRADE Approach in Systematic Reviews and Guidelines. *Br. J. Anaesth.* **2019**, *123*, 554–559. [CrossRef]
55. Costa, J.; Montero, J.; Serrano, S.; Albaladejo, A.; López-Valverde, A.; Bica, I. Accuracy in the Legal Age Estimation according to the Third Molars Mineralization among Mexicans and Columbians. *Atención Primaria* **2014**, *46*, 165–175. [CrossRef]
56. Markovic, E.; Marinkovic, N.; Zelic, K.; Milovanovic, P.; Djuric, M.; Nedeljkovic, N. Dental Age Estimation according to European Formula and Willems Method: Comparison between Children with and without Cleft Lip and Palate. *Cleft Palate Craniofacial J.* **2021**, *58*, 612–618. [CrossRef]
57. Shamim, T. Forensic Pediatric Dentistry. *J. Forensic Dent. Sci.* **2018**, *10*, 128. [CrossRef]
58. Rath, H.; Rath, R.; Mahapatra, S.; Debta, T. Assessment of Demirjian's 8-Teeth Technique of Age Estimation and Indian-Specific Formulas in an East Indian Population: A Cross-Sectional Study. *J. Forensic Dent. Sci.* **2017**, *9*, 45.
59. Jayaraman, J.; Wong, H.M.; King, N.; Roberts, G. The French–Canadian Data Set of Demirjian for Dental Age Estimation: A Systematic Review and Meta-Analysis. *J. Forensic Leg. Med.* **2013**, *20*, 373–381. [CrossRef]
60. Lee, S.-S.; Kim, D.; Lee, S.; Lee, U.-Y.; Seo, J.S.; Ahn, Y.W.; Han, S.-H. Validity of Demirjian's and Modified Demirjian's Methods in Age Estimation for Korean Juveniles and Adolescents. *Forensic Sci. Int.* **2011**, *211*, 41–46. [CrossRef]
61. Zaborowicz, K.; Biedziak, B.; Olszewska, A.; Zaborowicz, M. Tooth and Bone Parameters in the Assessment of the Chronological Age of Children and Adolescents Using Neural Modelling Methods. *Sensors* **2021**, *21*, 6008. [CrossRef]

62. Murray, P.E.; Stanley, H.R.; Matthews, J.B.; Sloan, A.J.; Smith, A.J. Age-Related Odontometric Changes of Human Teeth. *Oral Surg. Oral Med. Oral Pathol. Oral Radiol. Endod.* **2002**, *93*, 474–482. [CrossRef] [PubMed]
63. Verma, M.; Verma, N.; Sharma, R.; Sharma, A. Dental Age Estimation Methods in Adult Dentitions: An Overview. *J. Forensic Dent. Sci.* **2019**, *11*, 57. [CrossRef] [PubMed]
64. Zheng, Q.; Ge, Z.; Du, H.; Li, G. Age Estimation Based on 3D Pulp Chamber Segmentation of First Molars from Cone-Beam–Computed Tomography by Integrated Deep Learning and Level Set. *Int. J. Leg. Med.* **2020**, *135*, 365–373. [CrossRef] [PubMed]
65. Putra, R.H.; Doi, C.; Yoda, N.; Astuti, E.R.; Sasaki, K. Current Applications and Development of Artificial Intelligence for Digital Dental Radiography. *Dentomaxillofacial Radiol.* **2021**, *51*, 20210197. [CrossRef] [PubMed]
66. Demirjian, A.; Goldstein, H.; Tanner, J.M. A New System of Dental Age Assessment. *Hum. Biol.* **1973**, *45*, 211–227.

Disclaimer/Publisher's Note: The statements, opinions and data contained in all publications are solely those of the individual author(s) and contributor(s) and not of MDPI and/or the editor(s). MDPI and/or the editor(s) disclaim responsibility for any injury to people or property resulting from any ideas, methods, instructions or products referred to in the content.

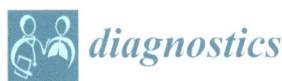

Review

Anatomical Factors of the Anterior and Posterior Maxilla Affecting Immediate Implant Placement Based on Cone Beam Computed Tomography Analysis: A Narrative Review

Milica Vasiljevic [1,†], Dragica Selakovic [2,†], Gvozden Rosic [2], Momir Stevanovic [1], Jovana Milanovic [1], Aleksandra Arnaut [1] and Pavle Milanovic [1,*]

1 Department of Dentistry, Faculty of Medical Sciences, University of Kragujevac, 34000 Kragujevac, Serbia
2 Department of Physiology, Faculty of Medical Sciences, University of Kragujevac, 34000 Kragujevac, Serbia
* Correspondence: pavle11@yahoo.com
† These authors contributed equally to this work.

Abstract: Background: The aim of this narrative review was to provide insights into the influence of the morphological characteristics of the anatomical structures of the upper jaw based on cone beam computed tomography (CBCT) analysis on the immediate implant placement in this region. Material and Methods: To conduct this research, we used many electronic databases, and the resulting papers were chosen and analyzed. From the clinical point of view, the region of the anterior maxilla is specific and can be difficult for immediate implant placement. Findings: Anatomical structures in the anterior maxilla, such as the nasopalatine canal and accessory canals, may limit and influence the implant therapy outcome. In addition to the aforementioned region, immediate implant placement in the posterior maxilla may be challenging for clinicians, especially in prosthetic-driven immediate implant placement procedures. Data presented within the recently published materials summarize the investigations performed in order to achieve more reliable indicators that may make more accurate decisions for clinicians. Conclusion: The possibility for immediate implant placement may be affected by the NPC shape in the anterior maxilla, while the presence of ACs may increase the incidence of immediate implant placement complications. The variations in IRS characteristics may be considered important criteria for choosing the implant properties required for successful immediate implant placement.

Keywords: morphometric analysis; anterior maxilla; posterior maxilla; immediate implant placement; cone beam computed tomography (CBCT)

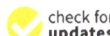

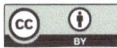

1. Introduction

The anatomical border between the anterior and posterior maxilla represents a bony ridge named the zygomaticoalveolar crest. The anterior maxilla is the region that extends from the first premolar on one side to the first premolar on the other side, the cranial border is represented by the anterior nasal opening (the piriform aperture), and the caudal border is the crestal bone [1]. The benefits of cone beam computed tomography (CBCT) usage in planning interventions in the anterior maxilla region have been confirmed in planning implant placement, especially regarding the existence and type of nasopalatine (NPC) and accessory canals (ACs). Also, the importance of CBCT image analyses has been reported in planning interventions in the maxillary molar region. The advantages of such a diagnostic procedure were highlighted in the sense of interradicular septum (IRS) morphological characteristics analysis, which allows for reliable planning of implant therapy.

The use of CBCT imaging in medicine evolved in the 1980s, which was followed by its introduction in dentistry during the 1990s [1]. CBCT is an extraoral radiographic technique that provides a precise 3D image of hard-tissue structures. CBCT imaging is based on the use of a rotating gantry carrying a source of X-ray radiation and a detector.

A divergent cone-shaped source of radiation passes directly across the field of interest, and the remaining attenuated radiation is beamed onto the X-ray detector surface on the other side [2,3]. In order to make full volume of the image, only one rotation around the patient is necessary [4]. It is well-known that a significant improvement in the analysis of this maxillary region was achieved by using CBCT. The use of CBCT has overcome the deficiencies of other radiological methods, such as the distortions and superimpositions of 2D radiography, poor resolution, the limited access of computed tomography, the high cost, difficulties in interpretation in dentistry, the longer scanning time, disturbances of metal artifacts, and the high radiation exposure of computed tomography and multi-sliced computed tomography [3]. The use of the CBCT methodology has already been proven to have remarkable characteristics for the subtle morphometric analysis of structures that may be of potential interest in planning the procedures accompanied by immediate implant placement [3,4].

The work's methodology results in multiplanar views of the dento-maxillofacial region [5]. Also, CBCT provides primary image reconstruction in three fundamental orthogonal planes (Figure 1), such as axial, sagittal, and coronal [6]. Furthermore, the advantages of CBCT analysis provide across-sectional (individual plane) evaluation. It has an importance in the estimation of non-symmetrical structures, such as maxillary sinus septa and alveolar ridge dimensions [7,8]. As the radiation dose in conventional CT and MSCT imaging is up to 10 times higher than in CBCT, CBCT has primacy in the examination of anatomical structures [9]. In addition to the mentioned preference, there are many other advantages, such as the sub-millimeter resolution (2 line pair/mm), images of higher diagnostic quality, shorter scanning times (~60 s), minimal distortion and reduced radiation dosage [2], as well as lower cost than the CT/MSCT [10].

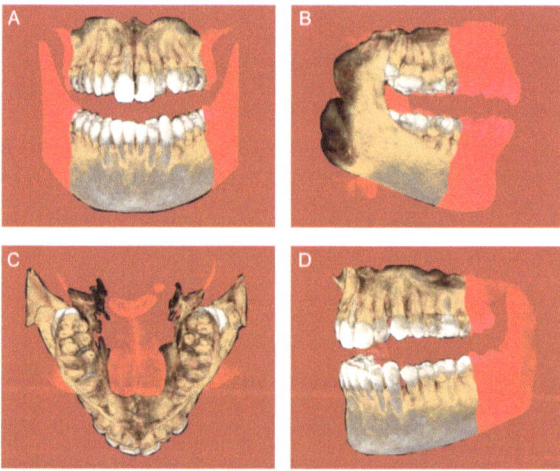

Figure 1. CBCT images with the orthogonal planes: (**A**) coronal, (**B**) sagittal, (**C**) axial, and (**D**) individual plane.

From the clinical point of view, knowledge of anatomical structures and their spatial relationships is crucial in medicine and dentistry for diagnosis and treatment planning [11,12]. Oral and maxillofacial surgery, implantology, orthodontic, ophthalmology, and otorhinolaryngology are fields with increased usage of CBCT [13–17]. The indications for using CBCT have been established by numerous international associations (the Swiss Association of Dentomaxillofacial Radiology and the American Academy of Oral and Maxillofacial Radiology [18,19]). The evaluation of nasopalatine canal (NPC) morphometric characteristics is highly recommended in immediate implant placement planning [20]. Furthermore, CBCT is a reliable radiographic tool used to simulate clinical situations (implant placement) using virtual implants so as to prevent complications [21,22]. Also, virtual planning in maxillofacial surgery is impossible without 3D imaging, and it has been confirmed that CBCT has become a pillar in the design of therapy and in the navigation-based guidance of surgeons during procedures [23–26]. Furthermore, CBCT scans could allow for navigation implantology, so it is currently considered the gold standard for implant site estimation and treatment planning [27]. The study by Nickenig and collaborators [28] has confirmed that navigation implant placement using CBCT and surgical guides may provide successful implant therapy. It leads to the following advantages: a more precise implantation site, the protection of anatomical structures, high geometrical accuracy, being less invasive, shorter treatment and surgery periods, flapless surgery, and, consequently, less possibility of swelling [29]. Furthermore, 3D bone estimation is recommended for numerous procedures, such as preoperative surgical planning for computed assisted surgeries of tumors and traumas, ridge preservation [30], sinus floor elevation [31,32], and implant placement with bone augmentation [33,34] or phased procedures following block grafts [35–38].

Therefore, the aim of this narrative review was to highlight recent findings regarding the advantages of using the CBCT methodology in the evaluation of the maxillary region and its specific morphometric characteristics with clinical importance.

2. Materials and Methods

Our investigation used the electronic scientific resources PubMed, Scopus, and additional sources, such as Google Scholar and major journals. The search was supplemented with a manual search based on the reference lists of the selected papers and other previous reviews including related journals. Inclusion criteria were studies discussing morphological and morphometric characteristics of NPC, ACs, and IRS using CBCT. Only English-language articles were reviewed. Exclusion criteria included studies with patients under the age of 18. Scientific data were searched during the period between 1 January 2008 and 1 July 2024 to identify primary articles utilizing keywords: "cone beam computed tomography" OR "cone beam CT" OR "CBCT" AND nasopalatine canal OR NPC, accessory canals OR ACs, interradicular septum OR interradicular septal bone OR IRS OR ISB, anterior maxilla OR premaxilla OR alveolar ridge OR posterior maxilla, maxillary central incisors OR MCIs. Those studies that fulfilled the selection criteria were processed for data extraction. After extensive searching, a total of 115 studies were identified and underwent title and abstract screening, and then 61 studies were selected for full-text screening. After full-text screening, 24 studies were excluded. Hence, a total of 37 studies that met our inclusion criteria were processed for data extraction (Figure 2).

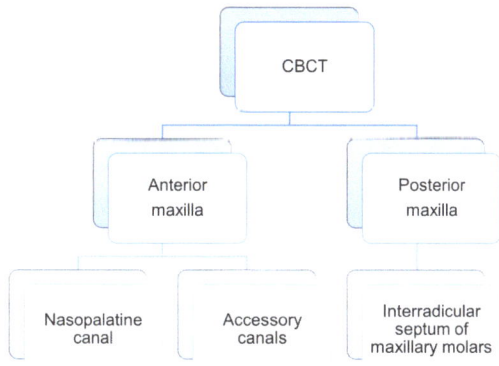

Figure 2. The scheme of the analyzed anatomical structures of the anterior and posterior maxilla through CBCT.

3. Benefits of CBCT Usage in Planning the Interventions in the Anterior Maxilla Region

Recent studies [13,14] performed using morphometric analyses of CBCT images in the anterior maxilla region performed in order to improve the planning of surgical interventions in that region identified NPC and ACs as potential morphological key structures for the final outcome.

It is well-known that the most prominent anatomical structure in the anterior maxilla is the NPC, the content of which is already described [21,39–42]. In addition, Mardinger and coworkers [43] classified NPC shapes in four categories, as follows: cylindrical-, funnel-, banana-, and hourglass-shaped.

Distribution of NPC shapes in the study by Mardingler and collaborators [43] was cylindrical, funnel, hourglass, and banana (Figure 3) (50.7, 30.9, 14.5, and 3.9%, respectively). However, Fukuda and coworkers [44] reported the following distribution: funnel, cylindrical, hourglass, and banana (50, 45, 5, and 0%, respectively). Gil-Markques and colleagues [45] noticed that 32.5% of NPCs were banana-shaped, while cylindrical and funnel shapes appeared in 23.5%, while hourglass was the least represented with 20%. In addition, de Lima and coworkers [46] found that the funnel NPC shape was the most frequent, followed by cylindrical, hourglass, and banana NPC shapes (34.1, 27.5, 25.1, and 13.3%, respectively). Recent studies by Milanovic [14] and Arnaut [13] described similar NPC shape distribution. Namely, Milanovic and colleagues [14] noticed that funnel was 35.4%, cylindrical 31%, hourglass 24.8%, and banana 8.8%. Furthermore, Arnaut and coworkers [13] reported that funnel was the dominant NPC shape (34.59%), followed by cylindrical, hourglass, and banana (28.57%, 24.89%, and 12.03%, respectively).

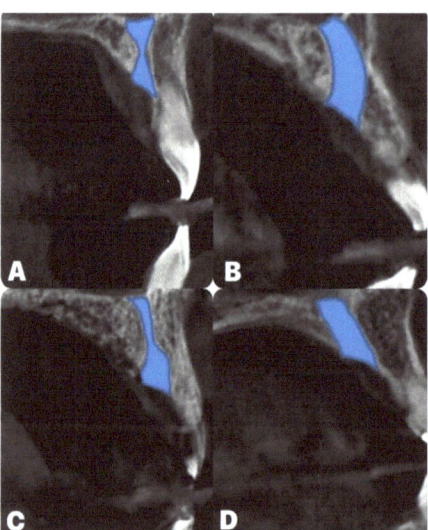

Figure 3. The different NPC types: (**A**) hourglass; (**B**) banana; (**C**) funnel; (**D**) cylindrical.

In addition, numerous studies [43–47] examined dimensions of NPC (NPC length, the diameter of incisive foramen, and the nasal foramen diameter). Thus, Mardingler and coworkers [43] noticed that the mean NPC length was 10.7 mm, while the diameters of the incisive foramen and the nasal foramen were 2.94 mm and 2.55 mm, respectively. Etoz and colleagues [47] reported that the mean NPC length and the incisive and the nasal foramen diameter were found at average levels of 12.59 mm, 5.06, and 3.09 mm, respectively. In addition, Fukuda and collaborators [44] quantified the NPC length and the incisive and the nasal diameters as 11.75 mm, 4.28 mm, and 2.84 mm, respectively. Similarly, de Lima and coworkers [46] presented an NPC length of 12.67 mm, while the incisive foramen and the nasal foramen diameters were 3.49 mm and 2.89 mm, respectively.

Furthermore, we analyzed studies that examined the horizontal dimension of the anterior maxilla at different levels that corresponded to postponed NPC [14,39,45]. Thus, Bornstein and colleagues [39] evaluated the horizontal dimension of the anterior maxilla at three consecutive levels. At the lowest level, they observed the minimal dimension of buccal bone wall (6.5 mm) that was followed by the dimension at the middle level (6.59 mm), while the highest thickness (7.6 mm) was observed at the highest level. Gil-Markques and coworkers [45] also measured the horizontal dimension of the anterior maxilla (central incisors region) at three levels and confirmed the same algorithm: the thickness of the buccal bone increased stepwise according to the level of elevation (6.8, 7.2, and 9.9 mm, respectively). On the other hand, Milanovic and collaborators [14] analyzed the horizontal dimension of the anterior maxilla at four consecutive levels (A, B, C, and D) and reported the nonlinear dimensions' increase (7.11, 7.03, 7.52, and 9.22 mm, respectively). However, only the study by Milanovic and coworkers [14] statistically evaluated the relationship between NPC shape and the horizontal dimension of the anterior maxilla. That methodological approach was used for defining the potential criteria for immediate implant placement in the region of the maxillary central incisors. Severe criteria for expected success are demanded in implant therapy, so it seems necessary to evaluate the morphometric characteristics of the implant site prior to intervention. Hence, Botermans and colleagues [48] recommended the criteria for immediate implant placement in the maxillary esthetic zone. Namely, they proposed that the minimum distances from the labial and palatal bone plates should be 2 mm each. Also, Milanovic and colleagues analyzed the anterior maxilla in the region of the central incisors and gave potential checkpoints in the immediate implant placement planning [14]. Furthermore, the most critical point (insufficient alveolar bone dimension) for the fulfillment of requirements for successful implant therapy was observed in the banana NPC shape. Following the minimal implant diameter (3 mm, [48]) for central incisors immediate implant placement, we present the available bone according to the NPC shape in Table 1.

Table 1. Available bone dimension for the implant placement in the anterior maxilla according to the NPC shape (in mm). Insufficient space (marked in red); minimal required dimensions (marked in yellow); sufficient space (marked in green).

The Horizontal Dimensions of the Anterior Maxilla at Different Levels	NPC Shape			
	Banana	Hourglass	Cylindrical	Funnel
Level A	2.3	3.2	2.9	3.5
Level B	1.4	3.4	3.2	3
Level C	1.6	4	3.6	3.7
Level D	2	5.9	5.7	5.8

Other neurovascular structures in the anterior maxilla analyzed for their potential importance in this narrative review were ACs. Numerous studies estimated morphological and morphometric characteristics of ACs [49–57]. However, the reported data for the presence of ACs were variable. Thus, Machado [51] reported an incidence of 52.1% and Vasiljevic [49] reported 49.23%, while Baena-Caldas [50] reported that ACs were present in all patients. On the other hand, de Oliveira-Santos [57] observed the presence of ACs in only 15.7%.

In addition, according to ACs' direction, von Arx and coworkers [52] described three AC shapes (Figure 4) and noticed that the incidence of the curved AC shape was 56.7%, while vertical and Y AC shapes were present in 41.79% and 1.51%, respectively. Tomrukcu and colleagues [53] reported that the curved shape was even more frequent (69.15%) when compared to vertical and Y AC shapes (26.16 and 4.67%). In a study by Vasiljevic and collaborators [49], the prevalence of AC shapes was 48.96%, 36.45%, and 14.58% (curved, vertical, and Y-shaped, respectively).

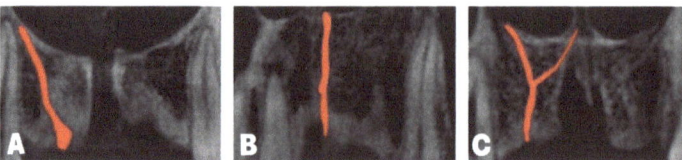

Figure 4. Accessory canal shapes: (**A**) curved; (**B**) vertical; (**C**) Y-shape.

Numerous studies estimated AC diameters [49,51,53,57] and confirmed that the mean diameter of ACs was approximately 1–1.5 mm. However, the evaluation of the distance between maxillary central incisors and ACs was performed only in the study by Vasiljevic and coworkers [49]. That analysis also provided insight into the relationship between NPC shape and the distance between ACs and maxillary central incisors.

As mentioned above, although not evaluated to the extent of NPC, another anatomical structure that could have an impact on immediate implant placement in the maxillary central incisors region is the AC. The recommended ideal implant position in the anterior maxillary extraction socket is the apico-palatal guiding slot technique (2 mm below the apex of the extraction socket [58]). At the same time, a proposed safety zone of 2 mm from the implant position to the bundle was recommended by Greenstein and colleagues [59]. According to the literature data, it is obvious that ACs' presence may be considered as a limiting factor for immediate implant placement in the region of maxillary central incisors [59–61]. In order to reach a compromise in the recommended data, it is clear that in Table 2 it is quantitatively confirmed that the existence of ACs should be considered as excluding criteria for the implant placement.

Table 2. Average palatal distance between accessory canals (ACs) and maxillary central incisors (MCIs) for implant placement according to NPC shape (in mm). Insufficient distance marked in red.

ACs–MCIs Distance at the Different Levels	NPC Shape			
	Banana	Hourglass	Cylindrical	Funnel
Level A	1.18	0.9	0.8	1.05
Level B	1.19	1.1	1.08	1.17
Level C	0.8	1.25	1.7	1.3

Finally, based on all morphometric measurements obtained from CBCT images in numerous studies [13,14,49], provisional guidelines were proposed for the immediate implant placement according to the NPC shape and ACs' presence (Figure 5).

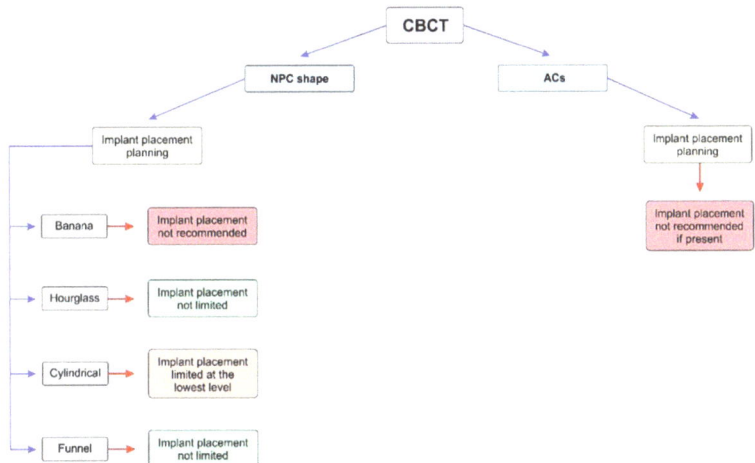

Figure 5. Proposed recommendations for implant placement according to the NPC shape and ACs present. Recommendations for implant placement are based only on the morphometric characteristics without additional interventions (ossedensificaton, bone grafting, and NPC exploration).

4. Benefits of CBCT Usage in Planning the Interventions in the Maxillary Molar Region

From the aspect of the posterior maxilla, IRS presents the ideal place for implant placement, and it is not surprising that numerous studies estimated morphological IRS characteristics [62–66].

A recent study considering IRS [62] presented morphological and morphometric IRS maxillary molar characteristics at the predefined levels using sagittal and axial CBCT slices. There were no significant differences (sagittal slices) reported between IRS characteristics of the maxillary molars (both) in bilateral comparison. The same confirmation was noticed using axial CBCT slices. In addition, differences between IRS characteristics of the first and second maxillary molars were evaluated. Namely, using sagittal CBCT slices, we concluded that the interradicular septum width of the first molars was significantly higher when compared to the second maxillary molars at all evaluated IRS height levels. The same results were reported for the interradicular furcation angle. On the other hand, the IRS height of the second molars was significantly higher than the IRS of the first molars (7 mm and 6.5 mm). Agostinelli and coworkers [66] reported a higher value for the IRS height of the first maxillary molars compared to the second (4.51 vs. 3.24 mm). Finally, no significant difference was shown in the distance between the IRS base and the sinus floor of the first and second molars.

Furthermore, using axial CBCT slices, the perimeter and IRS surface area of the first and second molars were estimated [63]. The average first maxillary molars' perimeter and surface area values were app. 11 mm and 5.5 mm^2 at the lowest level, with stepwise increases in perimeter (12.5, 14, and 16 mm) and surface area (8, 9, and 12.5 mm^2) in the higher sectors. The IRS perimeter and surface area of the second maxillary molars were significantly lower when compared to the first molars. Again, from the bottom to the top, a stepwise increase was observed both for the perimeter (7.5, 10, 11, and 13 mm) and the surface area (3, 4.5, 5.5. and 6.5 mm^2) of the second maxillary molars. A similar observation was reported by Agostinelli and colleagues [66].

Because a possible relationship between different anatomical structures was noticed in previous studies [13,14], the interconnection between the IR furcation angle and the IRS surface area/height at level A for both maxillary molars was estimated. Namely, the correlation between the IR furcation angle and the IRS surface area at level A was significantly positive, while it revealed a significant negative correlation between the IR furcation angle and the IRS height for both groups of molars [63].

This was soon followed by a recent study [63], which proposed the classification of the IRS structure into five different shapes (arrow-, boat-, drop-, palatal-convergence-, and buccal-convergence-shaped) based on coronal CBCT slice analysis (Figure 6). This classification resulted in predefined quantitative criteria for maxillary molars' IRS. The maxillary molars' IRS widths at the base level for the arrow, boat, palatal, and buccal convergence were ≥4 mm. In contrast, for the drop IRS shape, the IRS width was ≤4 mm, which was also the case for both maxillary molars. The second (and final) principal criterion for IRS shape classification was the IR furcation angle. The first molars' IR furcation angles for the arrow and palatal convergence shapes were ≤60° and ≤70°, respectively. On the other hand, the IR furcation angle of buccal convergence, drop, and boat IRS shapes were ≥60°, ≥70°, and ≥90°, respectively. Less variability in the IR furcation angle was shown in the second molars. Hence, the arrow, drop, palatal, and buccal convergence shapes presented IR furcation angles ≤70°, while in the boat IRS shape the angle was ≥70°. It was also noticed that the most frequent IRS shape was arrow (app. 45%), while the lowest frequency was observed for the drop-shaped IRS (app. 11.5%). Similar variability in IRS shapes' appearance was present in both the first and the second maxillary molars.

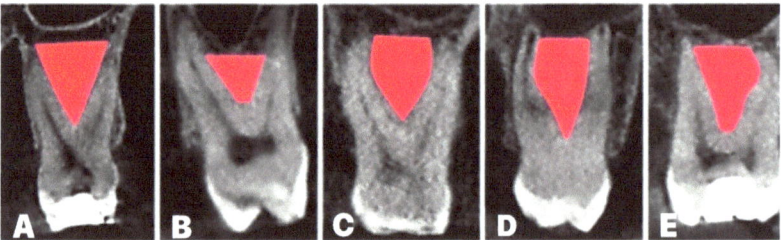

Figure 6. Maxillary molars' IRS shapes: (**A**) arrow; (**B**) boat; (**C**) drop; (**D**) palatal convergence; (**E**) buccal convergence.

In the same study [63], the IRS shape significantly affected all examined parameters (IRS width at the different levels, IR furcation angle, IRS height, distance between IRS base and sinus floor, distance between IR furcation and sinus floor, as well as IRS surface area at all estimated IRS levels). For the first maxillary molars, at all evaluated IRS levels obtained on the coronal view, palatal convergence showed the highest value for the IRS width, as well as height. Afterwards, the IR furcation angle expressed the highest values in the boat shape. This shape also expressed the smallest distance between the IR furcation and the sinus floor. For the second molars, the drop-shaped IRS presented the narrowest IRS at all estimated levels, but with the highest septum. The same was true for the first molars; the largest angle and the smallest distance between the IR furcation and the sinus floor were in the boatshape for the second molars.

Finally, the results obtained on axial slices [63] confirmed that the largest IRS surface area (at all estimated levels) was in the palatal convergence IRS shape for the first upper molars group. Interestingly, the results of the same study showed that the variations in the IRS surface area for the second molars were more prominent, as the highest values for the IRS surface area were observed at the different IRS heights for various IRS shapes.

Also, several authors gave recommendations for IRS dimensions (minimum width of 3 mm and height of 10 mm) for successful immediate implant placement [67,68]. According to this recommendation, we give a suggestion for immediate implant placement based on IRS shape morphometric characteristics [63] in Figure 7. On the other hand, some interventions, such as ossedensification and crestal sinus lift, can overcome this limitation. Namely, both IRS ossedensification and crestal sinus lift elevation can be performed in one-stage surgery. Numerous studies confirmed high rates of success of this intervention [69,70].

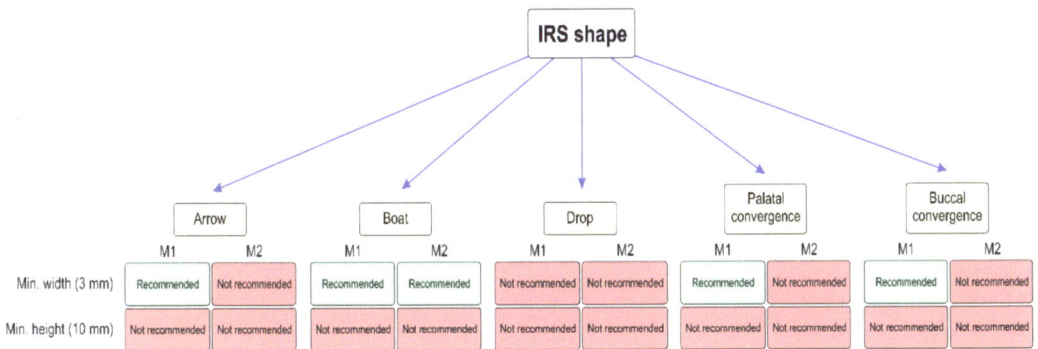

Figure 7. Proposed implant placement recommendations according to the morphometric characteristics depending on IRS shape (without additional surgical treatment).

In addition, following the even more rigorous criterion, based on the fact that the most commonly used implant diameter in the posterior maxilla is 4 mm [69,70], in Figure 8, an overview is presented confirming that none of IRS shapes provides sufficient space for reliable implant placement stability. The proposed analysis is in line with the previous report that described difficulties with immediate implant placement into IRS [71].

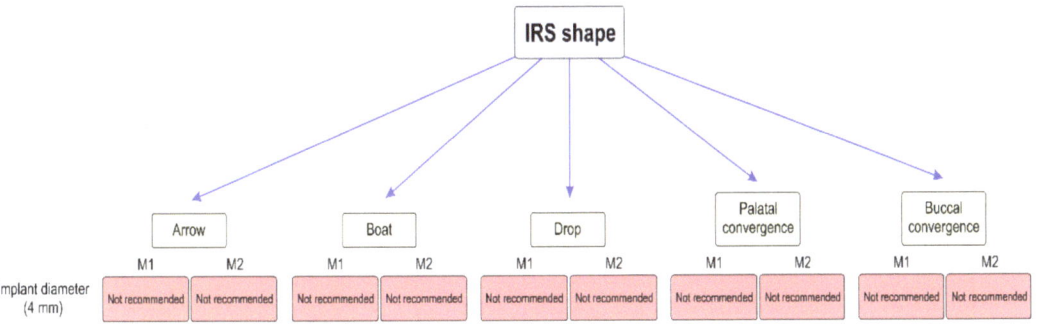

Figure 8. The analysis of IRS morphometric potentials required for reliable implant placement stability according to the IRS shape. (Proposed recommendations for the implant placement are based only on the IRS morphometric characteristics without additional surgical treatment).

5. Discussion

As it is already known, CBCT provides precise bone measurements in order to prevent complications during interventions in the anterior maxilla [13,14]. One of the main criteria for successful immediate implant placement in the region of maxillary central incisors is sufficient thickness of the labial alveolar bone [72]. Thus, some authors [73,74] reported that labial alveolar bone thickness should be at least 2 mm to avoid labial gingival recession and so that biological and esthetic outcomes are achieved. In addition, CBCT examination of the alveolar ridge inclination during implant planning therapy is highly recommended [20]. Namely, immediate implant placement in the region of the anterior maxilla, especially in the lateral incisors area, could be compromised by facial bone concavity [75–77].

On the other hand, it has been confirmed in recent studies that anatomical structures in the anterior maxilla, such as the NPC and accessory canals (ACs), could also compromise interventions in that region [21,49]. It is not surprising that numerous studies performed using CBCT images' morphometric analyses in the anterior maxilla region with the aim to improve the planning of surgical interventions in that region pointed to the NPC and ACs as potential morphological key structures for the final outcome [13,14].

Several NPC morphological classifications have been proposed in the current literature data [43,47,78,79]. Milanovic and collaborators evaluated the dimensions of the alveolar bone (as the common place for NPC and AC appearance) and the thickness at the four consecutive height levels and concluded that the inferior parts of the anterior maxilla presented a lesser dimension than the superior parts [14]. Their findings were in line with the previous observations by Güncü [80] and Lopez and collaborators [81]. A recent study [14] estimated the impact of NPC shape on the anterior maxilla dimensions and confirmed that the impact existed. Namely, except at the lowest level, patients with the banana NPC shape had the smallest horizontal dimension of the anterior maxilla [14].

In order to achieve adequate morphometric conditions for immediate implant placement, especially in patients with a banana NPC shape, several additional surgical interventions (such as bone augmentation and NPC exploration) have been proposed [82,83]. Also, using the NPC as an implant place can be considered [84]. Furthermore, it was suggested by Singhal and coworkers [85] to use surgical guides for precise implant placement into nasopalatine foramen. In patients with funnel NPC shapes, simultaneous use of surgical guides during implant insertion has been recommended [86].

In contrast to the commonly accepted opinion that the NPC is the only neurovascular structure in the anterior maxilla with clinical importance [87], the importance of the estimation of the additional existing channels was highlighted in recent studies [49,50]. A recent study [49] confirmed that the ACs were present in the region of the maxillary central incisors in 49.23% of patients, which is in line with von Arx and colleagues [52], while Wanzeler and collaborators found ACs in almost 90% [54]. Bilateral localization was reported as the most frequent in estimation of ACs' localization by Anatoly and coworkers [55], which is in accordance with our previous study [49]. On the other hand, Manhães and collaborators showed that the variations in AC distribution were side-dependent [56]. Machado [51] and Vasiljevic and coworkers [49] also evaluated ACs' diameter and showed that it was approximately 1 mm, while Oliveira Santos and colleagues [57] reported a slightly larger AC diameter.

Furthermore, there are numerous studies that assessed the interconnection between NPCs and ACs and related anatomical structures [14,49,88]. In addition, the specific relationship between those two vulnerable anatomical structures (NPCs and ACs) in anterior maxilla was estimated by Vasiljevic and coworkers [49], confirming that the described relationship significantly depends on the NPC shape.

It has been confirmed that the NPC's and ACs' localization could be a limiting factor for dental implant placement [14,89]. The orthognathic surgical interventions, such as Le Fort 1, require examination of anatomical structures and careful treatment planning to avoid neurovascular complications [90]. From the point of view of implantology, Botermans and coworkers reported that a secure zone between the NPC and the implant is required [48]. However, several virtual implant placement studies showed that it was difficult to achieve those recommendations [21,91]. Furthermore, Botermans and collaborators [48] noticed NPC perforation during virtual immediate implant placement in about 53% of cases, while Jia and colleagues [91] showed slightly above 16%. Also, the damage to ACs during implant placement is described in the literature [89]. It is confirmed that the damage to anatomical structures in the anterior maxilla could be followed by several complications, such as non-integration of a dental implant, mucosa necrosis, pain, paresthesia, hemorrhage, the sensation of the burning head in the occipital region, and neuropathy [89,92].

Summarizing the algorithm presented in Figure 5, it is obvious that the patients with a banana NPC shape represent the most vulnerable group for immediate implant placement. On the other hand, the morphometric characteristics of the anterior maxilla in subjects with a cylindrical NPC shape are considered to require additional interventions (such as bone grafting) in order to qualify for immediate implant placement. Hourglass and funnel shapes of the NPC, according to our previous results, allow sufficient operating space for surgical interventions. In order to achieve adequate morphometric conditions for the immediate implant placement, especially in patients with a banana NPC shape, several additional surgical interventions (such as bone augmentation and NPC exploration) have been proposed [82,83]. Also, it could be considered to use NPC as an implant place [83,84]. Furthermore, it was suggested by Singhal and coworkers [85] to use surgical guides for precise implant placement into nasopalatine foramen. In patients with a funnel NPC shape, simultaneous use of surgical guides during implant insertion has been recommended [86].

As seen in Figure 5, the presence of ACs should be considered as an absolute contraindication for immediate implant placement. So, the clinicians should follow Shelley's [93] recommendation that in those cases there is a need for other therapeutic options, such as a realistic fixed alternative (adhesive cantilever bridge), in order to avoid potentially damaging implant therapy

Because the posterior maxillary parts are often exposed to several [94–99] surgical interventions (such as implant placement therapy, Le Fort I osteotomy, sinus surgery and sinus lift elevation, cyst enucleation, tumor extirpation, surgical tooth extraction, and present donor site area), the accurate morphometric analysis of CBCT images is required for reliable planning.

The anatomical structures in posterior maxillary parts show high variability [100–102]. From the clinical point of view, IRS has been frequently evaluated as the ideal place for implants [63,103]. Numerous advantages of implant placement in maxillary molars IRS are described, such as the possibility of achieving primary implant stability, adequate force distribution, and plaque control [104,105]. On the other hand, anatomical challenges, as well as the differences between implant diameter and post-extractive alveoli, quality and quantity of bone, root length and configuration, the root trunk height, and roots' divergence, could make surgical interventions more difficult [67,106–109]. Several IRS classifications according to the different criteria have been offered in the literature [63,64]. Namely, Bleyan and collaborators [64] described four categories based on the IRS width (after tooth extraction), as follows: S-I—septum initial width above 4 mm; S-II—septum initial width 3–4 mm; S-III—septum initial width 2–3 mm; and S-IV—septum initial width below 2 mm or no septal bone present. On the other hand, Milenkovic and coworkers [63] defined five IRS shapes based on linear measurements and visual impressions (arrow-, boat-, drop-, palatal-convergence-, and buccal-convergence-shaped) by analyzing CBCT images. However, Smith and colleagues [65] estimated the relationship between the implant and the IRS and noticed three categories: type A sockets (alveoli have sufficient septal bone, which circumferentially surrounds the coronal implant part), type B sockets (the septal bone does not cover the total implant surface, but it is enough to achieve primary implant stability), and the least, type C (has an insufficient septal bone to stabilize the implant without engaging the socket wall).

In post-extractive alveoli, clinicians could also use one of the root cavities to insert the implant in order to achieve primary implant fixation, but it does not meet the requirements for the correct prosthetic implant position [110]. However, previous studies reported that IRS presents the ideal implant site from a prosthetic view [111]. It is not surprising that Rajkovic Pavlovic and coworkers [112] emphasized the importance of radiological IRS evaluation in implant placement planning due to the fact that primary implant stability is determined by the alveoli architecture [113]. In order to obtain better insights into IRS morphological characteristics, Milenkovic and coworkers [63] presented criteria for the classification of five IRS shapes. As presented in Figure 7, the minimal clinical margin for achieving the primary implant stability could not be established only for the drop-shaped IRS, according to the criterion of IRS width. In contrast, this indicator for the primary implant stability in the second molars was achieved only in the boat IRS shape. According to the implant height, as the criterion necessary to achieve implant stability, none of the IRS shapes allows for successful implant placement.

Although previous analyses do not look optimistic from the point of implant placement success, it should be noted that clinicians have a plethora of possibilities to achieve the final success of implant stability by applying additional interventions. Those interventions may be performed prior to implant placement, simultaneously, and/or following the standard implant placement procedure. Some of them are aimed at increasing the IRS width, while the others are recommended for the enlargement of the IRS height. As previously commented, both goals have to be achieved. However, the final success of those procedures accompanied with the implant placement is still under evaluation.

Considering the procedures for the enhancement of IRS width, it should be noticed that osseodensification is a novel method of biomechanical bone preparation in order to achieve improvement in better implant stability when compared to the standard drill [69]. Hence, in the clinical study conducted by Bleyan and coworkers [64], the osseodensification method to improve IRS dimensions was used. They reported the success of implant therapy by means of a 93.1% survival rate at the 12-month follow-up (135/145 implants). Another surgical technique that improves the post-extractive alveoli volume is socket grafting [114–117]. There are numerous materials for filling the gap between implants and alveoli described in the literature [118–120]. The clinical studies confirmed the success of implant therapy by substituting the insufficient implant sites [65,121].

In cases with insufficient bone height, the sinus lift procedure aims to improve vertical bone dimensions below the maxillary sinus in order to provide the possibility of implant placement [122]. Also, the sinus membrane perforation risk could be reduced through this procedure while simultaneously achieving primary implant stability [123]. On the other hand, the dimensions of membrane perforation play an important role in implant placement success [124,125] Thus, Lombardo and coworkers concluded that internal sinus lift presented a small risk of membrane perforation and stable bone around implants with a high rate of success at mid-term follow-up for atrophic maxilla [126].

The mentioned procedures aimed to enhance IRS width and IRS height, and in relation to the analysis presented in the study that analyzed IRS shapes, it is worth noting that CBCT images' morphometric analysis allows for the achievement of exact morphometric parameters that can lead to better planning of interventions in the maxillary molar region.

On the other hand, modern implant therapy includes short implants with wide threads, such as AnyRidge implants (Anyridge®, Megagen, South Korea) [127]. Numerous studies concluded that using this implant type may achieve high primary stability in immediate implant placement for the maxillary posterior region [128,129].

6. Conclusions

Taken altogether, the impact of the methodological approach based on CBCT image analysis of maxilla, as presented in this summary of our recent studies, is manifested by achieving more reliable recommendations for performing certain interventions in the maxillary region. Summarizing the proposed operating procedures, according to our recent investigations based on the potential usefulness of CBCT-based diagnostic procedures in planning some specific interventions in the described regions of interest, it seems that the following can be stated:

- The possibility for immediate implant placement may be affected by the NPC shape in the anterior maxilla, while the presence of ACs, in general, may increase the incidence of immediate implant placement complications;
- The variations in IRS characteristics may be considered important criteria for choosing the implant properties required for successful immediate implant placement.

The presented relationships of potential clinical importance may be considered as tentative factors for exclusion criteria under the described circumstances. Furthermore, in the case that there are no absolute contraindications for the interventions in this region, the use of the proposed methodology allows for better intervention planning by means of predefining optimal procedures and quantification of the extent of accompanied treatments.

7. Future Directions

The recent literature provides exact data on the anatomical configuration of the upper jaw that may affect implant placement. However, subsequent studies could be directed towards virtual implant placement in order to obtain more precise insight into the relationship between the implant and vulnerable anatomical structures, such as the NPC, ACs, and maxillary sinus membrane. Beside gold standards for implant macrodesign, using virtual planning software for implant surgery with a different macrodesign should also be examined, as well as the relationship between such a design and the aforementioned anatomical structure.

Author Contributions: Conceptualization: P.M., M.V., D.S. and G.R.; methodology—literature review: P.M., M.V., D.S. and G.R.; writing—original draft preparation: P.M., M.V., A.A., M.S., J.M., D.S. and G.R.; writing—review and editing: P.M., M.V., A.A., M.S., J.M., D.S. and G.R. All authors have read and agreed to the published version of the manuscript.

Funding: This research received no external funding.

Acknowledgments: This work was supported by the Faculty of Medical Sciences (JP 06/22), University of Kragujevac, Serbia.

Conflicts of Interest: The authors declare no conflicts of interest.

Abbreviations

CBCT	Cone beam computed tomography
NPC	Nasopalatine canal
ACs	Accessory canals
IRS	Interradicular septum

References

1. Von Arx, T.; Lozanoff, S. *Clinical Oral Anatomy*; Springer: Cham, Switzerland, 2017. [CrossRef]
2. Scarfe, W.C.; Farman, A.G. What is cone-beam CT and how does it work? *Dent. Clin. N. Am.* **2008**, *52*, 707–730. [CrossRef] [PubMed]
3. Kumar, M.; Shanavas, M.; Sidappa, A.; Kiran, M. Cone beam computed tomography—Know its secrets. *J. Int. Oral Health* **2015**, *7*, 64–68. [PubMed]
4. Hashimoto, K.; Kawashima, S.; Araki, M.; Iwai, K.; Sawada, K.; Akiyama, Y. Comparison of image performance between cone-beam computed tomography for dental use and four-row multidetector helical CT. *J. Oral Sci.* **2006**, *48*, 27–34. [CrossRef] [PubMed]
5. Shahbazian, M.; Vandewoude, C.; Wyatt, J.; Jacobs, R. Comparative assessment of panoramic radiography and CBCT imaging for radiodiagnostics in the posterior maxilla. *Clin. Oral Investig.* **2014**, *18*, 293–300. [CrossRef] [PubMed]
6. DeVos, W.; Casselman, J.; Swennen, G.R. Cone beam computerized tomography (CBCT) imaging of oral and maxillofacial region: A systemic review of literature. *Int. J. Oral Maxillofac. Surg.* **2009**, *38*, 609–625. [CrossRef] [PubMed]
7. Orhan, K.; KusakciSeker, B.; Aksoy, S.; Bayindir, H.; Berberoğlu, A.; Seker, E. Cone beam CT evaluation of maxillary sinus septa prevalence, height, location and morphology in children and an adult population. *Med. Princ. Pract.* **2013**, *22*, 47–53. [CrossRef] [PubMed]
8. Ortiz-Puigpelat, O.; Lázaro-Abdulkarim, A.; de Medrano-Reñé, J.M.; Gargallo-Albiol, J.; Cabratosa-Termes, J.; Hernández-Alfaro, F. Influence of Implant Position in Implant-Assisted Removable Partial Denture: A Three-Dimensional Finite Element Analysis. *J. Prosthodont.* **2019**, *28*, e675–e681. [CrossRef] [PubMed]
9. Loubele, M.; Bogaerts, R.; Van Dijck, E.; Pauwels, R.; Vanheusden, S.; Suetens, P.; Marchal, G.; Sanderink, G.; Jacobs, R. Comparison between effective radiation dose of CBCT and MSCT scanners for dentomaxillofacial applications. *Eur. J. Radiol.* **2009**, *71*, 461–468. [CrossRef] [PubMed]
10. Winter, A.A.; Pollack, A.S.; Frommer, H.H.; Koenig, L. Cone beam volumetric tomography vs. medical CT scanners. *N. Y. State Dent. J.* **2005**, *71*, 28–33.
11. Von Arx, T.; Lozanoff, S.; Bornstein, M.M. Extraoral anatomy in CBCT—A literature review. Part 1: Nasoethmoidal region. *Swiss Dent. J.* **2019**, *129*, 804–815. [CrossRef] [PubMed]
12. Hodez, C.; Griffaton-Taillandier, C.; Bensimon, I. Cone-beam imaging: Applications in ENT. *Eur. Ann. Otorhinolaryngol. Head Neck Dis.* **2011**, *128*, 65–78. [CrossRef] [PubMed]
13. Arnaut, A.; Milanovic, P.; Vasiljevic, M.; Jovicic, N.; Vojinovic, R.; Selakovic, D.; Rosic, G. The Shape of Nasopalatine Canal as a Determining Factor in Therapeutic Approach for Orthodontic Teeth Movement—A CBCT Study. *Diagnostics* **2021**, *11*, 2345. [CrossRef] [PubMed]
14. Milanovic, P.; Selakovic, D.; Vasiljevic, M.; Jovicic, N.U.; Milovanović, D.; Vasovic, M.; Rosic, G. Morphological Characteristics of the Nasopalatine Canal and the Relationship with the Anterior Maxillary Bone—A Cone Beam Computed Tomography Study. *Diagnostics* **2021**, *11*, 915. [CrossRef] [PubMed]

15. Bremke, M.; Leppek, R.; Werner, J.A. Die digitale Volumen tomographie in der HNO-Heilkunde [Digital volume tomography in ENT medicine]. *HNO* **2010**, *58*, 823–832. [CrossRef] [PubMed]
16. Tschopp, M.; Bornstein, M.M.; Sendi, P.; Jacobs, R.; Goldblum, D. Dacryocystography using cone beam CT in patients with lacrimal drainage system obstruction. *Ophthalmic Plast. Reconstr. Surg.* **2014**, *30*, 486–491. [CrossRef] [PubMed]
17. Gaêta-Araujo, H.; Alzoubi, T.; Vasconcelos, K.F.; Orhan, K.; Pauwels, R.; Casselman, J.W.; Jacobs, R. Cone beam computed tomography in dentomaxillofacial radiology: A two-decade overview. *Dentomaxillofac. Radiol.* **2020**, *49*, 20200145. [CrossRef] [PubMed]
18. Dula, K.; Benic, G.I.; Bornstein, M.M.; Dagassan Berndt, D.; Filippi, A.; Hicklin, S.; Kissling-Jeger, F.; Luebbers, H.T.; Sculean, A.; Sequeira-Byron, P.; et al. SADMFR guidelines for the use of cone beam computed tomography/digital volume tomography. *Swiss Dent. J.* **2015**, *125*, 945–953. [CrossRef] [PubMed]
19. Tyndall, D.A.; Price, J.B.; Tetradis, S.; Ganz, S.D.; Hildebolt, C.; Scarfe, W.C. Position statement of the American Academy of Oral and Maxillofacial Radiology on selection criteria for the use of radiology in dental implantology with emphasis on cone beam computed tomography. Oral Surg. *Oral Surg. Oral Med. Oral Pathol. Oral Radiol.* **2012**, *113*, 817–826. [CrossRef] [PubMed]
20. Buser, D.; Chappuis, V.; Belser, U.C.; Chen, S. Implant placement post extraction in esthetic single tooth sites: When immediate, when early, when late? *Periodontology 2000* **2016**, *73*, 84–102. [CrossRef] [PubMed]
21. Alkanderi, A.; Al Sakka, Y.; Koticha, T.; Li, J.; Masood, F.; Suárez-López Del Amo, F. Incidence of nasopalatine canal perforation in relation to virtual implant placement: A cone beam computed tomography study. *Clin. Implant Dent. Relat. Res.* **2020**, *22*, 77–83. [CrossRef] [PubMed]
22. Chan, H.L.; Garaicoa-Pazmino, C.; Suarez, F.; Monje, A.; Benavides, E.; Oh, T.J.; Wang, H.L. Incidence of implant buccal plate fenestration in the esthetic zone: A cone beam computed tomography study. *Int. J. Oral Maxillofac. Implants* **2014**, *29*, 171–177. [CrossRef] [PubMed]
23. Lin, H.H.; Lo, L.J. Three-dimensional computer-assisted surgical simulation and intraoperative navigation in orthognathic surgery: A literature review. *J. Formos. Med. Assoc.* **2015**, *114*, 300–307. [CrossRef] [PubMed]
24. Adolphs, N.; Haberl, E.J.; Liu, W.; Keeve, E.; Menneking, H.; Hoffmeister, B. Virtual planning for craniomaxillofacial surgery—7 Years of experience. *J. Cranio-Maxillofac. Surg.* **2014**, *42*, e289–e295. [CrossRef] [PubMed]
25. Zinser, M.J.; Mischkowski, R.A.; Dreiseidler, T.; Thamm, O.C.; Rothamel, D.; Zöller, J.E. Computer-assisted orthognathic surgery: Waferless maxillary positioning, versatility, and accuracy of an image-guided visualisation display. *Br. J. Oral Maxillofac. Surg.* **2013**, *51*, 827–833. [CrossRef] [PubMed]
26. Alkhayer, A.; Piffkó, J.; Lippold, C.; Segatto, E. Accuracy of virtual planning in orthognathic surgery: A systematic review. *Head Face Med.* **2020**, *16*, 34. [CrossRef] [PubMed]
27. Deporter, D.; EbrahimiDastgurdi, M.; Rahmati, A.; G Atenafu, E.; Ketabi, M. CBCT data relevant in treatment planning for immediate maxillary molar implant placement. *J. Adv. Periodontol. Implant Dent.* **2021**, *2*, 49–55. [CrossRef] [PubMed]
28. Nickenig, H.J.; Eitner, S. Reliability of implant placement after virtual planning of implant positions using cone beam CT data and surgical (guide) templates. *J. Craniomaxillofac. Surg.* **2007**, *4–5*, 207–211. [CrossRef] [PubMed]
29. Ramasamy, M.; Giri; Raja, R.; Subramonian; Karthik; Narendrakumar, R. Implant surgical guides: From the past to the present. *J. Pharm. Bioallied Sci.* **2013**, *1*, S98–S102. [CrossRef] [PubMed]
30. Abdelhamid, A.; Omran, M.; Bakhshalian, N.; Tarnow, D.; Zadeh, H.H. An open randomized controlled clinical trial to evaluate ridge preservation and repair using SocketKAPTM and SocketKAGETM: Part 2—Three-dimensional alveolar bone volumetric analysis of CBCT imaging. *Clin. Oral Implants Res.* **2015**, *27*, 631–639. [CrossRef] [PubMed]
31. Gorla, L.F.; Spin-Neto, R.; Boos, F.B.; Pereira Rdos, S.; Garcia Junior, I.R.; Hochuli-Vieira, E. Use of autogenous bone and beta-tricalcium phosphate in maxillary sinus lifting: A prospective, randomized, volumetric computed tomography study. *Int. J. Oral Maxillofac. Surg.* **2015**, *44*, 1486–1491. [CrossRef] [PubMed]
32. Markovic, A.; Misic, T.; Calvo-Guirado, J.L.; Delgado-Ruiz, R.A.; Janjic, B.; Abboud, M. Two-center prospective, randomized, clinical, and radiographic study comparing osteotome sinus floor elevation with or without bone graft and simultaneous implant placement. *Clin. Implant Dent. Relat. Res.* **2016**, *18*, 873–882. [CrossRef] [PubMed]
33. Kuchler, U.; Chappuis, V.; Gruber, R.; Lang, N.P.; Salvi, G.E. Immediate implant placement with simultaneous guided bone regeneration in the esthetic zone: 10-year clinical and radiographic outcomes. *Clin. Oral Implants Res.* **2016**, *27*, 253–257. [CrossRef] [PubMed]
34. Chen, S.T.; Buser, D. Esthetic outcomes following immediate and early implant placement in the anterior maxilla—A systematic review. *Int. J. Oral Maxillofac. Implants* **2014**, *29*, 186–215. [CrossRef] [PubMed]
35. Misch, C.M.; Jensen, O.T.; Pikos, M.A.; Malmquist, J.P. Vertical bone augmentation using recombinant bone morphogenetic protein, mineralized bone allograft, and titanium mesh: A retrospective cone beam computed tomography study. *Int. J. Oral Maxillofac. Implants* **2015**, *30*, 202–207. [CrossRef] [PubMed]
36. Spin-Neto, R.; Stavropoulos, A.; Coletti, F.L.; Pereira, L.A.; Marcantonio, E., Jr.; Wenzel, A. Remodeling of cortical and corticocancellous fresh-frozen allogenic block bone grafts—A radiographic and histomorphometric comparison to autologous bone grafts. *Clin. Oral Implants Res.* **2015**, *26*, 747–752. [CrossRef] [PubMed]
37. Cho, E.A.; Kim, S.J.; Choi, Y.J.; Kim, K.-H.; Chung, C.J. Morphologic evaluation of the incisive canal and its proximity to the maxillary central incisors using computed tomography images. *Angle Orthod.* **2015**, *86*, 571–576. [CrossRef] [PubMed]

38. Gull, M.A.B.; Maqbool, S.; Mushtaq, M.; Ahmad, A. Evaluation of Morphologic Features and Proximity of Incisive Canal to the Maxillary Central Incisors Using Cone Beam Computed Tomography. *IOSR J. Dent. Med. Sci.* **2018**, *17*, 46–50.
39. Bornstein, M.M.; Balsiger, R.; Sendi, P.; von Arx, T. Morphology of the nasopalatine canal and dental implant surgery: A radiographic analysis of 100 consecutive patients using limited cone-beam computed tomography. *Clin. Oral Implants Res.* **2011**, *22*, 295–301. [CrossRef] [PubMed]
40. Jacobs, R.; Lambrichts, I.; Liang, X.; Martens, W.; Mraiwa, N.; Adriaensens, P.; Gelan, J. Neurovascularization of the anterior jaw bones revisited using high-resolution magnetic resonance imaging. *Oral Surg. Oral Med. Oral Pathol. Oral Radiol. Endod.* **2007**, *103*, 683–693. [CrossRef] [PubMed]
41. Lake, S.; Iwanaga, J.; Kikuta, S.; Oskouian, R.J.; Loukas, M.; Tubbs, R.S. The Incisive Canal: A Comprehensive Review. *Cureus* **2018**, *10*, e3069. [CrossRef] [PubMed]
42. Keith, D.A. Phenomenon of mucous retention in the incisive canal. *J. Oral Surg.* **1979**, *37*, 832–834. [PubMed]
43. Mardinger, O.; Namani-Sadan, N.; Chaushu, G.; Schwartz-Arad, D. Morphologic Changes of the Nasopalatine Canal Related to Dental Implantation: A Radiologic Study in Different Degrees of Absorbed Maxillae. *J. Periodontol.* **2008**, *79*, 1659–1662. [CrossRef] [PubMed]
44. Fukuda, M.; Matsunaga, S.; Odaka, K.; Oomine, Y.; Kasahara, M.; Yamamoto, M.; Abe, S. Three-dimensional analysis of incisive canals in human dentulous and edentulous maxillary bones. *Int. J. Implant Dent.* **2015**, *1*, 12. [CrossRef] [PubMed]
45. Gil-Marques, B.; Sanchis-Gimeno, J.A.; Brizuela-Velasco, A.; Perez-Bermejo, M.; Larrazábal-Morón, C. Differences in the shape and direction-course of the nasopalatine canal among dentate, partially edentulous and completely edentulous subjects. *Anat. Sci. Int.* **2020**, *95*, 76–84. [CrossRef] [PubMed]
46. De Lima, A.C.N.M.; Peniche, D.A.; Coutinho, T.M.C.; Guedes, F.R.; Visconti, M.A.; Risso, P.A. The nasopalatine canal and its relationship with the maxillary central incisors: A cone-beam computed tomography study. *Res. Soc. Dev.* **2021**, *10*, e351101522978. [CrossRef]
47. Etoz, M.; Sisman, Y. Evaluation of the nasopalatine canal and variations with cone-beam computed tomography. *Surg. Radiol. Anat.* **2014**, *36*, 805–812. [CrossRef]
48. Botermans, A.; Lidén, A.; de Carvalho Machado, V.; Chrcanovic, B.R. Immediate Implant Placement in the Maxillary Aesthetic Zone: A Cone Beam Computed Tomography Study. *J. Clin. Med.* **2021**, *10*, 5853. [CrossRef] [PubMed]
49. Vasiljevic, M.; Milanovic, P.; Jovicic, N.; Vasovic, M.; Milovanovic, D.; Vojinovic, R.; Selakovic, D.; Rosic, G. Morphological and Morphometric Characteristics of Anterior Maxilla Accessory Canals and Relationship with Nasopalatine Canal Type-A CBCT Study. *Diagnostics* **2021**, *11*, 1510. [CrossRef] [PubMed]
50. Baena-Caldas, G.; Rengifo-Miranda, H.; Heerera-Rubio, A.; Peckham, X.; Zúñiga, J. Frequency of canalissinuosus and its anatomic variations in cone beam computed tomography images. *Int. J. Morphol.* **2019**, *37*, 852–857. [CrossRef]
51. Machado, V.C.; Chrcanovic, B.R.; Felippe, M.B.; Manhães Júnior, L.R.; de Carvalho, P.S. Assessment of accessory canals of the canalissinuosus: A study of 1000 cone beam computed tomography examinations. *Int. J. Oral Maxillofac. Surg.* **2016**, *45*, 1586–1591. [CrossRef] [PubMed]
52. Von Arx, T.; Lozanoff, S.; Sendi, P.; Bornstein, M.M. Assessment of bone channels other than the nasopalatine canal in the anterior maxilla using limited cone beam computed tomography. *Surg. Radiol. Anat.* **2013**, *35*, 783–790. [CrossRef] [PubMed]
53. Tomrukçu, D.N.; Köse, T.E. Assesment of accessory branches of canalissinuosus on CBCT images. *Med. Oral Patol. Oral Cir. Bucal.* **2020**, *25*, e124–e130. [CrossRef] [PubMed]
54. Wanzeler, A.M.; Marinho, C.G.; Alves Junior, S.M.; Manzi, F.R.; Tuji, F.M. Anatomical study of the canalissinuosus in 100 cone beam computed tomography examinations. *Oral Maxillofac. Surg.* **2015**, *19*, 49–53. [CrossRef] [PubMed]
55. Anatoly, A.; Sedov, Y.; Gvozdikova, E.; Mordanov, O.; Kruchinina, L.; Avanesov, K.; Vinogradova, A.; Golub, S.; Khaydar, D.; Hoang, N.G.; et al. Radiological and Morphometric Features of CanalisSinuosus in Russian Population: Cone-Beam Computed Tomography Study. *Int. J. Dent.* **2019**, *2019*, 2453469. [CrossRef] [PubMed]
56. Manhães Júnior, L.R.; Villaça-Carvalho, M.F.; Moraes, M.E.; Lopes, S.L.; Silva, M.B.; Junqueira, J.L. Location and classification of Canalissinuosus for cone beam computed tomography: Avoiding misdiagnosis. *Braz. Oral Res.* **2016**, *30*, e19. [CrossRef] [PubMed]
57. De Oliveira-Santos, C.; Rubira-Bullen, I.R.; Monteiro, S.A.; León, J.E.; Jacobs, R. Neurovascular anatomical variations in the anterior palate observed on CBCT images. *Clin. Oral Implants Res.* **2013**, *24*, 1044–1048. [CrossRef] [PubMed]
58. Hwang, K.G.; Park, C.J. Ideal implant positioning in an anterior maxillary extraction socket by creating an apico-palatal guiding slot: A technical note. *Int. J. Oral Maxillofac. Implants* **2008**, *23*, 121–122. [PubMed]
59. Greenstein, G.; Tarnow, D. The mental foramen and nerve: Clinical and anatomical factors related to dental implant placement: A literature review. *J. Periodontol.* **2006**, *77*, 1933–1943. [CrossRef] [PubMed]
60. Sharma, S.; Narkhede, S.; Sonawane, S.; Gangurde, P. Evaluation of Patient's Personal Reasons and Experience with Orthodontic Treatment. *J. Int. Oral Health* **2013**, *5*, 78–81. [PubMed]
61. Chung, C.J.; Nguyen, T.; Lee, J.; Kim, H. Incisive canal remodelling following maximum anterior retraction reduces apical root resorption. *Orthod. Craniofacial. Res.* **2021**, *24*, 59–65. [CrossRef] [PubMed]
62. Pavlovic, Z.R.; Milanovic, P.; Vasiljevic, M.; Jovicic, N.; Arnaut, A.; Colic, D.; Petrovic, M.; Stevanovic, M.; Selakovic, D.; Rosic, G. Assessment of Maxillary Molars Interradicular Septum Morphological Characteristics as Criteria for Ideal Immediate Implant Placement—The Advantages of Cone Beam Computed Tomography Analysis. *Diagnostics* **2022**, *12*, 1010. [CrossRef] [PubMed]

63. Milenkovic, J.; Vasiljevic, M.; Jovicic, N.; Milovanovic, D.; Selakovic, D.; Rosic, G. Criteria for the Classification of the Interradicular Septum Shape in Maxillary Molars with Clinical Importance for Prosthetic-Driven Immediate Implant Placement. *Diagnostics* **2022**, *12*, 1432. [CrossRef] [PubMed]
64. Bleyan, S.; Gaspar, J.; Huwais, S.; Schwimer, C.; Mazor, Z.; Mendes, J.J.; Neiva, R. Molar Septum Expansion with Osseodensification for Immediate Implant Placement, Retrospective Multicenter Study with Up-to-5-Year Follow-Up, Introducing a New Molar Socket Classification. *J. Funct. Biomater.* **2021**, *12*, 66. [CrossRef] [PubMed]
65. Smith, R.B.; Tarnow, D.P. Classification of molar extraction sites for immediate dental implant placement: Technical note. *Int. J. Oral Maxillofac. Implants* **2013**, *28*, 911–916. [CrossRef] [PubMed]
66. Agostinelli, C.; Agostinelli, A.; Berardini, M.; Trisi, P. Anatomical and Radiologic Evaluation of the Dimensions of Upper Molar Alveoli. *Implant Dent.* **2018**, *27*, 171–176. [CrossRef] [PubMed]
67. Padhye, N.; Shirsekar, V. Tomographic evaluation of mandibular molar alveolar bone for immediate implant placement—A retrospective cross-sectional study. *Clin. Oral Implants Res.* **2019**, *30*, 265. [CrossRef]
68. Nunes, L.S.; Bornstein, M.M.; Sendi, P.; Buser, D. Anatomical characteristics and dimensions of edentulous sites in the posterior maxillae of patients referred for implant therapy. *Int. J. Periodontics Restor. Dent.* **2013**, *33*, 337–345. [CrossRef] [PubMed]
69. Pai, U.Y.; Rodrigues, S.J.; Talreja, K.S.; Mundathaje, M. Osseodensification—A novel approach in implant dentistry. *J. Indian Prosthodont. Soc.* **2018**, *18*, 196–200. [CrossRef] [PubMed]
70. Alhayati, J.Z.; Al-Anee, A.M. Evaluation of crestal sinus floor elevations using versah burs with simultaneous implant placement, at residual bone height ≥2.0_<6.0 mm. A prospective clinical study. *Oral Maxillofac. Surg.* **2023**, *27*, 325–332. [CrossRef] [PubMed]
71. Demirkol, N.; Demirkol, M. The Diameter and Length Properties of Single Posterior Dental Implants: A Retrospective Study. *Cumhur. Dent. J.* **2019**, *22*, 276–282. [CrossRef]
72. Thirunavakarasu, R.; Arun, M.; Abhinav, R.P.; Ganesh, B.S. Commonly Used Implant Dimensions in the Posterior Maxilla—A Retrospective Study. *J. Long-Term Eff. Med. Implants* **2022**, *32*, 25–32. [CrossRef] [PubMed]
73. Ghoncheh, Z.; Zade, B.M.; Kharazifard, M.J. Root Morphology of the Maxillary First and Second Molars in an Iranian Population Using Cone Beam Computed Tomography. *J. Dent.* **2017**, *14*, 115–122.
74. Wang, H.M.; Shen, J.W.; Yu, M.F.; Chen, X.Y.; Jiang, Q.H.; He, F.M. Analysis of facial bone wall dimensions and sagittal root position in the maxillary esthetic zone: A retrospective study using cone beam computed tomography. *Int. J. Oral Maxillofac. Implants* **2014**, *29*, 1123–1129. [CrossRef] [PubMed]
75. Miyamoto, Y.; Obama, T. Dental cone beam computed tomography analyses of postoperative labial bone thickness in maxillary anterior implants: Comparing immediate and delayed implant placement. *Int. J. Periodontics Restor. Dent.* **2011**, *31*, 215–225.
76. Grunder, U.; Gracis, S.; Capelli, M. Influence of the 3-D bone-to-implant relationship on esthetics. *Int. J. Periodontics Restor. Dent.* **2005**, *25*, 113–119.
77. Zhan, W.; Skrypczak, A.; Weltman, R. Anterior maxilla alveolar ridge dimension and morphology measurement by cone beam computerized tomography (CBCT) for immediate implant treatment planning. *BMC Oral Health* **2015**, *15*, 65.
78. Safi, Y.; Moshfeghi, M.; Rahimian, S.; Kheirkhahi, M.; Manouchehri, M.E. Assessment of Nasopalatine Canal Anatomic Variations Using Cone Beam Computed Tomography in a Group of Iranian Population. *Iran. J. Radiol.* **2017**, *14*, e13480. [CrossRef]
79. Bahşi, I.; Orhan, M.; Kervancıoğlu, P.; Yalçın, E.D.; Aktan, A.M. Anatomical evaluation of nasopalatine canal on cone beam computed tomography images. *Folia. Morphol.* **2019**, *78*, 153–162. [CrossRef] [PubMed]
80. Güncü, G.N.; Yıldırım, Y.D.; Yılmaz, H.G.; Galindo-Moreno, P.; Velasco-Torres, M.; Al-Hezaimi, K.; Al-Shawaf, R.; Karabulut, E.; Wang, H.L.; Tözüm, T.F. Is there a gender difference in anatomic features of incisive canal and maxillary environmental bone? *Clin. Oral Implants Res.* **2013**, *24*, 1023–1026. [CrossRef] [PubMed]
81. Jornet, P.L.; Boix, P.P.; Perez, A.S.; Boracchia, A. Morphological Characterization of the Anterior Palatine Region Using Cone Beam Computed Tomography. *Clin. Implant Dent. Relat. Res.* **2014**, *17*, 459–464.
82. Chen, K.; Li, Z.; Liu, X.; Liu, Q.; Chen, Z.; Sun, Y.; Chen, Z.; Huang, B. Immediate Implant Placement with Buccal Bone Augmentation in the Anterior Maxilla with Thin Buccal Plate: A One-Year Follow-Up Case Series. *J. Prosthodont.* **2021**, *30*, 473–480. [CrossRef] [PubMed]
83. Bodereau, E.F.; Flores, V.Y.; Naldini, P.; Torassa, D.; Tortolini, P. Clinical Evaluation of the Nasopalatine Canal in Implant-Prosthetic Treatment: A Pilot Study. *Dent. J.* **2020**, *8*, 30. [CrossRef]
84. Scher, E.L. Use of the incisive canal as a recipient site for root form implants: Preliminary clinical reports. *Implant Dent.* **1994**, *1*, 38–41. [CrossRef] [PubMed]
85. Singhal, M.K.; Dandriyal, R.; Aggarwal, A.; Agarwal, A.; Yadav, S.; Baranwal, P. Implant Placement into the Nasopalatine Foramen: Considerations from Anatomical and Surgical Point of View. *Ann. Maxillofac. Surg.* **2018**, *2*, 347–351. [CrossRef] [PubMed]
86. Gargallo-Albiol, J.; Barootchi, S.; Marqués-Guasch, J.; Wang, H.L. Fully Guided Versus Half-Guided and Freehand Implant Placement: Systematic Review and Meta-analysis. *Int. J. Oral Maxillofac. Implants* **2020**, *35*, 1159–1169. [CrossRef] [PubMed]
87. Yeap, C.W.; Danh, D.; Chan, J.; Parashos, P. Examination of canalis sinuosus using cone beam computed tomography in an Australian population. *Aust. Dent. J.* **2022**, *67*, 249–261. [CrossRef] [PubMed]
88. Milanovic, P.; Vasiljevic, M. Gender Differences in the Morphological Characteristics of the Nasopalatine Canal and the Anterior Maxillary Bone—CBCT Study. *Serb. J. Exp. Clin. Res.* **2021**. [CrossRef]

89. Rosano, G.; Testori, T.; Clauser, T.; Massimo Del Fabbro, M. Management of a neurological lesion involving Canalis Sinuosus: A case report. *Clin. Implant Dent. Relat. Res.* **2021**, *23*, 149–155. [CrossRef] [PubMed]
90. Garg, S.; Kaur, S. Evaluation of Post-operative Complication Rate of Le Fort I Osteotomy: A Retrospective and Prospective Study. *J. Maxillofac. Oral Surg.* **2014**, *13*, 120–127. [CrossRef] [PubMed]
91. Jia, X.; Hu, W.; Meng, H. Relationship of central incisor implant placement to the ridge configuration anterior to the nasopalatine canal in dentate and partially edentulous individuals: A comparative study. *PeerJ* **2015**, *3*, e1315. [CrossRef] [PubMed]
92. McCrea, S.J.J. Aberrations Causing Neurovascular Damage in the Anterior Maxilla during Dental Implant Placement. *Case Rep. Dent.* **2017**, *2017*, 5969643. [CrossRef] [PubMed]
93. Shelley, A.; Tinning, J.; Yates, J.; Horner, K. Potential neurovascular damage as a result of dental implant placement in the anterior maxilla. *Br. Dent. J.* **2019**, *226*, 657–661. [CrossRef] [PubMed]
94. Salehinejad, J.; Saghafi, S.; Zare-Mahmoodabadi, R.; Ghazi, N.; Kermani, H. Glandular odontogenic cyst of the posterior maxilla. *Arch. Iran Med.* **2011**, *14*, 416–418. [PubMed]
95. Khojasteh, A.; Nazeman, P.; Tolstunov, L. Tuberosity-alveolar block as a donor site for localized augmentation of the maxilla: A retrospective clinical study. *Br. J. Oral Maxillofac. Surg.* **2016**, *54*, 950–955. [CrossRef] [PubMed]
96. Lim, A.A.; Wong, C.W.; Allen, J.C., Jr. Maxillary third molar: Patterns of impaction and their relation to oroantral perforation. *J. Oral Maxillofac. Surg.* **2012**, *70*, 1035–1039. [CrossRef] [PubMed]
97. Lorenz, J.; Blume, M.; Korzinskas, T.; Ghanaati, S.; Sader, R.A. Short implants in the posterior maxilla to avoid sinus augmentation procedure: 5-year results from a retrospective cohort study. *Int. J. Implant. Dent.* **2019**, *5*, 3. [CrossRef] [PubMed]
98. Cheung, L.K.; Fung, S.C.; Li, T.; Samman, N. Posterior maxillary anatomy: Implications for Le Fort I osteotomy. *Int. J. Oral Maxillofac. Surg.* **1998**, *27*, 346–351. [CrossRef] [PubMed]
99. Arul, A.S.; Verma, S.; Arul, A.S.; Verma, R. Infiltrative odontogenic myxoma of the posterior maxilla: Report of a case. *J. Nat. Sci. Biol. Med.* **2013**, *4*, 484–487. [CrossRef] [PubMed]
100. Benic, G.I.; Elmasry, M.; Hammerle, C.H. Novel digital imaging techniques to assess the outcome in oral rehabilitation with dental implants: A narrative review. *Clin. Oral Implants Res.* **2015**, *26*, 86–96. [CrossRef] [PubMed]
101. Whyte, A.; Boeddinghaus, R. The maxillary sinus: Physiology, development and imaging anatomy. *Dentomaxillofac. Radiol.* **2019**, *48*, 20190205. [CrossRef] [PubMed]
102. Stanley, J.N. Wheeler's Dental Anatomy. In *Physiology and Occlusion*, 9th ed.; Saunders Elsevier: St. Louis, MO, USA, 2010.
103. Rodriguez-Tizcareño, M.H.; Bravo-Flores, C. Anatomically guided implant site preparation technique at molar sites. *Implant Dent.* **2009**, *5*, 393–401. [CrossRef] [PubMed]
104. Prosper, L.; Crespi, R.; Valenti, E.; Capparé, P.; Gherlone, E. Five-year follow-up of wide-diameter implants placed in fresh molar extraction sockets in the mandible: Immediate versus delayed loading. *Int. J. Oral Maxillofac. Implants* **2010**, *25*, 607–612. [PubMed]
105. Iglesia-Puig, M.A.; Solana, F.J.; Holtzclaw, D.; Toscano, N. Immediate Implant Considerations for Interradicular Bone in Maxillary Molars: Case Reports. *J. Implant Adv. Clin. Dent.* **2012**, *4*, 19–31.
106. Atieh, M.A.; Payne, A.G.; Duncan, W.J.; de Silva, R.K.; Cullinan, M.P. Immediate placement or immediate restoration/loading of single implants for molar tooth replacement: A systematic review and meta-analysis. *Int. J. Oral Maxillofac. Implants* **2010**, *25*, 401–415. [PubMed]
107. Peñarrocha, M.; Uribe, R.; Balaguer, J. Immediate implants after extraction. A review of the current situation. A review of the current situation. *Med. Oral* **2004**, *9*, 234–242. [PubMed]
108. McAllister, B.S.; Haghighat, K. Bone augmentation techniques. *J. Periodontol.* **2007**, *78*, 377–396. [CrossRef] [PubMed]
109. Rominger, J.W.; Triplett, R.G. The use of guided tissue regeneration to improve implant osseointegration. *J. Oral Maxillofac. Surg.* **1994**, *52*, 106–112. [CrossRef] [PubMed]
110. Almog, D.M.; Sanchez, R. Correlation between planned prosthetic and residual bone trajectories in dental implants. *J. Prosthet. Dent.* **1999**, *81*, 562–567. [CrossRef] [PubMed]
111. Shokry, M.M.; Taalab, M.R. Immediate implant placement through inter-radicular bone drilling before versus after roots extraction in mandibular molar area (a randomized controlled clinical study). *Egypt. Dent. J.* **2022**, *68*, 1377–1388. [CrossRef]
112. Pavlovic, Z.R.; Petrovic, M. Morphological Characteristics of Maxillary Molars Interradicular Septum and Clinical Implications—What Do We Know So Far? *Serb. J. Exp. Clin. Res.* **2022**. [CrossRef]
113. Sayed, A.J.; Shaikh, S.S.; Shaikh, S.Y.; Hussain, M.A. Interradicular bone dimensions in primary stability of immediate molar implants—A cone beam computed tomography retrospective analysis. *Saudi Dent. J.* **2021**, *33*, 1091–1097. [CrossRef] [PubMed]
114. Avila-Ortiz, G.; Elangovan, S.; Kramer, K.W.; Blanchette, D.; Dawson, D.V. Effect of alveolar ridge preservation after tooth extraction: A systematic review and meta-analysis. *J. Dent. Res.* **2014**, *93*, 950–958. [CrossRef] [PubMed]
115. Ohba, S.; Sumita, Y.; Nakatani, Y.; Noda, S.; Asahina, I. Alveolar bone preservation by a hydroxyapatite/collagen composite material after tooth extraction. *Clin. Oral Investig.* **2019**, *23*, 2413–2419. [CrossRef] [PubMed]
116. Covani, U.; Giammarinaro, E.; Marconcini, S. Alveolar socket remodeling: The tug-of-war model. *Med. Hypotheses* **2020**, *142*, 109746. [CrossRef] [PubMed]
117. Covani, U.; Giammarinaro, E.; Panetta, D.; Salvadori, P.A.; Cosola, S.; Marconcini, S. Alveolar Bone Remodeling with or without Collagen Filling of the Extraction Socket: A High-Resolution X-ray Tomography Animal Study. *J. Clin. Med.* **2022**, *11*, 2493. [CrossRef]

118. Lekovic, V.; Camargo, P.M.; Klokkevold, P.R.; Weinlaender, M.; Kenney, E.B.; Dimitrijevic, B.; Nedic, M. Preservation of alveolar bone in extraction sockets using bioabsorbable membranes. *J. Periodontol.* **1998**, *69*, 1044–1049. [CrossRef] [PubMed]
119. Wu, D.; Zhou, L.; Lin, J.; Chen, J.; Huang, W.; Chen, Y. Immediate implant placement in anterior teeth with grafting material of autogenous tooth bone vs xenogenic bone. *BMC Oral Health* **2019**, *19*, 266. [CrossRef] [PubMed]
120. Zaki, J.; Yusuf, N.; El-Khadem, A.; Scholten, R.J.P.M.; Jenniskens, K. Efficacy of bone-substitute materials use in immediate dental implant placement: A systematic review and meta-analysis. *Clin. Implant Dent. Relat. Res.* **2021**, *23*, 506–519. [CrossRef] [PubMed]
121. Artzi, Z.; Parson, A.; Nemcovsky, C.E. Wide-diameter implant placement and internal sinus membrane elevation in the immediate postextraction phase: Clinical and radiographic observations in 12 consecutive molar sites. *Int. J. Oral Maxillofac. Implants* **2003**, *18*, 242–249. [PubMed]
122. Riben, C.; Thor, A. The Maxillary Sinus Membrane Elevation Procedure: Augmentation of Bone around Dental Implants without Grafts-A Review of a Surgical Technique. *Int. J. Dent.* **2012**, *2012*, 105483. [CrossRef] [PubMed]
123. Liu, H.; Liu, R.; Wang, M.; Yang, J. Immediate implant placement combined with maxillary sinus floor elevation utilizing the transalveolar approach and nonsubmerged healing for failing teeth in the maxillary molar area: A randomized controlled trial clinical study with one-year follow-up. *Clin. Implant Dent. Relat. Res.* **2019**, *21*, 462–472. [CrossRef] [PubMed]
124. Díaz-Olivares, L.A.; Cortés-Bretón Brinkmann, J.; Martínez-Rodríguez, N.; Martínez-González, J.M.; López-Quiles, J.; Leco-Berrocal, I.; Meniz-García, C. Management of Schneiderian membrane perforations during maxillary sinus floor augmentation with lateral approach in relation to subsequent implant survival rates: A systematic review and meta-analysis. *Int. J. Implant Dent.* **2021**, *7*, 91. [CrossRef] [PubMed]
125. Testori, T.; Weinstein, T.; Taschieri, S.; Wallace, S.S. Risk factors in lateral window sinus elevation surgery. *Periodontology 2000* **2019**, *81*, 91–123. [CrossRef] [PubMed]
126. Lombardo, G.; Signoriello, A.; Marincola, M.; Liboni, P.; Faccioni, P.; Zangani, A.; D'Agostino, A.; Nocini, P.F. Short and Ultra-Short Implants, in Association with Simultaneous Internal Sinus Lift in the Atrophic Posterior Maxilla: A Five-Year Retrospective Study. *Materials* **2022**, *15*, 7995. [CrossRef] [PubMed]
127. Bechara, S.; Lukosiunas, A.; Dolcini, G.A.; Kubilius, R. Fixed Full Arches Supported by Tapered Implants with Knife-Edge Thread Design and Nanostructured, Calcium-Incorporated Surface: A Short-Term Prospective Clinical Study. *Biomed. Res. Int.* **2017**, *2017*, 4170537. [CrossRef] [PubMed]
128. Hoekstra, J.W.M.; van Oirschot, B.A.; Jansen, J.A.; van den Beucken, J.J. Innovative implant design for continuous implant stability: A mechanical and histological experimental study in the iliac crest of goats. *J. Mech. Behav. Biomed. Mater.* **2021**, *122*, 104651. [CrossRef] [PubMed]
129. Baldi, D.; Lombardi, T.; Colombo, J.; Cervino, G.; Perinetti, G.; Di Lenarda, R.; Stacchi, C. Correlation between Insertion Torque and Implant Stability Quotient in Tapered Implants with Knife-Edge Thread Design. *Biomed. Res. Int.* **2018**, *2018*, 7201093. [CrossRef] [PubMed]

Disclaimer/Publisher's Note: The statements, opinions and data contained in all publications are solely those of the individual author(s) and contributor(s) and not of MDPI and/or the editor(s). MDPI and/or the editor(s) disclaim responsibility for any injury to people or property resulting from any ideas, methods, instructions or products referred to in the content.

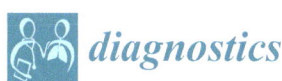

Article

Assessment of Reliability, Agreement, and Accuracy of Masseter Muscle Ultrasound Thickness Measurement Using a New Standardized Protocol

Mateusz Rogulski [1], Małgorzata Pałac [1,2], Tomasz Wolny [2], and Paweł Linek [1,2,*]

[1] Musculoskeletal Diagnostic and Physiotherapy—Research Team, The Jerzy Kukuczka Academy of Physical Education, 40-065 Katowice, Poland; rogulski21@interia.pl (M.R.); malgorzatapalac3@gmail.com (M.P.)
[2] Musculoskeletal Elastography and Ultrasonography Laboratory, Institute of Physiotherapy and Health Sciences, The Jerzy Kukuczka Academy of Physical Education, 40-065 Katowice, Poland; t.wolny@twreha.com
* Correspondence: linek.fizjoterapia@vp.pl; Tel.: +48-661-768-601

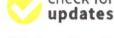

Citation: Rogulski, M.; Pałac, M.; Wolny, T.; Linek, P. Assessment of Reliability, Agreement, and Accuracy of Masseter Muscle Ultrasound Thickness Measurement Using a New Standardized Protocol. *Diagnostics* 2024, 14, 1771. https://doi.org/10.3390/diagnostics14161771

Academic Editor: Luis Eduardo Almeida

Received: 6 July 2024
Revised: 10 August 2024
Accepted: 12 August 2024
Published: 14 August 2024

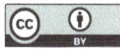

Copyright: © 2024 by the authors. Licensee MDPI, Basel, Switzerland. This article is an open access article distributed under the terms and conditions of the Creative Commons Attribution (CC BY) license (https://creativecommons.org/licenses/by/4.0/).

Abstract: There is no validated method of assessing masseter muscle thickness (MMT) by ultrasound imaging (US). However, this is important to ensure study and measurement quality of MMT by US in future studies, as MMT differs depending on the examined area. Thus, this study's aim was to present a new standardized method for assessing the MMT by US and to evaluate the reliability, consistency, and accuracy of its measurements. We also compared the results of MMT measurements obtained by US and computer tomography (CT). The study included nine healthy adults. The US and CT scans were collected in a supine rest position with the mandible in relaxed position. US measurements were determined according to a new standardized protocol (with precise probe location). The MMT measured by CT and US over a seven-day interval showed excellent intra-rater reliability. The mean MMT measured by CT was 12.1 mm (1.74) on the right side and 11.9 mm (1.61) on the left side. The mean MMT measured by US was 12.7 mm (2.00) on the right side and 11.5 mm (1.37) on the left side. The mean percent error in MMT measurement between CT and US was below 6%. A strong linear relationship was found between the CT and US measurements of the MMT on both body sides ($p < 0.001$, $r \geq 0.93$). The proposed method of MMT measurement using US demonstrated excellent reliability, yielding results similar to those obtained from CT images. We recommend the use of this standardization protocol in further studies where precise assessment of MMT by US is expected.

Keywords: masseter muscle; ultrasound imaging; reliability; computed tomography

1. Introduction

The masseter muscle is one of the muscles of mastication, playing a crucial role in the physiological movements and positioning of the mandible. It has also been associated with temporomandibular joint (TMJ) disorders, craniomandibular dysfunctions, bruxism, and orofacial pain [1–3]. Masseter muscle thickness is a parameter commonly analyzed in such studies, and is linked to certain features of the dental arches [4,5], anthropometry [6], and dental disorders [7]. The thickness of the masseter muscle has also been considered in the context of systemic diseases such as sarcopenia and osteoporosis [8–18].

Masseter muscle thickness is generally assessed using ultrasound imaging (US), a non-invasive, cost-effective procedure widely available for use in both children and adults [19]. More complex diagnostic tools such as computed tomography (CT) and magnetic resonance imaging (MRI) are also employed to assess the thickness of the masseter muscle. Although CT and MRI scans provide accurate and reliable cross-sectional images of muscles, including the masseter, they are not routinely used due to their variable availability and relatively high costs [20].

Recently, Gawriołek et al. [21] confirmed that masseter muscle thickness significantly differs depending on the area examined, and strongly suggested the necessity of examining the masseter muscle in specified areas with both coronal and axial projections to achieve objective and repeatable results. To the best of our knowledge, no standardized and precisely validated method for assessing masseter muscle thickness using US currently exists in the literature [7,20,22–25]. Blicharz et al. [26] reviewed various methods for measuring and assessing masseter muscle thickness using US, highlighting that none of these procedures have been fully verified in terms of reliability and accuracy. Given the important role of the masseter muscle in clinical and research settings, there is a clear need for standardization in US measurement of its thickness. The absence of such standardization, alongside a lack of information on measurement reliability, agreement, and accuracy, could significantly undermine the quality of future studies involving US measurements of masseter muscle thickness. Therefore, the aim of this study is to present a new standardized method for assessing the masseter muscle thickness and to evaluate the reliability, consistency, and accuracy of its US measurements in adults. We also aim to cross-reference the results of masseter muscle thickness measurements obtained via US and CT. We believe this could contribute to the introduction of a unified method for assessing masseter muscle thickness in both scientific research and clinical practice.

2. Materials and Methods

2.1. Setting and Study Design

US measurements were performed in the Musculoskeletal Elastography and Ultrasonography Laboratory at the Jerzy Kukuczka Academy of Physical Education. CT scans were collected from the Radiology Department at an outpatient clinic. US measurements (thickness) were recorded by two experienced physiotherapists. CT scan measurements were performed by two medical doctors (a radiologist and a dentist) separately. Initially, the CT scan was taken, and then the US was performed within a period of 7 days. The study was authorized by the Bioethics Committee for Scientific Studies at the Academy of Physical Education in Katowice on 21 April 2022 (Decision No. 2a/2022). Procedures and methods were performed in accordance with the relevant guidelines and regulations. All participants gave their signed and informed consent to participate.

2.2. Participants

Participants were recruited at the dental clinic from June to September 2022 from among patients referred for CT to exclude dentogenic infection foci. Participants were eligible for inclusion if they (1) had not received any dental treatment during the study period (between CT and US); (2) had no history of craniofacial trauma, orthodontic treatment, genetic diseases, craniofacial tumors, masticatory organ dysfunction; (3) had full dental arches (excluding teeth 8); (4) had no abnormalities on CT scans; (5) did not exhibit dysfunctions and parafunctions of a craniofacial nature or of the TMJ.

2.3. Ultrasound Measurements

An Aixplorer ultrasound scanner (Product Version 12.2.0, Sofware Version 12.2.0.808, Supersonic Imagine, Aix-en-Provence, France) coupled with a linear transducer array (2–10 MHz; SuperLinear 10-2, Vermon, Tours, France) was used to assess masseter muscle thickness. The US scans were collected in supine rest position with the mandible in a relaxed position.

Prior to the US measurements, for each participant, the precise location of the probe was determined by a dentist and a trained assistant (a physiotherapy student). The precise location of the US probe was based on previous analysis of anatomical preparations and the authors' own experience. The proposed procedure was as follows (Figure 1A). (a) The distance on the subject's skin between the lateral edge of the orbit in the pupil line and the point where the mandibular angle transitions into the mandibular body was determined and drawn, called the mandible–eyelid (M-E) distance; (b) the determined M-E distance was measured with a digital caliper in millimeters; (c) the value of 40% of the M-E distance was calculated, and this value was then measured from the transition point of the mandibular angle into the mandibular body; (d) the obtained point indicates the position of the center of the US probe; (e) this center of the US probe was marked. This procedure allows precise and reproducible positioning of the US probe in the frontal and sagittal plane while considering probe rotation (Figure 1B). The center of the probe is placed at the 40% point (the center of probe position) while the entire probe was placed parallel to the M-E distance (Figure 1B). A US image was taken 3 times by each physiotherapist, on both sides of the face, respectively.

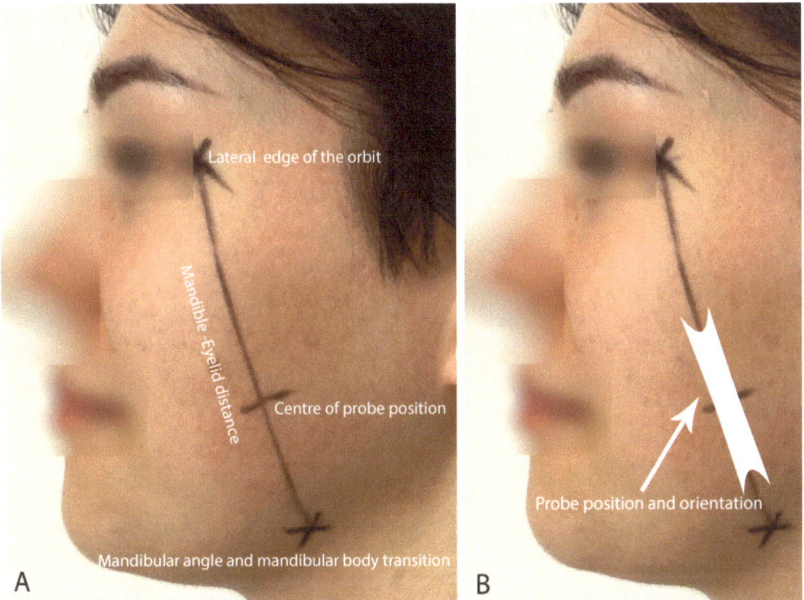

Figure 1. Determination of probe placement (**A**). Final probe position and orientation (**B**).

2.4. Computed Tomography

CT (Device Observer Manufacturer: PNMS, Device Observer Model Name: NeuViz 16, Device Observer Serial Number: N16E100009; Shenyang, China) was performed in the supine position. All subjects were instructed by the dentist to maintain a resting mandibular position during the CT scan procedure. The CT scan was performed with an accuracy of N*T [mm] 0.75 mm.

2.5. Data Analysis

2.5.1. Ultrasound Parameters

The US images were saved on an external drive in DICOM format and transferred to a computer where they were further processed using RadiAnt DICOM Viewer (Medixant, Poznań, Poland) to assess masseter muscle thickness. Thickness measurements were taken at 3 locations: (A) in the middle of the picture (this refers to the center of the probe position point); (B) an additional 2 locations 0.5 cm to the left and 0.5 cm to the right from point A, respectively (Figure 2). In further analyses, the average thickness value from these three locations indicated the mean masseter muscle thickness for a given image.

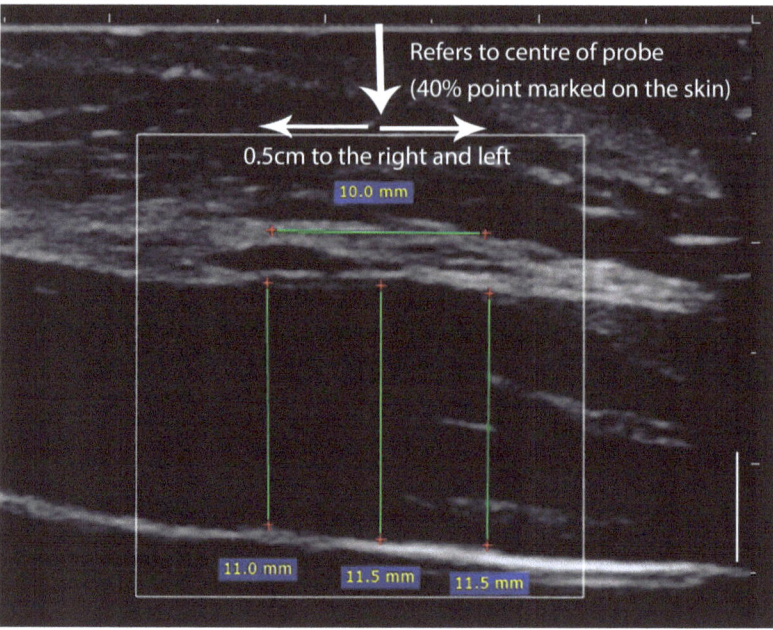

Figure 2. Illustration of ultrasound measurements of masseter muscle.

2.5.2. Computed Tomography

CT scans were saved on an external drive in DICOM format and transferred to a computer where they were further processed using RadiAnt DICOM Viewer (Medixant, Poznań, Poland) to assess masseter muscle thickness and M-E distance. First of all, length measurement of the M-E distance was performed on a 3D Virtual Reality (VR) scan between two referential points (mandible, eyelid) using the first Bone and Skin mode. This procedure involved viewing the patient from a profile perspective. Secondly, the M-E distance was determined by connecting the following points: the lateral edge of the orbit at the pupil line and the point where the mandibular angle transitions into the mandibular body. Furthermore, a point was marked 40% of the distance from the lower end of the segment defining the center of the masseter muscle and the area of the maxillary tubercle (Figure 3a). Afterwards, a soft tissue window was selected and a multiplanar reformated reconstruction (MPR) mode was activated. On the MPR, the image was adjusted according to the anatomical planes as follows: horizontal plane—the point passing between the anterior and posterior nasal spines; (Figure 3b) sagittal plane—the line between the anterior and posterior nasal spike; (Figure 3c) frontal plane—the thickness of the masseter muscle measured at the level of the maxillary cusp (this position was equivalent to 40% of the M-E distance). Finally, two thickness measurements were taken 0.5 cm up and 0.5 cm down from a predetermined point on the external surface of the masseter muscle (Figure 3d) In further analyses, the mean thickness value from these three locations indicated the mean masseter muscle thickness for a given body side. All measurements were taken on the right and left sides of the face.

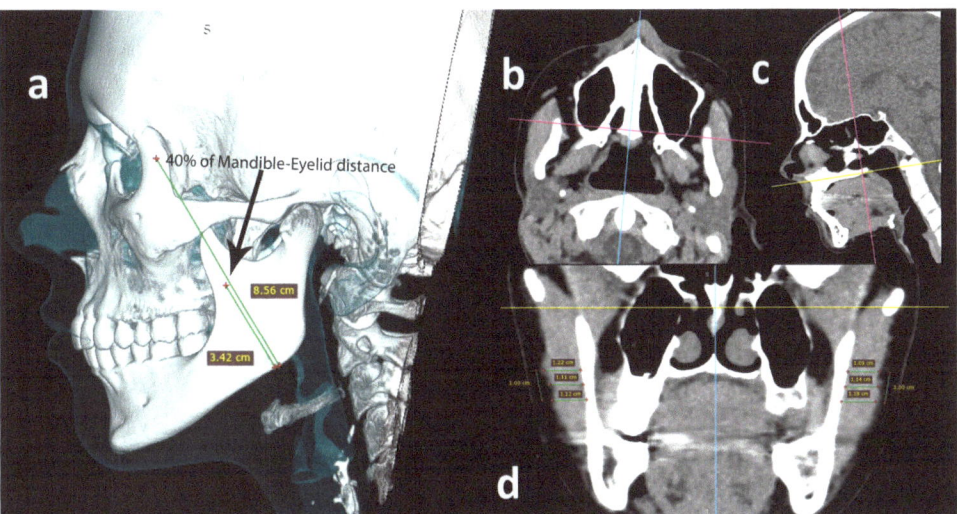

Figure 3. Presentation of masseter muscle thickness measurements by computer tomography. (**a**) 3D VR image; (**b**) horizontal plane; (**c**) sagittal plane; (**d**) frontal plane.

2.6. Statistical Analyses

For the calculation of intra- and inter-rater reliability, Intraclass Correlation Coefficient (ICC) type 3,1 and type 2,2 were used, respectively. The ICC was interpreted as follows: 1.00–0.75 (excellent), 0.74–0.60 (moderate), 0.59–0.40 (fair), and below 0.40 (poor reliability) [27]. The agreement was calculated by assessing (1) the standard error of measurement (SEM = SD × $\sqrt{(1 - ICC)}$, with SD representing the standard deviation of the measure; and (2) the results of the Bland and Altman test (BA). The BA test was performed by plotting the difference between the two measurement techniques against their average in order to identify potential systematic errors. The accuracy was calculated as a percent error using the following formula: [(CT measurement − US measurement)/CT measurement] × 100. Additionally, correlation between the two measurement techniques was evaluated using the Pearson correlation coefficient. The Pearson correlation coefficient was graded as r < 0.2 for very weak, 0.20–0.39 for weak, 0.40–0.59 for moderate, 0.60–0.79 for strong, and ≥0.8 for very strong correlation [14].

3. Results

3.1. Participants

Finally, the study included nine participants (three men and six women; mean age: 25.4 years; mean body mass: 63.5 kg; mean body height: 172.8; BMI: 21.4 kg/m^2) who met the inclusion criteria.

3.2. Masseter Muscle Thickness (Reliability and Agreement)

The masseter muscle thickness measured by CT over a seven-day interval received excellent intra-rater reliability with a coefficient of variation (CV) below 1.5%. The BA test revealed systematic error in the masseter muscle measured on the right side by a radiologist, meaning that during the second measurement, this muscle was slightly thinner (bias 0.21 mm) compared to the first measurement. The inter-rater reliability for the first CT measurement of the masseter muscle was excellent, with a CV below 1.5%. The BA test showed no systematic error (Table 1).

Table 1. Reliability and validity of masseter muscle thickness measurement by computer tomography and ultrasonography.

		Masseter Muscle Thickness	
		Right Side	Left Side
Computer Tomography			
Intra-rater reliability Radiologist (seven-day interval)	$ICC_{3.1}$ (95% CI) [1]	0.99 (0.97–0.99)	0.98 (0.93–0.99)
	SEM (mm)	0.17	0.22
	CV (%)	1.22	0.81
	Bias [3] (mm)	−0.21 [2]	−0.14
Intra-rater reliability Dentist (seven-day interval)	$ICC_{3.1}$ (95% CI) [1]	0.98 (0.91–0.99)	0.97 (0.89–0.99)
	SEM (mm)	0.27	0.26
	CV (%)	0.28	0.40
	Bias [3] (mm)	0.05	0.07
Inter-rater reliability	$ICC_{2.1}$ (95% CI) [1]	0.88 (0.60–0.97)	0.98 (0.92–0.99)
	SEM (mm)	0.63	0.22
	CV (%)	1.33	0.89
	Bias [3] (mm)	−0.23	−0.22
Ultrasonography			
Intra-session reliability First physiotherapist	$ICC_{3.1}$ (95% CI) [1]	0.85 (0.47–0.96)	0.87 (0.53–0.97)
	SEM (mm)	0.68	0.56
	CV (%)	1.97	3.59
	Bias [3] (mm)	−0.36	−0.60
Intra-session reliability Second physiotherapist	$ICC_{3.1}$ (95% CI) [1]	0.98 (0.93–0.97)	0.94 (0.76–0.99)
	SEM (mm)	0.25	0.41
	CV (%)	0.30	0.55
	Bias [3] (mm)	0.05	0.09
Inter-rater reliability	$ICC_{2.1}$ (95% CI) [1]	0.92 (0.71–0.98)	0.87 (0.44–0.97)
	SEM (mm)	0.54	0.53
	CV (%)	1.48	2.93
	Bias [3] (mm)	0.26	−0.48

CV—coefficient of variation; ICC—intraclass correlation coefficient; SEM—standard error of the mean; [1] the 95% confidence interval; [2] systematic error as the line of equality is not in the 95% confidence interval; [3] Bland–Altman Test.

The masseter muscle thickness measured by US received excellent intra-session reliability (with a 15 min interval between measurements). The corresponding CV values varied from 2 to 4% for the first assessor, whereas the CV value for the second assessor was below 1%. The inter-rater reliability for the first US measurements performed over a seven-day interval were also excellent, with corresponding CV below 3%. The BA test form US measurements showed no systematic error (Table 1).

3.3. Mandible–Eyelid Distance

The mean M-E distance measured by CT was 87.6 mm (4.34) and 87.7 mm (3.80) on the right and left sides, respectively. The mean M-E distance measured by digital caliper was 88.3 mm (4.00) and 87.5 mm (3.41) on the right and left sides, respectively. Mean percent error in the M-E distance measurement between CT and the digital caliper was below 1.4% regardless of body side. The exact percent error varied from 0.05% to 3% within the examined population. The Bland–Altman analysis has shown that the bias for the M-E distance measurement by CT and digital caliper was close to zero with no systematic error (Figure 4A). A significant linear relationship was shown between the CT and digital caliper measurements on both body sides ($p < 0.001$, $r \geq 0.93$, Figure 4B).

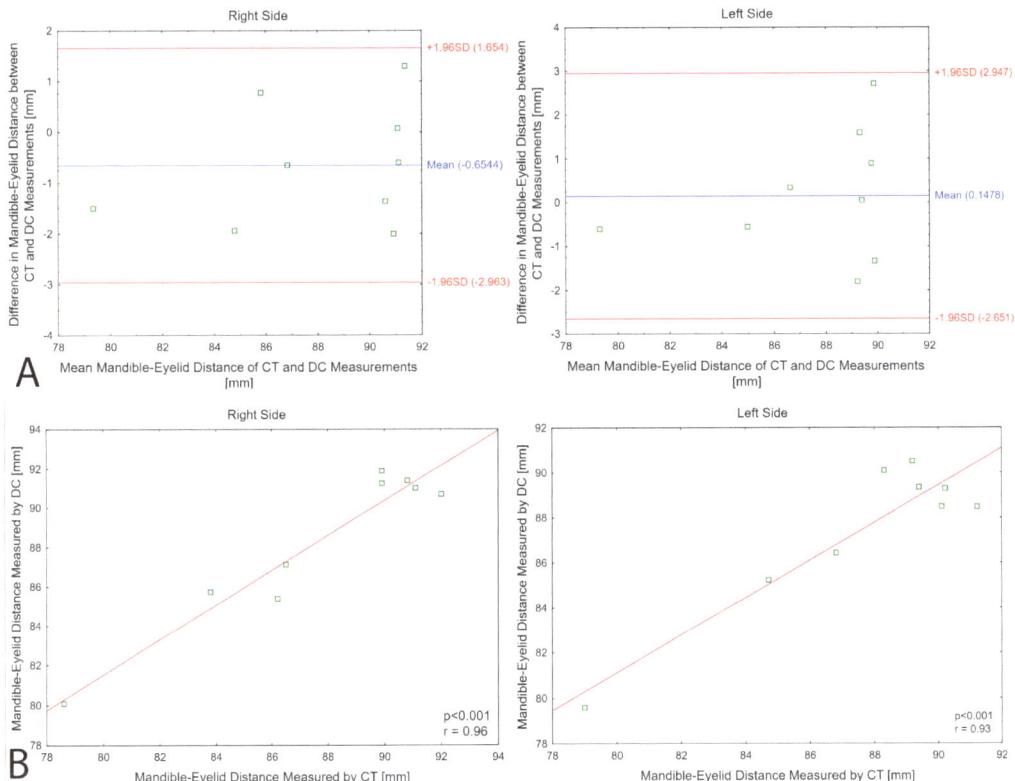

Figure 4. Analysis between computer tomography (CT) and digital caliper (DC) measurements of the mandible–eyelid distance: (**A**) Bland–Altman plot; (**B**) Pearson correlation.

3.4. Masseter Muscle Thickness (CT versus US)

The mean masseter muscle thickness measured by CT was 12.1 mm (1.74) and 11.9 mm (1.61) on the right and left sides, respectively. In turn, the mean masseter muscle thickness measured by US was 12.7 mm (2.00) and 11.5 mm (1.37) on the right and left sides, respectively. Mean percent error in masseter muscle thickness measurement between CT and US was below 6% regardless of body side. The exact percent error varied from 0% to 12.7% within the examined population. The Bland–Altman analysis has shown that the mean bias for the masseter muscle thickness measurement by CT and US was 0.4–0.6 mm, with systematic error detected on the right side (Figure 5A). A strong linear relationship was found between the CT and US measurements on both body sides ($p < 0.001$, $r \geq 0.93$, Figure 5B).

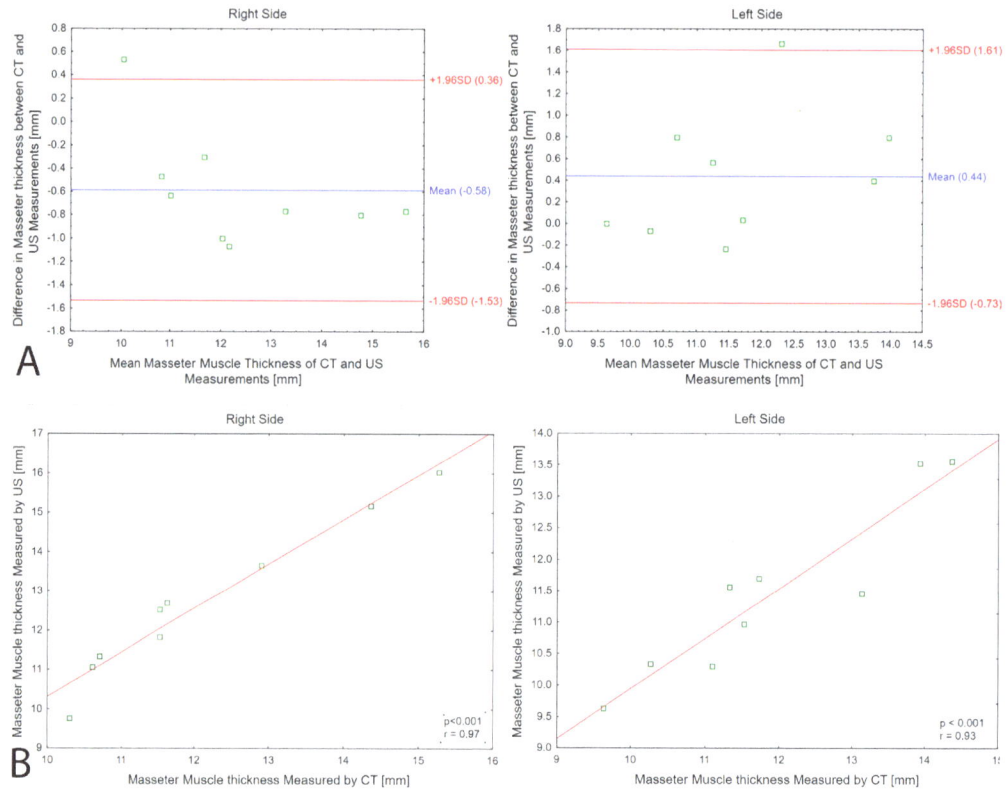

Figure 5. Analysis between computer tomography (CT) and ultrasound (US) measurements of the masseter muscle: (**A**) Bland–Altman plot; (**B**) Pearson correlation.

4. Discussion

The purpose of this study was to evaluate the reliability, agreement, and accuracy of masseter muscle thickness measurements. This study was undertaken due to the lack of a detailed and validated method for assessing masseter muscle thickness using US. Such validation is necessary to ensure the quality of studies and measurements in future research involving US measurement of masseter muscle thickness, as the masseter muscle is linked to various craniomandibular dysfunctions [1–3] and systemic diseases [8–18]. Taking this into account, we have demonstrated in the present study that the proposed method for measuring masseter muscle thickness using US achieved excellent reliability, yielding results similar to those obtained from CT images in healthy adults. Thus, the results obtained allow us to claim that the developed method of assessing the thickness of the masseter muscle using US can be implemented and verified on patients with some craniofacial conditions.

The systematic review by Blicharz et al. [26] presented various scientific reports that describe different methods for measuring and assessing masseter muscle thickness using US. However, as the authors concluded, none of these procedures have been fully verified for reliability and accuracy. To the best of our knowledge, we have found only a few different methods in the literature for examining the masseter muscle with US [7,18,21,23–26,28]. Volk et al. [25] positioned the US transducer perpendicular to the skin surface and transverse to the segment of the zygomatic bone arch and mandibular angle. Satiroglu et al. [24] positioned the US transducer on the skin surface in the middle of the mandibular branch, without taking into consideration the actual middle (center) position. Strini et al. [7] positioned the US transducer perpendicular to the course of the muscle fibers of the masseter muscle in the midsection between the zygomatic arch and the angle of the mandible based solely on palpation. Park et al. [23], in contrast to the mentioned works, has possibly presented the most reproducible methodology for examining the masseter muscle thickness by US. Park et al. [23] positioned the ultrasound probe perpendicular to the course of the masseter muscle at a level that coincided with the occlusal plane of the studied subjects. However, it seems that the intraoral line (occlusal plane) and the extraoral line (probe position) will not match in each subject. Ispir et al. [28] positioned the ultrasound probe perpendicular to the masseter muscle in the anteroposterior direction, and the measurement was taken at the widest point in the transverse section. In turn, González-Fernández M. et al. [18] positioned the transducer perpendicular to the external edge of the muscle (between the intertragic fissure and the oral commissure, parallel to the Frankfort plane).

Thus, taking all mentioned studies into consideration [7,18,23–26,28], it should be pointed out that the location of the US probe placement was not precise, and the examiners had some freedom in probe position. Therefore, in the present study, it was decided to determine the position of the US transducer with the greatest possible precision by drawing lines on the subject's skin. Certainly, this method extends the duration of the examination, but enables highly reproducible US probe placement (imposes a precise probe alignment in all directions). This approach has not been used in other scientific studies on the US measurement of the masseter muscle. Our novel method of examining the masseter muscle with US could be highly relevant, especially for repeated measurements of muscle thickness at intervals in clinical trials. In addition, in the proposed method, the probe is positioned along the muscle fibers, which may be particularly useful in shear wave elastography of the masseter muscle.

In scientific research, an important aspect is the reliability of the methods used to evaluate tissues (US of masseter muscle thickness in this study). In this regard, the methods proposed by Strini et al. [7] and Volk et al. [25] were not validated. Park et al. [23] only presented reliability results for one and two repeated measurements, where ICC results of 0.7–0.9 were obtained. In none of the mentioned works were accuracy and agreement assessed. In our study, we presented an assessment of the reliability, agreement, and accuracy of US measurements of the masseter muscle and compared the US results with CT results. The results have shown that in the US evaluation of the masseter muscle, the ICC value exceeds 0.8, there were no systematic errors, and the results were highly correlated with CT.

Implications and Limitations

In this present study, we demonstrated that the emerging new method of masseter muscle US assessment can be validated on clinical material and then used in clinical studies to evaluate changes in masseter muscle thickness, or in observational studies of masseter muscle thickness variability in different populations. It might also be possible to study the effect of additional factors, i.e., pharmacotherapy, physiotherapy, and surgical treatment, on the thickness of the masseter muscle by using such a method.

The present study has several limitations. First of all, the study included only nine healthy adults. Thus, the results should be considered as preliminary and cannot be extrapolated to children, adolescents, or patients with specific conditions. Second, measurements were collected in the supine rest position, whereas body position can affect the masseter muscle measurements. Furthermore, we do not know if this proposed method will be suitable for assessing the masseter muscle in contraction. Lastly, reliability of the proposed method is still affected by the palpation needed while determining the proper probe positioning. Hence, the person drawing lines on the face in our study received 10 h of hands-on training.

5. Conclusions

The proposed method of masseter muscle thickness measurement using US has demonstrated excellent reliability with similar results to those obtained from CT images in a healthy adult population. The results allow us to conclude that the developed method of assessing the thickness of the masseter muscle using US can be implemented and verified on patients with some craniofacial conditions. Therefore, we recommend investigating this method in further studies, where precise assessment of the masseter muscle by US is expected.

Author Contributions: Conceptualization, M.R. and P.L.; methodology, M.R., M.P., P.L. and T.W.; formal analysis, M.R., M.P. and T.W.; investigation, M.R., M.P., P.L. and T.W.; resources, M.R.; writing—original draft preparation, M.R.; writing—review and editing, M.P., P.L. and T.W.; visualization, M.P.; supervision, M.P. and P.L.; project administration, P.L.; funding acquisition, P.L. All authors have read and agreed to the published version of the manuscript.

Funding: This research received no external funding.

Institutional Review Board Statement: The study was conducted in accordance with the Declaration of Helsinki and approved by Bioethics Committee for Scientific Studies at the Academy of Physical Education in Katowice (Decision No. 2a/2022, 21 April 2022).

Informed Consent Statement: Informed consent was obtained from all subjects involved in the study.

Data Availability Statement: The raw data supporting the conclusions of this article will be made available by the authors on request.

Conflicts of Interest: The authors declare no conflicts of interest.

References

1. Iguchi, H.; Magara, J.; Nakamura, Y.; Tsujimura, T.; Ito, K.; Inoue, M. Changes in jaw muscle activity and the physical properties of foods with different textures during chewing behaviors. *Physiol. Behav.* **2015**, *152 Pt A*, 217–224. [CrossRef] [PubMed]
2. Lin, C.-S.; Wu, C.-Y.; Wu, S.-Y.; Chuang, K.-H.; Lin, H.-H.; Cheng, D.-H.; Lo, W.-L. Age- and sex-related differences in masseter size and its role in oral functions. *J. Am. Dent. Assoc.* **2017**, *148*, 644–653. [CrossRef]
3. Mapelli, A.; Machado, B.C.Z.; Giglio, L.D.; Sforza, C.; De Felício, C.M. Reorganization of muscle activity in patients with chronic temporomandibular disorders. *Arch. Oral Biol.* **2016**, *72*, 164–171. [CrossRef] [PubMed]
4. Ariji, Y.; Ariji, E. Magnetic resonance and sonographic imagings of masticatory muscle myalgia in temporomandibular disorder patients. *Jpn. Dent. Sci. Rev.* **2017**, *53*, 11–17. [CrossRef] [PubMed]
5. Hara, K.; Namiki, C.; Yamaguchi, K.; Kobayashi, K.; Saito, T.; Nakagawa, K.; Ishii, M.; Okumura, T.; Tohara, H. Association between myotonometric measurement of masseter muscle stiffness and maximum bite force in healthy elders. *J. Oral Rehabil.* **2020**, *47*, 750–756. [CrossRef] [PubMed]
6. Ramazanoglu, E.; Turhan, B.; Usgu, S. Evaluation of the tone and viscoelastic properties of the masseter muscle in the supine position, and its relation to age and gender. *Dent. Med. Probl.* **2021**, *58*, 155–161. [CrossRef] [PubMed]
7. Strini, P.J.S.A.; Barbosa, T.d.S.; Gavião, M.B.D. Assessment of thickness and function of masticatory and cervical muscles in adults with and without temporomandibular disorders. *Arch. Oral Biol.* **2013**, *58*, 1100–1108. [CrossRef] [PubMed]
8. Aldemir, K.; Üstüner, E.; Erdem, E.; Demiralp, A.S.; Oztuna, D. Ultrasound evaluation of masseter muscle changes in stabilization splint treatment of myofascial type painful temporomandibular diseases. *Oral Surgery Oral Med. Oral Pathol. Oral Radiol.* **2013**, *116*, 377–383. [CrossRef]
9. Chakarvarty, A.; Panat, S.R.; Sangamesh, N.C.; Aggarwal, A.; Jha, P.C. Evaluation of masseter muscle hypertrophy in oral submucous fibrosis patients -an ultrasonographic study. *J. Clin. Diagn. Res.* **2014**, *8*, ZC45. [CrossRef]
10. Kant, P.; Bhowate, R.R.; Sharda, N. Assessment of cross-sectional thickness and activity of masseter, anterior temporalis and orbicularis oris muscles in oral submucous fibrosis patients and healthy controls: An ultrasonography and electromyography study. *Dentomaxillofacial Radiol.* **2014**, *43*, 20130016. [CrossRef]
11. Bhoyar, P.S.; Godbole, S.R.; Thombare, R.U.; Pakhan, A.J. Effect of complete edentulism on masseter muscle thickness and changes after complete denture rehabilitation: An ultrasonographic study. *J. Investig. Clin. Dent.* **2012**, *3*, 45–50. [CrossRef]
12. Müller, F.; Hernandez, M.; Grütter, L.; Aracil-Kessler, L.; Weingart, D.; Schimmel, M. Masseter muscle thickness, chewing efficiency and bite force in edentulous patients with fixed and removable implant-supported prostheses: A cross-sectional multicenter study. *Clin. Oral Implant. Res.* **2012**, *23*, 144–150. [CrossRef]
13. Sathasivasubramanian, S.; Venkatasai, P.M.; Divyambika, C.V.; Mandava, R.; Jeffrey, R.; Jabeen, N.A.N.; Kumar, S.S. Masseter muscle thickness in unilateral partial edentulism: An ultrasonographic study. *J. Clin. Imaging Sci.* **2017**, *7*, 44. [CrossRef]

14. Schimmel, M.; Loup, A.; Duvernay, E.; Gaydarov, N.; Muller, F. The effect of mandibular denture abstention on masseter muscle thickness in a 97-year-old patient: A case report. *Int. J. Prosthodont.* **2010**, *23*, 418–420. [PubMed]
15. Trawitzki, L.V.; Dantas, R.O.; Elias-Júnior, J.; Mello-Filho, F.V. Masseter muscle thickness three years after surgical correction of class III dentofacial deformity. *Arch. Oral Biol.* **2011**, *56*, 799–803. [CrossRef]
16. Umeki, K.; Watanabe, Y.; Hirano, H.; Edahiro, A.; Ohara, Y.; Yoshida, H.; Obuchi, S.; Kawai, H.; Murakami, M.; Takagi, D.; et al. The relationship between masseter muscle thickness and appendicular skeletal muscle mass in Japanese community-dwelling elders: A cross-sectional study. *Arch. Gerontol. Geriatr.* **2018**, *78*, 18–22. [CrossRef]
17. Vasconcelos, P.B.; Palinkas, M.; De Sousa, L.G.; Regalo, S.C.H.; Santos, C.M.; De Rossi, M.; Semprini, M.; Scalize, P.H.; Siessere, S. The influence of maxillary and mandibular osteoporosis on maximal bite force and thickness of masticatory muscles. *Acta Odontol. Latinoam.* **2015**, *28*, 22–27. [CrossRef]
18. González-Fernández, M.; Perez-Nogueras, J.; Serrano-Oliver, A.; Torres-Anoro, E.; Sanz-Arque, A.; Arbones-Mainar, J.M.; Sanz-Paris, A. Masseter Muscle Thickness Measured by Ultrasound as a Possible Link with Sarcopenia, Malnutrition and Dependence in Nursing Homes. *Diagnostics* **2021**, *11*, 1587. [CrossRef]
19. Emshoff, R.; Emshoff, I.; Rudisch, A.; Bertram, S. Reliability and temporal variation of masseter muscle thickness measurements utilizing ultrasonography. *J. Oral Rehabil.* **2003**, *30*, 1168–1172. [CrossRef] [PubMed]
20. Serra, M.D.; Gavião, M.B.D.; Uchôa, M.N.d.S. The use of ultrasound in the investigation of the muscles of mastication. *Ultrasound Med. Biol.* **2008**, *34*, 1875–1884. [CrossRef] [PubMed]
21. Gawriołek, K.; Klatkiewicz, T.; Przystańska, A.; Maciejewska-Szaniec, Z.; Gedrange, T.; Czajka-Jakubowska, A. Standardization of the ultrasound examination of the masseter muscle with size-independent calculation of records. *Adv. Clin. Exp. Med.* **2021**, *30*, 441–447. [CrossRef]
22. Price, R.R.; Jones, T.B.; Goddard, J.; James, A.E., Jr. Basic concepts of ultrasonic tissue characterization. *Radiol. Clin. N. Am.* **1980**, *18*, 21–30. [CrossRef] [PubMed]
23. Park, K.-M.; Choi, E.; Kwak, E.-J.; Kim, S.; Park, W.; Jeong, J.-S.; Kim, K.-D. The relationship between masseter muscle thickness measured by ultrasonography and facial profile in young Korean adults. *Imaging Sci. Dent.* **2018**, *48*, 213–221. [CrossRef]
24. Şatıroğlu, F.; Arun, T.; Işık, F. Comparative data on facial morphology and muscle thickness using ultrasonography. *Eur. J. Orthod.* **2005**, *27*, 562–567. [CrossRef]
25. Volk, G.F.; Sauer, M.; Pohlmann, M.; Guntinas-Lichius, O. Reference values for dynamic facial muscle ultrasonography in adults. *Muscle Nerve* **2014**, *50*, 348–357. [CrossRef] [PubMed]
26. Blicharz, G.; Rymarczyk, M.; Rogulski, M.; Linek, P. Methods of Masseter and Temporal Muscle Thickness and Elasticity Measurements by Ultrasound Imaging: A Literature Review. *Curr. Med. Imaging* **2021**, *17*, 707–713. [CrossRef]
27. Cicchetti, D.; Sparrow, S. Developing criteria for establishing interrater reliability of specific items—Applications to assessment of adaptive-behavior. *Am. J. Ment. Defic.* **1981**, *86*, 127–137. [PubMed]
28. Ispir, N.G.; Toraman, M. The relationship of masseter muscle thickness with face morphology and parafunctional habits: An ultrasound study. *Dentomaxillofacial. Radiol.* **2022**, *51*, 20220166. [CrossRef]

Disclaimer/Publisher's Note: The statements, opinions and data contained in all publications are solely those of the individual author(s) and contributor(s) and not of MDPI and/or the editor(s). MDPI and/or the editor(s) disclaim responsibility for any injury to people or property resulting from any ideas, methods, instructions or products referred to in the content.

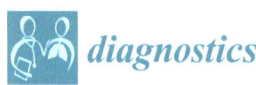 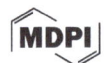

Article

The Occurrence and Risk Factors of Black Triangles Between Central Incisors After Orthodontic Treatment

Ji-Song Jung [1,†], Ho-Kyung Lim [2,†], You-Sun Lee [3,*] and Seok-Ki Jung [4,*]

1. Department of Orthodontics, Graduate School of Clinical Dentistry, Korea University, Seoul 02841, Republic of Korea; maerypaw@naver.com
2. Department of Oral and Maxillofacial Surgery, Korea University Guro Hospital, Seoul 08308, Republic of Korea; ungassi@korea.ac.kr
3. Department of Orthodontics, Korea University Anam Hospital, Seoul 02841, Republic of Korea
4. Department of Orthodontics, Korea University Guro Hospital, Seoul 08308, Republic of Korea
* Correspondence: kumc_ortho@korea.ac.kr (Y.-S.L.); jgosggg@korea.ac.kr (S.-K.J.)
† These authors contributed equally to this work.

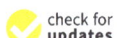

Citation: Jung, J.-S.; Lim, H.-K.; Lee, Y.-S.; Jung, S.-K. The Occurrence and Risk Factors of Black Triangles Between Central Incisors After Orthodontic Treatment. *Diagnostics* 2024, 14, 2747. https://doi.org/10.3390/diagnostics14232747

Academic Editors: Luis Eduardo Almeida and Francesco Inchingolo

Received: 30 September 2024
Revised: 24 November 2024
Accepted: 4 December 2024
Published: 6 December 2024

Copyright: © 2024 by the authors. Licensee MDPI, Basel, Switzerland. This article is an open access article distributed under the terms and conditions of the Creative Commons Attribution (CC BY) license (https://creativecommons.org/licenses/by/4.0/).

Abstract: Background/Objectives: To assess the incidence of and risk factors for black triangles between the central incisors after orthodontic treatment; Methods: Ninety-seven post-treatment patients (29 men and 68 women; mean age, 22.7 years) were retrospectively divided into two groups based on the presence or absence of black triangles, using intraoral photographs. Based on the Jemt Index, the black triangle occurrence group was further classified into mild, moderate, and severe groups. Parameters from periapical radio graphs, lateral cephalograms, and study models were compared between the occurrence and the non-occurrence groups by using independent *t*-tests. Logistic regression analysis was performed to identify the risk factors for black triangles; Results: The incidence of black triangles between the central incisors was 51% and 64% in the maxilla and in the mandible, respectively. The factors significantly associated with the occurrence of black triangles were age, treatment duration, the lingual inclination of the maxillary incisors in the maxilla, and age in the mandible ($p < 0.05$); Conclusions: This study showed the diverse risk factors associated with black triangles between central incisors after orthodontic treatment and revealed that the formation of black triangles is relatively common. Considering these risk factors during orthodontic diagnosis and treatment planning can help minimize the occurrence of black triangles.

Keywords: black triangle; open gingival embrasure; orthodontic treatment

1. Introduction

Over the past few decades, the goals of patients seeking orthodontic treatment have continuously evolved. In the 1980s and 1990s, patients primarily aimed to resolve malocclusion or restore normal occlusal function through orthodontic treatment. However, recent patients place a significant emphasis not only on functional occlusal recovery but also on aesthetic improvement [1–3].

Orthodontic treatment can induce unwanted side effects on periodontal tissues, such as root resorption, bone dehiscence, gingival recession, and the formation of black triangles, which may reduce patient satisfaction with the treatment [2,4,5]. A black triangle is an empty space beneath the contact area between teeth due to the loss of the interdental papilla [6]. This issue not only affects aesthetics but can also lead to periodontal problems by chronically trapping food debris and making plaque control more difficult. Therefore, a thorough understanding of the etiology and pathogenesis of black triangles, as well as appropriate orthodontic diagnosis and treatment, is required [7].

Previous studies have identified various factors contributing to the development of black triangles, including patient age, history of periodontitis, the distance between the interproximal contact and the alveolar crest, gingival biotype, and morphological characteristics of teeth [8]. However, there is still a lack of consensus regarding the relationship between orthodontic treatment and black triangles. Some studies have reported a high incidence of black triangles in patients who have undergone orthodontic treatment [9–16], while others have suggested that orthodontic treatment can stimulate the formation of interdental papillae, thus reducing the incidence of black triangles [17–19]. Consequently, a definitive conclusion about the relationship between orthodontic treatment and black triangles has yet to be reached. In addition, it should be distinguished from the case where black triangles occur when orthodontic treatment is performed on normal periodontal tissue with reduced periodontal support.

Risk factors associated with black triangle formation after orthodontic treatment include age, treatment duration, tooth shape, the amount of tooth movement, root angulation after treatment, the degree of crowding, the distance between the alveolar crest and the interproximal contact after treatment, traumatic brushing, the occurrence of periodontitis, and gingival biotype [20–26]. However, most previous studies have evaluated the impact of risk factors on black triangle formation in a unidimensional manner, which limits the understanding of how these factors might interact during orthodontic treatment. Therefore, comprehensive investigation of associations among various risk factors is necessary.

The purpose of this study was to examine the association between the occurrence of black triangles during orthodontic treatment and factors such as age, gender, bracket type, and extraction status. The null hypothesis of this study is that there is no correlation between the occurrence of black triangles during orthodontic treatment and factors such as age, gender, bracket type, and extraction status.

2. Materials and Methods

2.1. Subjects

Patients who completed orthodontic treatment at the Department of Orthodontics, Korea University Guro Hospital were selected for this study. Among them, patients without a black triangle between the maxillary and mandibular central incisors, as assessed by a Jemt Index score of 3 from intraoral photographs taken before orthodontic treatment, were included. Patients with periodontitis, anterior tooth loss, a history of previous orthodontic treatment, prosthetic restorations of the maxillary or mandibular central incisors, or those who underwent interproximal reduction (stripping) during orthodontic treatment were excluded from the study. A total of 300 patients who underwent orthodontic treatment between January 2020 and March 2022 were evaluated, and after applying the exclusion criteria, 97 patients (58 adults and 39 adolescents, 47 extraction and 50 non-extraction) who had pre- and post-treatment intraoral photographs, lateral cephalograms, periapical radiographs, and study models were selected for this retrospective study.

For age classification, adolescents were defined as patients aged 9 to under 20 years, and adults were defined as those aged 20 to under 55 years based on pre-treatment age. The extraction group consisted of patients who underwent the extraction of the first premolars in both the maxilla and mandible. The orthodontic appliances used for treatment were the 0.022-inch slot metal ligating brackets (Formula-R, Tomy Inc, Fukushima, Japan), self-ligating brackets (Clippy-C, Tomy Inc, Fukushima, Japan), and lingual brackets (Fujita, Succeeding Co, Morioka, Japan).

2.2. Measurement Methods

2.2.1. Classification of Black Triangles According to Severity

Intraoral frontal photographs of the maxillary and mandibular central incisors were taken within one week after the completion of orthodontic treatment. Intraoral photographs were taken from the front using standardized camera settings (shutter speed 1/125, ISO 200, F22) after drying the area with air. A parallel line was drawn from the gingival zenith (the most cervical point of the crown) and the most cervical point of the interproximal contact area, followed by a bisecting line through the midpoint of these two parallel lines, dividing the interdental papilla area into four sections. Based on the Jemt Index, patients were classified into two groups: the non-occurrence group (Score 3, the papilla fills up the entire proximal space) and the occurrence group, which was further subdivided into Score 2 (mild, half or more of the height of the papilla is present), Score 1 (moderate, less than half of the height of the papilla is present), and Score 0 (severe, no papilla is present) (Figure 1).

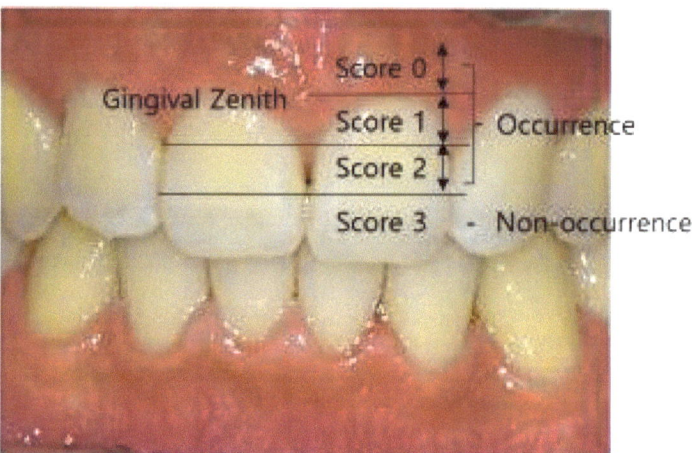

Figure 1. Classification of black triangles according to Jemt Index.

2.2.2. Measurements of Tooth Movement on Lateral Cephalograms

The angular and anteroposterior, as well as vertical, changes in the maxillary and mandibular central incisors before and after orthodontic treatment were measured using lateral cephalometric radiographs. Each radiograph was taken in a natural head position. Additionally, all subjects were instructed to stand still, hold their breath, swallow briefly before imaging, and refrain from swallowing while the radiographs were being taken. For the maxillary central incisors, the angular change was assessed by measuring the difference in the angle between the upper incisor and the SN plane (ΔU1 to SN), and for the mandibular central incisors, the difference in the incisor mandibular plane angle (ΔIMPA) was measured relative to the mandibular plane before and after orthodontic treatment.

The horizontal movement of the maxillary central incisors was measured as calculating the change in the distance between the perpendicular line drawn from the tip of the maxillary central incisor crown to the SN plane and the distance from this point to the Sella (S) (ΔTH = TH2 − TH1). The vertical movement of the maxillary central incisors was calculated by measuring the change in the perpendicular distance from the tip of the maxillary central incisor crown to the SN plane (ΔTV = TV2 − TV1) (Figure 2a).

For the mandibular central incisors, the horizontal movement was assessed by measuring the change in the straight-line distance between the tip of the mandibular central incisor crown and the perpendicular line drawn from the mandibular plane to the Pogonion (ΔTH = TH2 − TH1). The vertical movement was calculated by measuring the change in the perpendicular distance from the tip of the mandibular central incisor crown to the mandibular plane (ΔTV = TV2 − TV1) (Figure 2b).

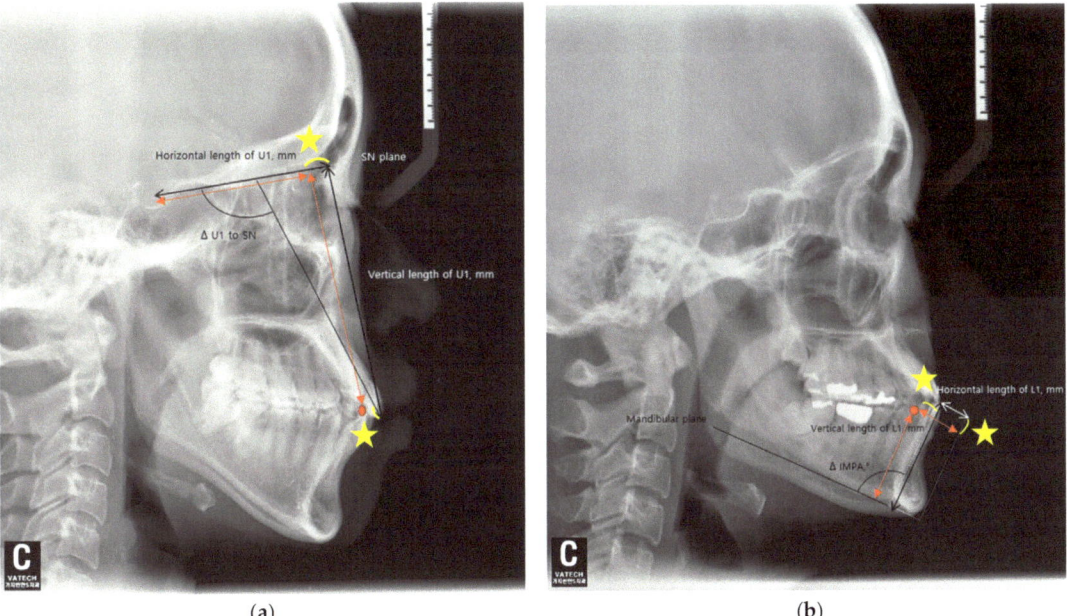

(a) (b)

Figure 2. Lateral cephalograms show measurements of tooth movement. (**a**) SN, Sella–Nasion; U1, the maxillary central incisor; Δ U1 to SN refer to the changes in measurements between before (T1) and after (T2) treatment (Δ = T2 − T1). (**b**) L1, the mandibular central incisor; IMPA, incisor mandibular plane angle. Δ IMPA refers to the changes in measurements between before (T1) and after (T2) treatment (Δ = T2 − T1).

2.2.3. The Tooth Shape and the Height of Alveolar Bone

In periapical radiographs taken before orthodontic treatment, the long axis of the maxillary and mandibular central incisors was established. The ratio of the perpendicular distance from the long axis to the mesial contact point of the crown (1) to the perpendicular distance from the long axis to the mesial CEJ (cemento–enamel junction) (2) was calculated (crown ratio = (1)/(2)) [27].

To minimize errors due to magnification or distortion in periapical radiographs, the clinical average crown lengths of the central incisors were used as reference values, and the amount of alveolar bone height change (ΔTA = TA2 − TA1) was measured [28]. The distance from the contact point (or the most cervical point of the contact surface) of the maxillary and mandibular central incisors to the alveolar crest was measured, keeping the measurement parallel to the long axis of the left central incisor, and the difference in distance before and after orthodontic treatment was compared. If there was a space between the teeth without a contact point, the distance from the narrowest point between the mesial surfaces of both crowns and the alveolar crest was measured. The angle between the roots of the left and right maxillary and mandibular central incisors was measured in patients after completing orthodontic treatment (Figure 3).

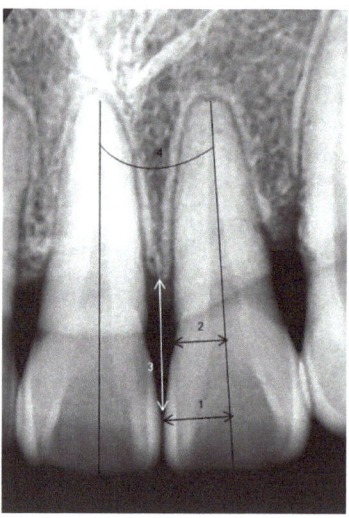

Figure 3. Periapical radiographic measurements. 1, perpendicular distance from the mesial interproximal contact to the tooth long axis; 2, perpendicular distance from the mesial CEJ to the tooth long axis; 3, distance of alveolar bone–interproximal contact; 4, post-treatment root angulation classification of black triangle according to Jemt Index.

2.2.4. Measurements of Crowding on Study Models

In pre-treatment study model photographs, the anteroposterior and mesiodistal crowding of the maxillary and mandibular central incisors was measured. The plane connecting the central incisors and the first molars was set as the occlusal plane, and the photographs were taken perpendicular to this occlusal plane. The midpalatal raphe in the maxilla and a perpendicular line bisecting the line connecting the mesial surfaces of the first molars in the mandible were used as the reference lines. Anteroposterior overlap was measured by the length of the line connecting the most mesial points of the left and right central incisors, drawn parallel to the reference line. Mesiodistal overlap was measured by the length of the perpendicular line drawn from the most mesial points of the left and right central incisors to the reference line. The angle change between the crowns of the left and right central incisors ($\Delta TR = TR2 - TR1$) was measured using occlusal surface photographs of the study models before and after orthodontic treatment. (Figure 4).

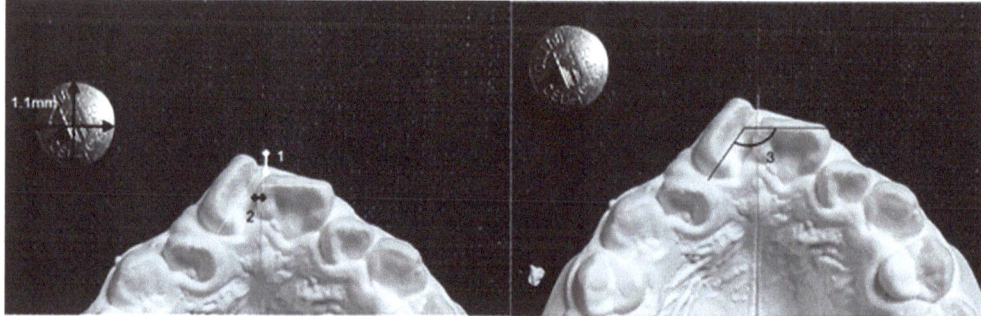

Figure 4. Measurements of the anteroposterior and transverse overlap of the two central incisors and the angle formed by the incisal edges. 1, degree of vertical overlap; 2, degree of horizontal overlap; 3, amount of crown rotation.

2.3. Statistical Analysis

Statistical analysis was performed using PASW Statistics version 18.0.0 (SPSS Inc., Chicago, IL, USA). The target sample size was determined based on a review of existing literature and calculations using the G Power program version 3.1.9.7. To confirm the association between the incidence rates and contributing factors in the two groups, the statistically significant minimum sample size was calculated to be 40 participants per group based on age, requiring a total of at least 80 participants. All measurements were conducted by a single examiner, who randomly selected and reanalyzed 25 patients at one-week intervals. The degree of black triangle occurrence after orthodontic treatment was assessed, and the association between black triangle occurrence and variables such as age, gender, bracket type, and extraction versus non-extraction groups was examined using the Chi-square test and Fisher's exact test.

For the occurrence and non-occurrence groups of black triangles, mean values and standard deviations were analyzed and compared using the independent t-test for variables such as treatment duration, age, tooth shape, pre- and post-treatment angle differences of the maxillary and mandibular incisors, horizontal and vertical movement changes of the maxillary and mandibular incisors, pre- and post-treatment differences in alveolar bone height, post-treatment angle between the roots of the left and right central incisors, anteroposterior and mesiodistal crowding of the maxillary and mandibular central incisors before treatment, and crown rotation changes before and after treatment.

Additionally, the independent t-test was performed to compare mean values for age (pediatric/adolescent versus adult) and extraction status (extraction versus non-extraction), which were identified as risk factors associated with black triangle occurrence in the Chi-square test. Simple logistic regression analysis was conducted to assess the association between risk factors and the occurrence of black triangles in the maxillary and mandibular central incisors during orthodontic treatment, followed by multiple logistic regression analysis to further analyze the combined risk factors and calculate the odds ratios. Statistical significance was set at a p-value of less than 0.05.

3. Results

3.1. Association Between Black Triangle Occurrence and Each Group

The number distribution of subjects in each group is presented in Table 1. The intraclass correlation coefficient (ICC) was used to determine the intra-examiner reliability of the measurements, which were scored as follows: ICC < 0.4, poor reliability; 0.4 < ICC < 0.75, moderate reliability; ICC > 0.75, excellent reliability. The ICC values in this study ranged from 0.93 to 0.99, demonstrating excellent reliability. Among the 97 patients, black triangles occurred in 51% of the maxillary incisors and 64% of the mandibular incisors after orthodontic treatment (Table 2). When comparing the occurrence of black triangles between adolescents and adults, adolescents showed a black triangle occurrence rate of 17.9% in the maxilla and 38% in the mandible, while adults had rates of 74% in the maxilla and 82% in the mandible, indicating a significant association between age and black triangle occurrence (Table 3). Among the extraction and non-extraction groups, only the maxilla in the extraction group showed a significant association with black triangle occurrence, while the type of bracket used did not show a significant difference in black triangle formation (Tables 4 and 5).

Table 1. Number distribution of subjects with each group.

Group		Subjects, n (%)
Gender	Male	29 (30%)
	Female	68 (70%)
Age	Young	39 (40%)
	Adult	58 (60%)

Table 1. *Cont.*

Group		Subjects, n (%)
Extraction	Extraction	47 (48%)
	Non-Extraction	50 (52%)
Brackets	Ligating	51 (53%)
	Self-ligating	36 (37%)
	Lingual	10 (10%)

Table 2. Incidence of black triangle ($n = 97$).

	Non-Occurrence	Occurrence		
		Mild	Moderate	Severe
Maxilla	47 (48%)	49 (51%)	1 (1%)	0 (0%)
Mandible	34 (35%)	59 (61%)	4 (4%)	0 (0%)

Table 3. Comparison of black triangle incidence between young and adult in the occurrence group [†].

	Young	Adult	Significance
Maxilla	7 (14%)	43 (86%)	***
Mandible	15 (24%)	48 (76%)	***

[†] Chi-square test was used to compare the incidence between young and adult. * $p < 0.05$; ** $p < 0.01$; *** $p < 0.001$.

Table 4. Comparison of black triangle incidence between extraction and non-extraction in the occurrence group [†].

	Extraction	Non-extraction	Significance
Maxilla	32 (64%)	18 (36%)	**
Mandible	32 (51%)	31 (49%)	NS

[†] Chi-square test was used to compare the incidence between extraction and non-extraction. NS, not significant; * $p < 0.05$; ** $p < 0.01$; *** $p < 0.001$.

Table 5. Comparison of black triangle incidence between bracket types in the occurrence group [†].

	Ligating	Self-Ligating	Lingual	Significance
Maxilla	24 (48%)	18 (36%)	8 (16%)	NS
Mandible	29 (46%)	26 (41%)	8 (13%)	NS

[†] Chi-square test was used to compare the incidence between bracket types. NS, not significant; * $p < 0.05$; ** $p < 0.01$; *** $p < 0.001$.

3.2. Comparison of Mean Values Between the Black Triangle Occurrence and Non-Occurrence Groups

When comparing the mean values between the black triangle occurrence and non-occurrence groups using the independent *t*-test, significant differences were observed in the maxilla for treatment duration, age, and the angle change of the central incisors before and after orthodontic treatment, and in the mandible for age. In the maxilla, the treatment duration was significantly longer in the occurrence group (40.00 ± 19.21 months) than in the non-occurrence group (29.96 ± 11.48 months). Additionally, the mean age in the occurrence group (28.14 ± 10.88 years) was significantly higher than that in the non-occurrence group (16.94 ± 5.92 years). In terms of the angle change of the maxillary central incisors relative to the SN plane, the occurrence group showed more lingual inclination (9.18 ± 1.10°) compared to the non-occurrence group (2.12 ± 1.29°) (Table 6).

When comparing the mean values between adolescents and adults in the maxilla using the independent *t*-test, adults showed a relatively longer treatment duration and greater lingual inclination of the maxillary central incisors (Table 7). Additionally, when comparing the extraction and non-extraction groups, the extraction group exhibited greater lingual inclination of the maxillary central incisors (Table 8).

Table 6. Comparison of black triangle incidence between the occurrence and non-occurrence groups in the maxilla and mandible (means ± SD) [†].

	Maxilla			Mandible		
	Occurrence	Non-Occurrence	Significance	Occurrence	Non-Occurrence	Significance
Treatment period, month	40.00 ± 19.21	9.96 ± 11.48	*	37.29 ± 17.42	31.15 ± 14.39	NS
Age, y	28.14 ± 10.88	16.94 ± 5.92	***	26.21 ± 10.65	16.24 ± 6.10	***
Tooth shape	1.24 ± 0.12	1.48 ± 1.90	NS	1.27 ± 0.14	1.27 ± 0.11	NS
ΔU1 to SN /ΔIMPA, °	−9.18 ± 1.10	−2.12 ± 1.29	***	2.19 ± 1.17	3.96 ± 2.86	NS
Horizontal movement of U1/L1, mm	−0.45 ± 0.66	−0.33 ± 1.05	NS	−0.11 ± 2.02	−0.37 ± 1.40	NS
Vertical movement of U1/L1, mm	1.64 ± 12.87	1.62 ± 13.33	NS	1.82 ± 13.08	−0.06 ± 1.00	NS
Δ Distance from ICP to ABC, mm	−0.64 ± 0.76	−0.50 ± 0.30	NS	−0.86 ± 1.28	0.46 ± 0.24	NS
Root angulation at T2, °	4.03 ± 1.69	4.04 ± 2.03	NS	3.81 ± 2.44	5.04 ± 1.72	NS
A-P overlapped distance, mm	0.10 ± 0.20	0.04 ± 0.01	NS	0.09 ± 0.28	0.61 ± 0.17	NS
Transverse overlapped distance, mm	−0.51 ± 0.23	−0.02 ± 0.17	NS	0.01 ± 0.04	−0.00 ± 0.04	NS
Rotation, °	11.49 ± 9.60	13.57 ± 6.10	NS	13.08 ± 9.84	11.93 ± 3.55	NS

[†] B Independent t-tests were used to compare between the occurrence and non-occurrence groups, and Bonferroni correction was performed. U1, maxillary incisor; L1, mandibular incisor; SN, Sella–Nasion; IMPA, incisor mandibular plane angle; T1, before treatment; T2, after treatment; Δ, T2-T1; ICP, interproximal contact point; ABC, alveolar bone crest; A-P, anteroposterior; NS, not significant; * $p < 0.05$; ** $p < 0.01$; *** $p < 0.001$.

Table 7. Comparison of black triangle incidence between the young and adult groups in the maxilla and mandible (means ± SD) [†].

	Maxilla			Mandible		
	Young	Adult	Significance	Young	Adult	Significance
Treatment period, month	30.23 ± 12.30	38.43 ± 18.39	*	30.23 ± 12.30	38.43 ± 18.39	*
Tooth shape	1.54 ± 2.08	1.23 ± 0.11	NS	1.28 ± 0.15	1.28 ± 0.19	NS
ΔU1 to SN /ΔIMPA, °	−2.88 ± 10.49	−7.69 ± 10.37	*	−0.21 ± 20.15	−4.30 ± 10.50	NS
Horizontal movement of U1/L1, mm	−0.37 ± 1.15	−0.41 ± 0.62	NS	0.30 ± 1.32	0.14 ± 2.10	NS
Vertical movement of U1/L1, mm	4.38 ± 20.32	−0.21 ± 1.43	NS	−0.08 ± 0.93	−1.97 ± 13.63	NS
Δ Distance from ICP to ABC, mm	−0.60 ± 0.57	−0.56 ± 1.24	NS	0.68 ± 0.52	0.76 ± 1.19	NS
Root angulation at T2, °	5.03 ± 3.37	5.26 ± 2.75	NS	5.47 ± 3.73	5.29 ± 3.41	NS
A-P overlapped distance, mm	0.02 ± 0.06	0.11 ± 0.42	NS	0.09 ± 0.23	0.08 ± 0.27	NS
Transverse overlapped distance, mm	−0.03 ± 10.19	−0.38 ± −0.22	NS	0.00 ± 0.04	0.01 ± 0.048	NS
Rotation, °	−12.78 ± 24.30	−12.31 ± 30.48	NS	−14.33 ± 19.16	−11.58 ± 32.08	NS

[†] B Independent t-tests were used to compare between the young and adult groups, and Bonferroni correction was performed. U1, maxillary incisor; L1, mandibular incisor; SN, Sella–Nasion; IMPA, incisor mandibular plane angle; T1, before treatment; T2, after treatment; Δ, T2-T1; ICP, interproximal contact point; ABC, alveolar bone crest; A-P, anteroposterior; NS, not significant; * $p < 0.05$; ** $p < 0.01$; *** $p < 0.001$.

Table 8. Comparison of means (±SD) between the extraction and non-extraction groups in the maxilla and mandible [†].

	Maxilla			Mandible		
	Extraction	Non-Extraction	Significance	Extraction	Non-Extraction	Significance
Treatment period, month	35.98 ± 15.80	34.34 ± 17.51	NS	36.98 ± 18.26	33.40 ± 17.80	NS
Age, y	1.51 ± 1.90	1.22 ± 0.08	NS	1.28 ± 1.15	1.27 ± 0.10	NS
Tooth shape	−9.77 ± 11.13	−1.99 ± 8.67	***	−5.35 ± 18.53	−0.99 ± 11.04	NS
ΔU1 to SN /ΔIMPA, °	−0.51 ± 0.59	−0.28 ± 1.62	NS	0.12 ± 1.37	0.27 ± 2.18	NS
Horizontal movement of U1/L1, mm	1.85 ± 13.20	1.42 ± 13.00	NS	−0.13 ± 0.58	−2.21 ± 14.70	NS
Vertical movement of U1/L1, mm	−0.38 ± 0.87	−0.76 ± 1.13	NS	−0.90 ± 1.08	−0.55 ± 0.83	NS
Δ Distance from ICP to ABC, mm	5.39 ± 3.17	4.95 ± 2.85	NS	5.43 ± 3.13	5.28 ± 3.90	NS
Root angulation at T2, °	0.09 ± 0.44	0.05 ± 0.17	NS	0.10 ± 0.32	0.06 ± 0.15	NS
A-P overlapped distance, mm	−0.04 ± 0.24	−0.03 ± −0.17	NS	0.008 ± 0.04	0.006 ± −0.04	NS
Transverse overlapped distance, mm	−16.14 ± 34.13	−9.051 ± 20.51	NS	−18.13 ± 29.18	−7.56 ± 25.12	NS
Rotation, °	35.98 ± 15.80	34.34 ± 17.51	NS	36.98 ± 18.26	33.40 ± 17.80	NS

[†] B Independent t-tests were used to compare between the extraction and non-extraction groups, and Bonferroni correction was performed. U1, maxillary incisor; L1, mandibular incisor; SN, Sella–Nasion; IMPA, incisor mandibular plane angle; T1, before treatment; T2, after treatment; Δ, T2-T1; ICP, interproximal contact point; ABC, alveolar bone crest; A-P, anteroposterior; NS, not significant; * $p < 0.05$; ** $p < 0.01$; *** $p < 0.001$.

3.3. Association Between Black Triangles and Risk Factors

The association between expected risk factors and the occurrence of black triangles was examined using simple regression analysis. In the maxilla, treatment duration, age, and the angle change of the maxillary central incisors before and after orthodontic treatment were identified as significant risk factors, while in the mandible, age was found to be a significant risk factor. Multiple regression analysis was then conducted to reanalyze these risk factors collectively. The results indicated that age and the angle change of the central incisors before and after orthodontic treatment were significant contributing factors in the maxilla, while age remained a significant factor in the mandible. In the maxilla, age showed an odds ratio of 1.087, and the angle change of the central incisors showed an odds ratio of 0.940. In the mandible, age had an odds ratio of 1.197 (Tables 9 and 10).

Table 9. Relationship between severity of black triangle and parameters related to treatment by simple logistic regression analysis [†].

	Maxilla			Mandible		
	B	SE	Significance	B	SE	Significance
Treatment period, month	0.045	0.016	**	0.026	0.015	NS
Age, y	0.189	0.044	***	0.180	0.045	***
Tooth shape	−0.200	−0.289	NS	0.052	1.602	NS
ΔU1 to SN /ΔIMPA, °	−0.070	0.022	**	0.006	0.014	NS
Horizontal movement of U1/L1, mm	−0.166	0.243	NS	−0.079	0.124	NS
Vertical movement of U1/L1, mm	0.062	0.203	NS	−0.235	0.316	NS
Δ Distance from ICP to ABC, mm	−0.138	0.208	NS	0.049	0.260	NS
Root angulation at T2, °	0.027	0.048	NS	−0.058	0.047	NS
A-P overlapped distance, mm	0.697	0.891	NS	0.725	1.125	NS
Transverse overlapped distance, mm	−0.698	1.083	NS	6.914	5.014	NS
Rotation, °	0.003	0.007	NS	−0.002	0.008	NS

[†] B Independent *t*-tests were used to compare between the extraction and non-extraction groups, and Bonferroni correction was performed. U1, maxillary incisor; L1, mandibular incisor; SN, Sella–Nasion; IMPA, incisor mandibular plane angle; T1, before treatment; T2, after treatment; Δ, T2-T1; ICP, interproximal contact point; ABC, alveolar bone crest; A-P, anteroposterior; NS, not significant; * $p < 0.05$; ** $p < 0.01$; *** $p < 0.001$.

Table 10. Main contributing factors to black triangle in the maxilla by multiple logistic regression analysis [†].

	B	SE	Significance	OR
Treatment period, month	0.030	0.018	NS	1.030
Age, y	0.172	0.044	***	1.087
Δ U1 to SN	−0.062	0.027	*	0.940

[†] Multiple logistic regression analysis was used. B indicates beta coefficient; SE, standard error; OR, odds ratio; U1, maxillary incisor; SN, Sella–Nasion; Δ, T2-T1; L1, mandibular incisor; NS, not significant; * $p < 0.05$; ** $p < 0.01$; *** $p < 0.001$.

4. Discussion

In this study, the incidence of black triangles after orthodontic treatment was found to be between 51% and 64%. This is higher than the previously reported rates of 38% to 58%, which can be attributed to differences in study design, sample size, age distribution, and methods for assessing black triangles [7,9,29]. The study confirmed a significant association between the occurrence of black triangles during orthodontic treatment and factors such as age and extraction status. Previous studies that highlighted the advantages of non-extraction treatment have reported that post-extraction orthodontic treatment leads to a significant reduction in the width of keratinized gingiva in the anterior region compared to non-extraction patients [2]. This suggests that extraction treatment may have a negative impact on periodontal tissues. However, as with other studies analyzing the effects of bracket type and bonding location on microbial distribution and periodontal health [30–32], this study found no significant association between the type of brackets or their bonding location and the occurrence of black triangles.

When comparing the mean values of various risk factors between patients with and without black triangles, the study found significant differences in the maxilla regarding treatment duration, age, and pre- and post-treatment incisor angulation changes. In the mandible, only age showed a significant difference. Previous studies have reported a significant increase in periodontal disease risk, such as inflammatory gingival hyperplasia, with longer orthodontic treatment durations due to increased plaque accumulation on appliances like brackets and power chains, as well as poor oral hygiene habits [33,34]. However, Ko-Kimura et al. [22] reported no significant statistical correlation between the duration of orthodontic treatment and the occurrence of black triangles. In this study, the occurrence of black triangles in the maxillary anterior region was significantly higher in patients with longer treatment durations than those without black triangles.

The direction of tooth movement has also been identified in previous studies as a risk factor for the formation of black triangles during orthodontic treatment. Specifically, numerous studies have reported that labial horizontal or labial angular movements of the maxillary anterior teeth increase the likelihood of gingival recession or black triangle formation due to thin labial alveolar bone [35,36]. In this study, of the 97 patients, only 27 exhibited labial angular movement during orthodontic treatment, and only 8 of these patients developed mild black triangles, scoring 2 on the Jemt Index. The remaining 19 patients did not develop black triangles. Therefore, no significant association was found between labial angular movement and black triangle formation, contrary to previous studies. However, the results of the multiple regression analysis showed that the likelihood of black triangle formation increased as the maxillary incisors underwent lingual angulation relative to the SN plane. The odds ratio for changes in maxillary incisor angulation was 0.940, indicating that for each degree of lingual angulation, the risk of black triangle formation increased by a factor of 1.06. This finding aligns with An et al. [7], who reported a significant association between black triangle formation and lingual horizontal movement of the maxillary incisors during orthodontic treatment.

The multiple regression analysis also revealed a significant association between age and the occurrence of black triangles during orthodontic treatment in both the maxilla and mandible. The odds ratios were 1.087 for the maxilla and 1.197 for the mandible, indicating that for each year of age, the risk of black triangle formation increased by 1.087 times in the maxilla and 1.197 times in the mandible. While age is commonly associated with an increased risk of periodontal disease, the occurrence of black triangles in older patients is not solely due to poor oral hygiene over time. As aging progresses, the reduction in oral epithelial keratinization, decreased interdental papilla height, and increased interdental space contribute to gingival recession and a higher likelihood of black triangles in adults [22,24]. These effects are particularly pronounced in adults over the age of 20 who undergo orthodontic treatment, as the ability of the papilla to regenerate and fill interdental spaces appears to diminish with age, exacerbating the condition during orthodontic interventions.

Tarnow et al. [21] reported a correlation between the distance from the contact point to the alveolar crest and the occurrence of black triangles. When the distance exceeds 5 mm, the interdental papilla cannot fill the black triangle, but when the distance is less than 5 mm, the papilla can re-fill the space. This study measured only the relative distance changes between the contact point and the alveolar crest before and after orthodontic treatment, and no significant association with black triangle formation was found. However, it was observed that alveolar bone height generally decreased in patients, regardless of whether black triangles developed. This suggests that age-related changes, typically associated with aging, were evident during the course of orthodontic treatment.

Future studies should classify patients according to the type and severity of malocclusion and their ability to maintain oral hygiene to investigate black triangle occurrence rates. Additionally, selecting a control group of patients who did not undergo orthodontic treatment for comparative analysis would be beneficial. The relationship between black triangle formation and gingival biotype should also be examined, as gingival phenotype plays a crucial role in determining susceptibility to black triangles. Thin gingival phenotypes are particularly prone to gingival recession and papilla loss, which can exacerbate black triangle formation. Evaluating these factors in future studies could enhance clinical decision-making. Furthermore, while this study did not directly compare fixed and removable appliances, future investigations should explore their respective impacts on black triangle formation to develop clearer guidelines for appliance selection. The risk factors associated with black triangles after orthodontic treatment are diverse. Being aware of these factors and predicting potential risks during diagnosis and treatment planning can help prevent or minimize the occurrence of black triangles.

Once black triangles form, various approaches can be considered for correction depending on the severity and underlying cause. Orthodontic techniques, such as controlled tipping or closing interdental spaces, can help reduce black triangle visibility, while interproximal stripping can minimize interdental spacing by reducing tooth size. Restorative approaches, including composite resins or veneers, may also be employed to address aesthetic concerns. Interdisciplinary collaboration between orthodontics, periodontics, and prosthodontics is necessary to reduce or eliminate black triangles that develop after orthodontic treatment.

5. Conclusions

This study showed that the occurrence of black triangles was significantly associated with age and extraction status, with a higher incidence observed in adults compared to adolescents and in extraction cases compared to non-extraction cases. In the maxilla, age, changes in incisor angulation relative to the SN plane, and treatment duration showed significant associations with the occurrence of black triangles after orthodontic treatment. In the mandible, only age was significantly associated.

Author Contributions: Conceptualization, J.-S.J. and H.-K.L.; methodology, J.-S.J.; software, J.-S.J.; validation, H.-K.L., Y.-S.L. and S.-K.J.; formal analysis, Y.-S.L.; investigation, S.-K.J.; resources, H.-K.L.; data curation, Y.-S.L.; writing—original draft preparation, J.-S.J and H.-K.L.; writing—review and editing, Y.-S.L. and S.-K.J.; visualization, J.-S.J.; supervision, S.-K.J.; project administration, Y.-S.L.; funding acquisition, S.-K.J. All authors have read and agreed to the published version of the manuscript.

Funding: This study was funded by National Research Foundation of Korea (NRF) grant funded by the Korean government (MSIT) (No. 2022R1F1A1066543).

Institutional Review Board Statement: The study was conducted according to the guidelines of the Declaration of Helsinki and approved by the Institutional Review Board of Korea University Guro Hospital (2022GR0461, 17 October 2022).

Informed Consent Statement: Patient consent was waived because the X-ray images were taken for treatment use, and there was no identifiable patient information.

Data Availability Statement: The data presented in this study are available upon request to the corresponding author due to the protection of patient privacy.

Conflicts of Interest: The authors declare no conflicts of interest.

References

1. Proffit, W.R.; Fields, H., Jr.; Moray, L. Prevalence of malocclusion and orthodontic treatment need in the United States: Estimates from the NHANES III survey. *Int. J. Adult Orthod. Orthognath. Surg.* **1998**, *13*, 97–106.
2. Abdelhafez, R.S. The effect of orthodontic treatment on the periodontium and soft tissue esthetics in adult patients. *Clin. Exp. Dent. Res.* **2022**, *8*, 410–420. [CrossRef]
3. Patano, A.; Malcangi, G.; Inchingolo, A.D.; Garofoli, G.; De Leonardis, N.; Azzollini, D.; Latini, G.; Mancini, A.; Carpentiere, V.; Laudadio, C.; et al. Mandibular Crowding: Diagnosis and Management—A Scoping Review. *J. Pers. Med.* **2023**, *13*, 774. [CrossRef]
4. Baysal, A. Evaluation of root resorption following rapid maxillary expansion using cone-beam computed tomography. *Angle Orthod.* **2012**, *82*, 488–494. [CrossRef]

5. Fuhrmann, R. Three-dimensional interpretation of periodontal lesions and remodeling during orthodontic treatment. Part III. *J. Orofac. Orthop.* **1996**, *57*, 224–237. [CrossRef] [PubMed]
6. Pugliese, F.; Hess, R. Preventing their occurrence, managing them when prevention is not practical. *Semin. Orthod.* **2019**, *25*, 175–186. [CrossRef]
7. An, S.S.; Choi, Y.J. Risk factors associated with open gingival embrasures after orthodontic treatment. *Angle Orthod.* **2018**, *88*, 267–274. [CrossRef]
8. Ziahosseini, P. Management of gingival black triangles. *Br. Dent. J.* **2014**, *217*, 559–563. [CrossRef]
9. Kurth, J.R. Open gingival embrasures after orthodontic treatment in adults: Prevalence and etiology. *Am. J. Orthod. Dentofac. Orthop.* **2001**, *120*, 116–123. [CrossRef]
10. Melsen, B. Tissue reaction following application of extrusive and intrusive forces to teeth in adult monkeys. *Am. J. Orthod.* **1986**, *89*, 469–475. [CrossRef]
11. Murakami, T. Periodontal changes after experimentally induced intrusion of the upper incisors in *Macaca fuscata* monkeys. *Am. J. Orthod. Dentofac. Orthop.* **1989**, *95*, 115–126. [CrossRef] [PubMed]
12. Melsen, B.; Agerbaek, N.; Markenstam, G. Intrusion of incisors in adult patients with marginal bone loss. *Am. J. Orthod. Dentofac. Orthop.* **1989**, *96*, 232–241. [CrossRef] [PubMed]
13. Duncan, W.J. Realignment of periodontally-affected maxillary teeth—A periodontist's perspective. Part II: Case reports. *N. Z. Dent. J.* **1997**, *93*, 117–123. [PubMed]
14. Rabie, A.B. Adjunctive orthodontic treatment of periodontally involved teeth: Case reports. *Quintessence Int.* **1998**, *29*, 13–19.
15. Cardaropoli, D.; Re, S.; Corrente, G.; Abundo, R. Intrusion of migrated incisors with infra bony defects in adult periodontal patients. *Am. J. Orthod. Dentofac. Orthop.* **2001**, *120*, 671–675. [CrossRef]
16. Re, S.; Corrente, G.; Abundo, R.; Cardaropoli, D. The use of orthodontic intrusive movement to reduce infra bony pockets in adult periodontal patients: A case report. *Int. J. Periodontics Restor. Dent.* **2002**, *22*, 365–371.
17. Dorsey, J.; Korabik, K. Social and psychological motivations for orthodontic treatment. *Am. J. Orthod.* **1977**, *72*, 460. [CrossRef]
18. Kilpeläinen, P.V.; Phillips, C.; Tulloch, J.F. Anterior tooth position and motivation for early treatment. *Angle Orthod.* **1993**, *63*, 171–174.
19. Cardaropoli, D.; Re, S. Interdental papilla augmentation procedure following orthodontic treatment in a periodontal patient. *J. Periodontol.* **2005**, *76*, 655–661. [CrossRef]
20. Oliveira, C.M.; Storrer, A.M. Papillary regeneration: Anatomical aspects and treatment approaches. *RSBO* **2012**, *9*, 448–456. [CrossRef]
21. Tarnow, D.P.; Magner, A.W.; Fletcher, P. The effect of the distance from the contact point to the crest of bone on the presence or absence of the interproximal dental papilla. *J. Periodontol.* **1992**, *63*, 995–996. [CrossRef]
22. Ko-Kimura, N.; Kimura-Hayashi, M.; Yamaguchi, M.; Ikeda, T.; Meguro, D.; Kanekawa, M.; Kasai, K. Some factors associated with open gingival embrasures following orthodontic treatment. *Aust. Orthod. J.* **2003**, *19*, 19–24. [CrossRef] [PubMed]
23. Tanaka, O.M.; Furquim, B.D.; Pascotto, R.C. The dilemma of the open gingival embrasure between maxillary central incisors. *J. Contemp. Dent. Pract.* **2008**, *9*, 92–98.
24. Chang, L.C. The association between embrasure morphology and central papilla recession. *J. Clin. Periodontol.* **2007**, *34*, 432–436. [CrossRef]
25. Ikeda, T.; Yamaguchi, M.; Meguro, D. Prediction and causes of open gingival embrasure spaces between the mandibular central incisors following orthodontic treatment. *Aust. Orthod. J.* **2004**, *20*, 87–92. [CrossRef]
26. Kozai, Y.; Tamaki, Y.; Nomura, Y.; Kaida, K. The factors of open gingival embrasure space between central incisors after orthodontic treatment in adult patients. *Orthod. Waves* **2010**, *69*, 39. [CrossRef]
27. Taylor, R.M. Variation in form of human teeth: An anthropologic and forensic study of maxillary incisors. *J. Dent. Res.* **1969**, *48*, 5–16. [CrossRef]
28. Song, J.W. Analysis of crown size and morphology, and gingival shape in the maxillary anterior dentition in Korean young adults. *J. Adv. Prosthodont.* **2017**, *9*, 315–320. [CrossRef]
29. Rashid, Z.J.; Gul, S.S. Incidence of Gingival Black Triangles following Treatment with Fixed Orthodontic Appliance: A Systematic Review. *Healthcare* **2022**, *10*, 1373. [CrossRef]
30. Sfondrini, M.F. Influence of lingual bracket position on microbial and periodontal parameters in vivo. *J. Appl. Oral. Sci.* **2012**, *20*, 357–361. [CrossRef]
31. Anhoury, P.; Nathanson, D.; Hughes, C.V.; Socransky, S.; Feres, M.; Chou, L.L. Microbial profile on metallic and ceramic bracket materials. *Angle Orthod.* **2002**, *72*, 338–343. [PubMed]
32. Van Gastel, J.; Quirynen, M.; Teughels, W.; Coucke, W.; Carels, C. Influence of bracket design on microbial and periodontal parameters in vivo. *J. Clin. Periodontol.* **2007**, *34*, 423–431. [CrossRef] [PubMed]
33. Pinto, A.S. Gingival enlargement in orthodontic patients: Effect of treatment duration. *Am. J. Orthod. Dentofac. Orthop.* **2017**, *152*, 477–482. [CrossRef] [PubMed]
34. Al-Abdaly, M.; Asiri, A.; Al-Abdaly, G.; Ghabri, M.; Alqaysi, M.; Aljathnan, A.; Al Naser, Y.; Alshahrani, N. Evaluation of the Influence of Fixed Orthodontic Treatment Duration on the Severity of Inflammatory Gingival Enlargement (Fixed Orthodontic Induced Gingival Enlargements) and Some Properties of Saliva. *Int. J. Clin. Med.* **2022**, *2*, 132–146. [CrossRef]

35. Kandasamy, S.; Goone Wardene, M.; Tennant, M. Changes in interdental papillae heights following alignment of anterior teeth. *Aust. Orthod. J.* **2007**, *23*, 16–23. [CrossRef]
36. Han, J.Y.; Jung, G.U. Labial and lingual and palatal bone thickness of maxillary and mandibular anteriors in human cadavers in Koreans. *J. Periodontal. Implant Sci.* **2011**, *41*, 60–66. [CrossRef]

Disclaimer/Publisher's Note: The statements, opinions and data contained in all publications are solely those of the individual author(s) and contributor(s) and not of MDPI and/or the editor(s). MDPI and/or the editor(s) disclaim responsibility for any injury to people or property resulting from any ideas, methods, instructions or products referred to in the content.

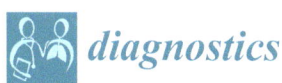

Systematic Review

The Frequency of Risk Factors for Cleft Lip and Palate in Mexico: A Systematic Review

Sandra López-Verdín [1], Judith A. Solorzano-López [1], Ronell Bologna-Molina [2,3], Nelly Molina-Frechero [4], Omar Tremillo-Maldonado [3], Victor H. Toral-Rizo [5] and Rogelio González-González [3,*]

1. Health Science Center, Research Institute of Dentistry, Universidad de Guadalajara, Guadalajara 44100, Mexico; sandra.lverdin@academicos.udg.mx (S.L.-V.); judith.solorzano6225@alumnos.udg.mx (J.A.S.-L.)
2. Molecular Pathology Area, School of Dentistry, Universidad de la República, Montevideo 11400, Uruguay; ronellbologna@odon.edu.uy
3. Department of Research, School of Dentistry, Universidad Juárez del Estado de Durango, Durango 34070, Mexico; omar.tremillo@ujed.mx
4. Department of Health Care, Universidad Autónoma Metropolitana Xochimilco, México City 04960, Mexico; nmolina@correo.xoc.uam.mx
5. School of Dentistry, National Autonomous University of Mexico, Toluca de Lerdo 50000, Mexico; vhtoralr@uaemex.mx
* Correspondence: rogelio.gonzalez@ujed.mx

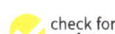

Abstract: Background: Cleft lip and palate is an anomaly that affects both women and men. It is considered to be among the most frequent congenital abnormalities and is related to modifications in chromosomal DNA and multiple genetic alterations. This anomaly can also be associated with various environmental factors, such as tobacco and alcohol consumption, medication use, and exposure to different environmental and industrial toxic substances. The objective of this study was to document the frequency of risk factors related to cleft lip and palate through a systematic review of Mexican studies. Methods: In this systematic review, a bibliographic search was conducted following PRISMA guidelines in the databases Scielo, ScienceDirect, PubMed, and EBSCO. Keywords related to cleft lip and palate, epidemiology, and risk factors were used. In all, 3 independent reviewers (J.A.S.L., S.L.V., and N.M.F.) selected and evaluated a total of 17 articles included in this analysis, achieving a coefficient of κ = 0.84. Results: The analysis revealed that the highest frequency of conducted studies was in the State of Mexico. The most common risk factors identified were environmental, pharmacological, consumption habits, and gynecological factors. Conclusions: Identifying the main risk factors for cleft lip and palate in the Mexican population will enable the implementation of preventive measures aimed at reducing exposure to these factors. Additionally, early intervention can improve the quality of life for individuals affected by this condition.

Keywords: cleft lip and palate; risk factors; Mexican population; toxic substances

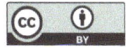

1. Introduction

Cleft lip and palate is the most frequent congenital malformation worldwide. This anomaly is produced by partial or complete fusion in the facial process during embryonic development. Both genetic variants and environmental etiologies may be involved in this failure, and it occurs with a prevalence of 1 per 1000 or 1500 births [1–3]. This congenital malformation was identified in the 4th century B.C [1]. The multifactorial nature of this condition makes prevention difficult and makes it challenging to determine a therapeutic target [4].

These clefts, along with other defects and syndromes that involve cleft lip and palate as one of their symptoms, amount to more than 400 different syndromes [5,6]. This is because of the chromosomal aberrations or monogenic diseases that can occur in 30% of cases [7].

Unlike non-syndromic cleft lip and palate, which is derived from the interaction between genetic and environmental factors, representing around 70% of cases, non-modifiable factors (sex, race, family history, etc.) and modifiable factors (diet, health status, medication, etc.) can exert an effect for a period of up to two months after conception [8].

Various studies carried out in recent years have identified several risk factors related to cleft lip and palate, including socio-economic factors, tobacco consumption, alcohol, drugs, maternal factors, infections by viruses and bacteria, genetic alterations and mutations, as well as occupational exposure [1,9–11].

However, the study of cleft lip and palate in the Mexican population is not applicable or insufficient to adequately characterize it. This is due to the frequency of risk factors, as well as their geographical distribution, which have been studied little.

Although the Ministry of Health in Mexico estimates a rate of 1 per 750 births, the prevalence of cleft lip and palate in this country is more complex and depends on the state in which the study was conducted [12,13].

Therefore, the purpose of this study was to carry out a systematic review to determine the frequency of risk factors associated with cleft lip and palate.

2. Material and Methods

2.1. Research Design

A descriptive and retrospective review of science articles published for the elaboration of this systematic review was carried out to resolve the question "What are the common risk factors associated with the development of cleft lip and palate in Mexican states?".

2.2. Search Strategy

A search was conducted in the Scielo, Science Direct, PubMed, and EBSCO databases without restrictions based on the year of publication and applying language filters to English and Spanish. Key search terms included "cleft lip and palate" AND "risk factors" AND "epidemiology OR epidemiological". The studies were screened for inclusion using predefined criteria. The selected items were organized into eight regions: northwest, northeast, west, east, northcentral, southcentral, southwest, and southeast. To enhance understanding of the factors, they were grouped into five categories: (1) socio-economic; (2) hereditary family history; (3) gynecological and perinatal; (4) habits and medicines; and (5) environmental factors.

2.3. Eligibility Criteria

The population, intervention, comparison, and outcome (PICO) synthesis tool was utilized to evaluate the eligibility criteria, which were defined as the following:

patient = patient diagnosed with cleft lip and palate in Mexico; intervention/exposure = systematic review and analysis of existing research to evaluate the cleft lip and palate associated with risk factors in Mexico; comparison = evaluate and compare risk factors and epidemiological characteristics across different regions in Mexico; outcome = identification of risk factors and epidemiological characteristics associated with cleft lip and palate in different regions of Mexico.

Inclusion criteria: Studies with patients diagnosed with left clip and palate, without restriction with gender and age; studies that evaluated human participants; and studies conducted only in Mexican states. The studies evaluated included the following: (i) studies reporting patients diagnosed with cleft lip and palate; (ii) studies including maternal, paternal, and neonatal epidemiological characteristics associated with cleft lip and palate; (iii) prospective or retrospective studies; (iv) studies specifying the state or city within Mexico where they were conducted; and (v) studies reporting frequencies of risk factors associated with cleft lip and palate.

Exclusion criteria: Studies were excluded if they met the following criteria: (i) had inadequate information; (ii) included other countries or if they were studies which included Mexico and other countries; (iii) were studies which did not include risk factors included in the search strategy; (iv) studied cleft lip and palate associated with other syndromes; (v) were review articles, meta-analyses, letters to the editor, or original research articles that did not report on cleft lip and palate or were not directly related to the review's purposes.

2.4. Data Extraction and Evaluation

Three independent authors (J.A.S.L., S.L.V., and N.M.F.) selected and evaluated studies that were deemed relevant for the complete text evaluation. After discussion and consensus among the three authors, the articles with pertinent content were chosen. A total of 20 articles were included in this analysis, achieving a coefficient of κ = 0.84. After selection of the articles, two authors (O.T.M and VH.T.R) individually extracted the quantitative and qualitative data from the selected articles. Standardized forms were used to facilitate the analysis of the information. The extracted information included the following data items: title, authors, year of publication, Mexican states in which data were collected, type of cleft present, number of participants including controls, as well as participants' age range.

A third reviewer (R.G.G.) was consulted in cases of disagreement between the two authors. The PRISMA guide was used for item selection according to inclusion and eligibility criteria. The term "Mexico" was used to exclude items pertaining to other countries. The review followed the PRISMA chart (Figure 1), with peer review of abstracts and full texts to verify compliance with the pre-established inclusion criteria.

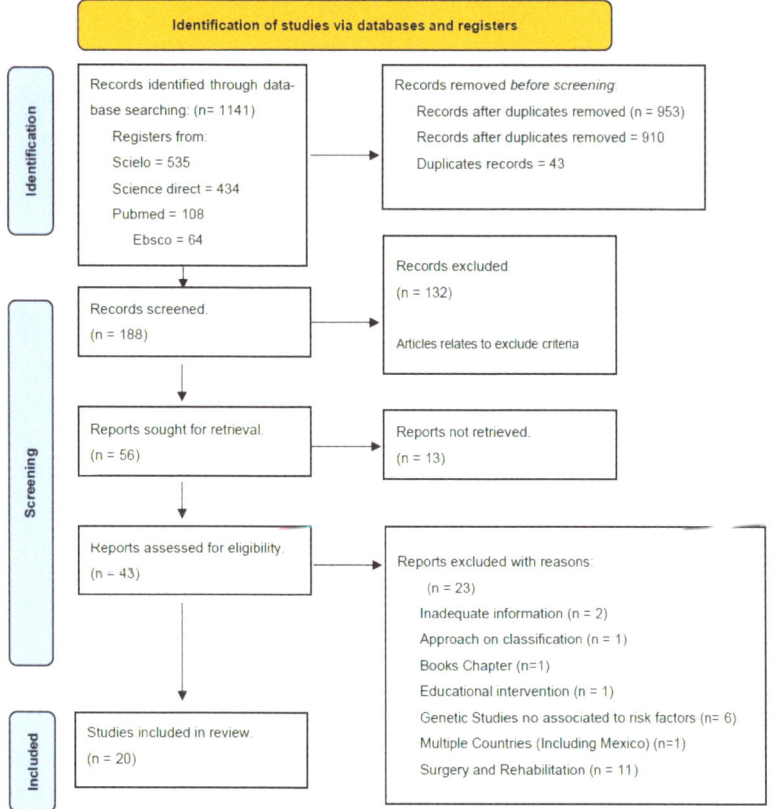

Figure 1. Four-phase PRISMA chart for searching and selecting items. PRISMA flow chart for the systematic review. Of the 1141 articles found in the 4 databases included in the search, 20 (1.75%) studies were selected for analysis. Following this, the articles underwent a title and abstract review, with the exception of any articles displayed.

Risk of bias was reviewed according to the Methodological Index for Non-Randomized Studies (MINORS), in which the global ideal score is 16 for non-comparative studies and 24 for comparative studies [14]. The data analyzed from each article were collected in Excel (Microsoft Excel 365, version 16.87, Microsoft 2024. Ciudad Santa Fe, MX) in the following order: study authors, year, place, presence or absence of cleft lip and palate, and risk factors associated with cleft lip and palate.

3. Results

Out of the total of 1141 (100%) results in the databases, only 20 (1.75%) articles that studied risk factors associated with cleft lip and palate, published between the years 2003 and 2023, were included. According to the MINORS instrument (Figure 2), all studies had a clear aim (I1), the majority included consecutive patients (I2), had unambiguous explanation of the criteria used to evaluate the main outcome (I4), and included all patients in the study without a loss less than 5% (I7). The principal weaknesses (yellow) were prospective collection data (I3), the fact that blinding evaluation was absent in all, and the prospective calculation of the study. Because of the lack of case–control studies, I9, I10, and I11 showed more yellow spaces. The mean global score for non-comparative studies was 12, and it was 21 for comparative studies (Figure 2, references in blue).

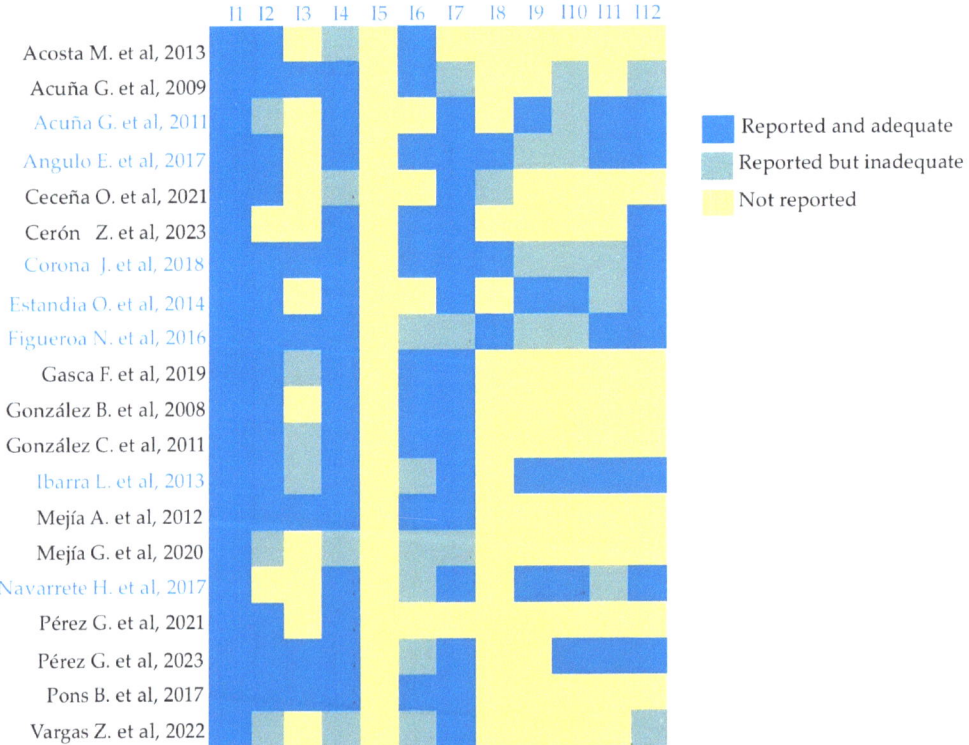

Figure 2. MINORS heat map. Items (I): I1—a clearly stated aim; I2—inclusion of consecutive patients; I3—prospective collection of data; I4—endpoints appropriate to the aim of the study; I5—unbiased assessment of the study endpoint; I6—follow-up period appropriate to the aim of the study; I7—loss to follow-up less than 5%; I8—prospective calculation; I9—an adequate control group; I10—contemporary groups; I11—baseline equivalence of groups; I12—adequate statistical analyses [9,13,15–32].

The states in which these studies were conducted were Baja California [15], Sinaloa [16], Nuevo León [17], Jalisco [18,19], Querétaro [20], Guerrero [21], Campeche [9,22], Puebla [23], Mexico State [24–26], and Mexico City [27–30]. Three of the studies were conducted throughout the entire republic [13,31,32]. The state of Mexico stands out among the 36,493 samples of cleft lip and palate patients with a total of 3174 cases, followed by the state of Jalisco, with 2008 cases, and Mexico City (CDMX), with 1244 cases accumulated over a period of 20 years (2003–2023). Similarly, the state of Colima has the lowest incidence of cases, accumulating only 21 cases in the same period.

Furthermore, the categories of factors were charted according to the region of Mexico in which they were examined (Figure 3). We note that the most analyzed factors in the northwest region, as well as in the northcentral, southwest, and southeast regions, were those in the habits and medicines category. The northeast region has a higher frequency of environmental factors, as it was the region that assessed all of these factors. Studies conducted in the western and eastern regions found that socio-economic factors had a high frequency; the same was observed in the southcentral region with gynecological and perinatal factors. On the contrary, hereditary–family background factors showed low frequencies in all regions of the country. It is important to note that not all studies assessed all categories.

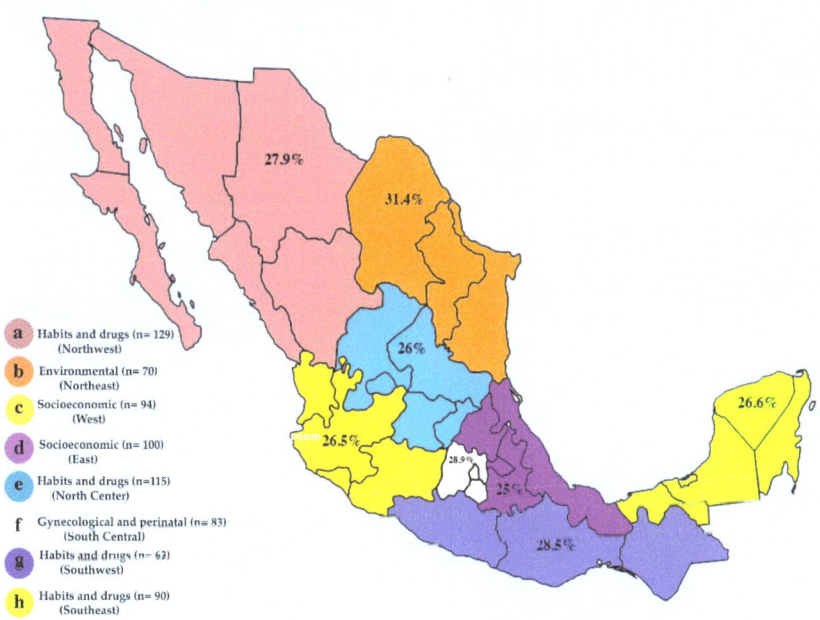

Figure 3. Map of the most common risk factor categories by region. (a) Lower California, Baja California, Sonora, Durango, Sinaloa; (b) Coahuila, Nuevo León, Tamaulipas; (c) Nayarit, Jalisco, Colima, Michoacán; (d) Hidalgo, Tlaxcala, Puebla, Veracruz; (e) Zacatecas, Aguascalientes, San Luis Potosí, Guanajuato, Querétaro; (f) State of Mexico, Mexico City, Morelos; (g) Guerrero, Oaxaca, Chiapas; (h) Tabasco, Campeche, Yucatán, Quintana Roo.

Next, in the category of socio-economic factors, risk factors were subsequently gathered that were studied in 14 of the 15 articles; among them, the following are highlighted: "mother's age" in 9 articles, "father's level of education" in 5 articles, and "fathers' age" in 4 articles. The highest incidence of cleft lip and palate cases was found in mothers under the age of 30 (84.5%). The predominant age of mothers was in the range of 24–26 (26.1, SD ± 1.39, min 24.5, max 28) years, while the father's age was 25–29 years (27.4, SD ± 2.7, min 23, max 30.3). The studies by Perez-González A [29,30] and Pons-Bonals A [20] divided mothers into age groups, with ages 20 to 29, 21 to 25, and 26 to 30 years showing the highest frequency. Pons-Bonals divided the father's age into groups, and the 21- to 25-year-old group showed the highest frequency of cases [20] (Figure 4a). Parents who only completed primary school were classified as possessing a low level of education (45.18%). The percentage of mothers and fathers who completed senior high school was 4.19% and 2.48%, respectively. The percentage of parents who completed senior high school and university studies was low (1.29% and 1.14% for mothers and fathers, respectively). A total of 10.34% did not have any academic background (Figure 4b).

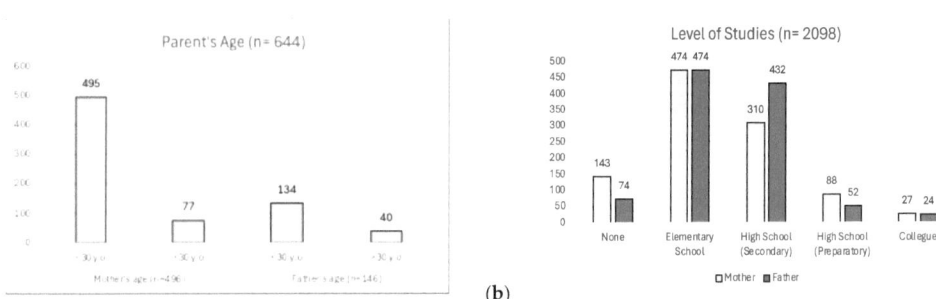

Figure 4. Socio-economic risk factors related to cleft lip and palate: (**a**) risk factors associated with parents' age; (**b**) risk factors related to education level.

In the category of gynecological and perinatal factors, 12 articles analyzed showed a total of 16 factors, with the "sex" factor being the most studied due to its presence in all of them. Meanwhile, six articles focused on the "prenatal care" factor, and seven articles discussed "folic acid consumption". Folic acid use and prenatal care were prevalent in most cases. These factors were followed in terms of frequency by being overweight and having previously undergone an abortion (Figure 5a).

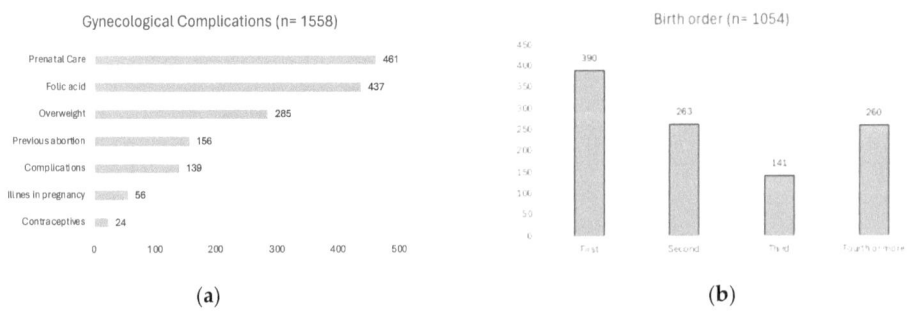

Figure 5. Gynecological and perinatal factors in Mexico: the category graphs depict the most common cases of (**a**) gynecological complications and (**b**) birth order.

From the perinatal factors present in cases of cleft lip and palate, it was observed that, regarding the order of birth, it is highlighted that, in most cases, the patient is the firstborn of the family (Figure 5b). Regarding the sex factor, 34,092 cases were evaluated, of which 58% of the cases were male and 42% were female, a ratio of 1.4:1.

Similarly, the category of habits and drug factors gathers 8 risk factors, analyzed in 12 articles, highlighting the medicine intake factor with/without prescription as the most analyzed, as it was present in 9 articles, a frequency of 24.4%. However, regarding frequencies, the highest percentage was the alcohol factor in the father, present in 24.7% of cases, followed by 20.6% of cases that identified the tobacco factor in the father (Figure 6).

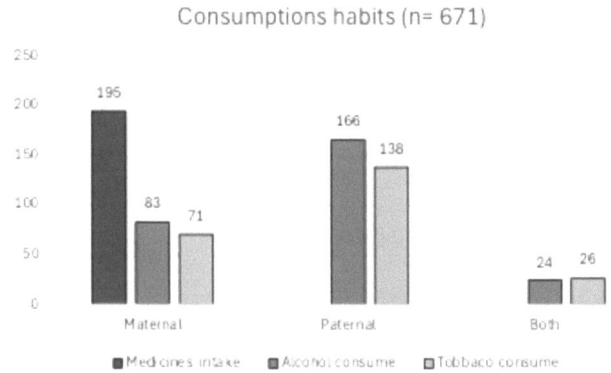

Figure 6. Frequencies of risky habits and medicine intake: fathers consumed alcohol and tobacco more frequently than mothers, and only a small percentage of both mothers and fathers used these substances simultaneously.

Industrial pollutants were observed in 333 cases (7 articles) that were presented within the areas of low, medium, and high concentrations of industrial pollutants, of which 63.9% of the cases were exposed to high concentrations of cyanides. For polluting metals, 69% of cases occurred in areas with low concentrations of metals. As for halogenated organic pollutants, a higher prevalence of cases was found in areas of high (49.8%) and medium (49.2%) concentrations, with a difference of only two cases between the two. A total of 60.9% of patients were exposed to medium concentrations of aromatic compounds, and 78% of cases were identified in areas with medium concentrations of greenhouse gases (Figure 7).

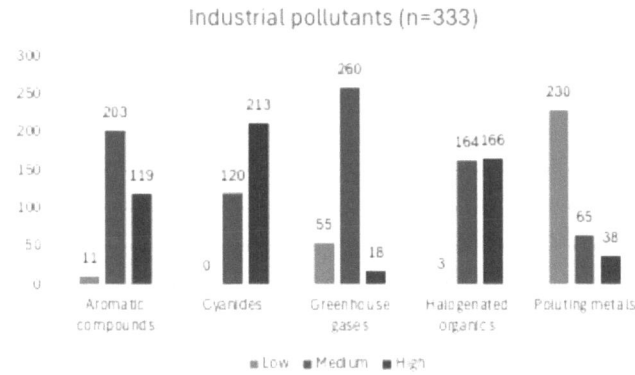

Figure 7. Frequency of cases related to industrial pollutant concentrations.

Finally, two works, in addition to reporting the frequency of some risk factors, evaluated the interaction of folic acid intake with polymorphisms in the methylenetetrahydrofolate (MTHFR) gene in the mestizo Mexican population. Ibarra-López et al., 2013 [21], found that mothers with 677CT or 677TT genotypes had a higher risk of having a child with cleft lip and palate, and in the case of the latter genotype, the risk increased with a lack of folate supplementation during the first trimester of pregnancy. Estandia-Ortega et al., 2014 [28], concluded that intake of folic acid and the TT genotype with the MTHFR C677T polymorphism in children independently reduced the risk of cleft lip and palate.

4. Discussion

On several occasions, the risk factors associated with lip and palate fissure and their inter-relationship with the socio-demographic, socio-economic, and pollution characteristics of different areas around the world have been studied in detail; however, most use information of Anglo-Saxon (European or North American) or Asian origin, which, due to racial and environmental differences, cannot be applicable or accurate for the Mexican population. In addition, the associated risk factors depend on the methodological design of the research.

Epidemiological studies suggest that maternal risk factors play an important role in the development of different birth defects where the parent's conditions are not the same, according to data that are little studied and often unknown. It is noteworthy that most of the frequencies in this paper indicate only maternal characteristics, because studies are generally oriented to identify exposure to risk factors during pregnancy [9,15,16,20,25,26]. However, some authors consider that paternal influence can be exerted before conception through toxicant transmission in semen or even genetic mutations; e.g., paternal smoking could interfere with the genesis of the male gamete [10] or other epigenetic changes in the nucleic acids of spermatozoa could be produced by the influence of environmental factors [33]. For this reason, Nguyen et al., 2007, evaluated the occupation of parents of children with isolated oral clefts in Norway, a variable missing in the studies included [34].

In this review, throughout the investigations, it was found that within the category of socio-economic factors, the age of the mother exerted the strongest influence. Nevertheless, at present, its place in terms of association has been diminished, and it is increasingly less frequently analyzed. Surprisingly, a higher proportion of parents (father and mother) under the age of 30 was found in several manuscripts [9,15,18,20,24,26], as opposed to the findings of previous research, where the influence of age on the risk of cleft lip and palate increases with the aging of one of the parents and decreases if one of the parents is young [30,35]. Similar results were obtained in a Nigerian population [36].

As a result of our findings, we concur with the assertions of Corona R. et al. regarding the parents' educational attainment: primary school education serves as the highest level of education in the majority of cases and consistently reflects a low socio-economic status [18].

Hereditary family history was recorded for most of the articles; however, it was not specified whether it was maternal or paternal history, leaving aside the branch of genealogy affected by this malformation. For this reason, little can be achieved in terms of prevention and genetic counseling. The data from the articles were collected from the areas of gynecology and obstetrics, which is why the focus granted to the paternal genealogy branch is minimal. Thus, in these cases, it is unknown whether the father had a child(s) with cleft lip and palate prior to the one identified in the current study [16,18,20,24,25,30]. A study by Muñoz et al. reported in 2001 that cases of cleft lip and palate are twice as common in families with a hereditary family history of malformations [6].

Undoubtedly, the consumption of folic acid is internationally recognized as a preventive measure for birth defects. In our results, we can observe that most of the mothers consumed folic acid and attended their prenatal care appointments; despite this, their son presented with cleft lip and palate. As set out in NOM-034-SSA2-201325, a daily intake of 4 mg of folic acid is recommended for pregnant women and their partners with a family or personal history of malformations or living in the geographical areas with the highest incidence of cases (Secretaria de Salud, 2023) [12]. Similarly, it is important to emphasize that this measure should be applied during the preconception period, which is three months before pregnancy and lasts until the 12th week of gestation. Thus, regularly, the mother starts consuming folic acid at the time when she is diagnosed with pregnancy; that is, when the pregnancy is advanced by a month or more and when the folic acid may no longer be as effective [9,26]. Interestingly, Ibarra et al., 2013, found an association between a lack of folic acid supplementation and the combination of the genotype variants 677TT and 677CT in the maternal MTHFR gene. Opposite results have been found in Norwegian [37] and French [38] populations. We did not find other genes evaluated in conjunction with risk factors in the Mexican population.

Body mass index (BMI) was only studied in mothers, and we can observe a clear association with cleft lip and palate and BMI, as most mothers were overweight or obese before, during, and after the pregnancy in question [16,18,26].

On the other hand, in our study, a higher frequency of cases was found for the firstborn child [20,24], contrary to what was stated by other authors, who found that the risk of cleft lip and palate increases when the number of offspring increases [9,16,19,26].

Tobacco and alcohol consumption are the factors that have the highest association with cleft lip and palate; however, these previous studies focused mainly on the mother, with few studies reporting this habit in both parents [9,20,27]. Nevertheless, these factors appeared with higher frequency in parents of children with cleft lip and palate, according to a study by Martinelli et al. in 2020 [11]. They claimed that the use of tobacco in men prior to insemination increases the risk of non-syndromic orofacial fissures [11].

In the same context, several authors pointed out that the pattern and severity of malformations caused by the use of medication depend on the dose, time, and duration of exposure, with the first trimester of pregnancy being the stage of highest risk. The risk of having a child with cleft lip and palate is five times higher when medications are consumed during pregnancy; our results were in agreement with this observation: this factor was found in more than half of the mothers [1,10,35,39].

Environmental risk factors were the least analyzed throughout the country; however, parents exposed to pollution were predisposed to having children with this malformation. Several authors found that increased exposure to solid urban waste raised the rate of cleft lip and palate, as did exposure to toxic substances in the environment and at work, such as wood smoke, chlorinated solvents, fertilizers, and pesticides [15,26,30,31]. While there was not a direct link between the two, Gasca et al. showed that there was a geographical proximity between cases of cleft lip and palate and exposure to environmental pollutants such as carbon dioxide, arsenic, mercury, nickel, lead, cadmium, and cyanide [17]. These pollutants are linked to birth defects and are found in moderate-to-high amounts in urban areas.

Importantly, this birth defect has a great deal of different causes; thus, it is difficult to determine a foolproof way to prevent it. This problem is related to a fusion of the palatine and labial processes that happen at a time during pregnancy when the mother usually does not know she is pregnant [11].

Regarding limitations, the differences in methods used to evaluate each variable studied complicate the homogeneity of results presented in this study. Another important limitation is related to the fact that the majority of the studies in this systematic review met the inclusion criteria but lacked evaluations of paternal risk factors. These risk factors, which include age, educational level, substance use, and exposure to industrial pollutants, could potentially be linked to the father's occupational characteristics. However, the reviewed articles do not fully document this connection.

5. Conclusions

It is important to highlight that the parental influence is related to exposure to toxic agents associated with consumption and/or a polluted environment, including alcohol and tobacco consumption, in which the influence of the father stands out more. This influence may be linked to a higher risk of cleft lip and palate in newborns. This review of risk factors for cleft lip and palate in Mexico not only helps with early diagnosis but also enables preventive measures and improved prenatal care. Early intervention and timely treatment can significantly improve the quality of life for children born with cleft lip and palate, emphasizing the importance of ongoing research and increased efforts to reduce the impact of these risk factors and, ultimately, to improve the well-being of affected individuals and their families. In addition, it is crucial to emphasize that more research is needed in Mexico to evaluate contaminating risk factors. Finally, additional genetic studies of parents of children with cleft lip and palate must be carried out in order to gain a deeper understanding of the factors that influence this condition.

Author Contributions: J.A.S.-L., S.L.-V. and N.M.-F. performed the digital search, selection, analysis, and extraction of the information. O.T.-M., V.H.T.-R. and R.G.-G. conducted the analysis and extraction of the information. All the authors contributed to the evaluation of risk bias using the MINORS instrument. J.A.S.-L., S.L.-V. and O.T.-M. prepared the tables and figures. All authors have read and agreed to the published version of the manuscript.

Funding: This research was financed by the Universidad de Guadalajara and Universidad Juárez del Estado de Durango (No. 101463).

Institutional Review Board Statement: Not applicable.

Informed Consent Statement: Not applicable.

Data Availability Statement: No new data were created or analyzed in this study.

Conflicts of Interest: The authors declare no conflicts of interest.

References

1. Suazo, J. Environmental factors in non-syndromic orofacial clefts: A review based on meta-analyses results. *Oral Dis.* **2022**, *28*, 3–8. [CrossRef] [PubMed]
2. Hao, Y.; Tian, S.; Jiao, X.; Mi, N.; Zhang, B.; Song, T.; An, L.; Zheng, X.; Zhuang, D. Association of Parental Environmental Exposures and Supplementation Intake with Risk of Nonsyndromic Orofacial Clefts: A Case-Control Study in Heilongjiang Province, China. *Nutrients* **2015**, *7*, 7172–7184. [CrossRef]
3. NIH. El Labio Leporino y el Paladar Hendido. Instituto Nacional de Investigación Dental y Craneofacial [Citado Enero 2021]. Available online: https://www.nidcr.nih.gov/espanol/temas-de-salud/labio-leporino-paladar-hendido (accessed on 10 June 2024).
4. Han, J.; Shimizu, T.; Shimizu, K.; Maeda, T. Detection of informative markers for searching a causative gene(s) of cleft lip with palate in a/wysn mice. *Pediatr. Dent. J.* **2005**, *15*, 72–78. [CrossRef]
5. Babai, A.; Irving, M. Orofacial Clefts: Genetics of Cleft Lip and Palate. *Genes* **2023**, *9*, 1603. [CrossRef]
6. Muñoz, J.; Bustos, I.; Quintero, C.; Giraldo, A. Factores de riesgo para algunas anomalías congénitas en población colombiana. *Rev. Salud Pública* **2001**, *3*, 268–282.
7. Rogers, B.O. Treatment of Cleft Lip and Palate during The Revolutionary War: Bicentennial Reflections (An Invited Article). *Cleft Palate J.* **1976**, *13*, 371–390.
8. Mossey, P.A.; Little, J.; Munger, R.G.; Dixon, M.J.; Shaw, W.C. Cleft lip and palate. *Lancet* **2009**, *374*, 1773–1785. [CrossRef]
9. Acuña-González, G.; Escoffie-Ramírez, M.; Medina-Solis, C.E.; Casanova-Rosado, J.F.; Pontigo-Loyola, A.P.; Villalobos-Rodelo, J.J.; de Márquez-Corona, M.L.; Granillo, H.I. Caracterización epidemiológica del labio y/o paladar hendido no sindrómico Estudio en niños de 0–12 años de edad en Campeche e Hidalgo. *Rev. ADM* **2009**, *66*, 50–58.
10. Altoé, S.R.; Borges, A.H.; Campos Neves, A.T.S.; Fábio Aranha, A.M.; Meireles Borba, A.; Martinez Espinosa, M.; Ricci Volpato, L.E. Influence of Parental Exposure to Risk Factors in the Occurrence of Oral Clefts. *J. Dent.* **2020**, *21*, 119–126. [CrossRef]
11. Martinelli, M.; Palmieri, A.; Carinci, F.; Scapoli, L. Non-syndromic Cleft Palate: An Overview on Human Genetic and Environmental Risk Factors. *Front. Cell Dev. Biol.* **2020**, *8*, 1155. [CrossRef]
12. Secretaría de Salud. NORMA Oficial Mexicana NOM. 034-SSA2-2013. 2013. Available online: http://www.salud.gob.mx/unidades/cdi/nom/034ssa202.html (accessed on 13 October 2023).
13. Navarrete-Hernández, E.; Canún-Serrano, S.; Valdés-Hernández, J.; Reyes-Pablo, A.E. Prevalencia de labio hendido con o sin paladar hendido en recién nacidos vivos. México, 2008–2014. *Rev. Mex. Ped.* **2017**, *84*, 101–110.
14. Slim, K.; Nini, E.; Forestier, D.; Kwiatwoski, F.; Panisi, Y.; Chipponi, J. Methodological index for non-randomized studies (MINORS): Development and validation of a new imstrument. *ANZ J. Surg.* **2003**, *73*, 712–716. [CrossRef] [PubMed]
15. Figueroa, N.P.F.; Acosta, H.F.M.; Espinoza, M.E.N.; Higuera, N.A.S.; Partida, E.A.B.; Espinoza, M.A.I. Evaluación de factores de riesgo maternos y ambientales asociados a labio y paladar hendidos durante el primer trimestre de embarazo. *Rev. Mex. Cir. Bucal Maxilofac.* **2016**, *12*, 93–98.

16. Angulo-Castro, E.; Acosta-Alfaro, L.F.; Guadron-Llanos, A.M.; Canizalez-Román, A.; Gonzalez-Ibarra, F.; Osuna-Ramírez, I.; Murillo-Llanes, J. Maternal Risk Factors Associated with the Development of Cleft Lip and Cleft Palate in Mexico: A Case-Control Study. *Iran. J. Otorhinolaryngol.* **2017**, *29*, 189–195. [CrossRef] [PubMed]
17. Gasca-Sanchez, F.M.; Santos-Guzman, J.; Elizondo-Dueñaz, R.; Mejia-Velazquez, G.M.; Ruiz-Pacheco, C.; Reyes-Rodriguez, D.; Vazquez-Camacho, E.; Hernandez-Hernandez, J.A.; Lopez-Sanchez, R.d.C.; Ortiz-Lopez, R.; et al. Spatial Clusters of Children with Cleft Lip and Palate and Their Association with Polluted Zones in the Monterrey Metropolitan Area. *Int. J. Environ. Res. Public Health* **2019**, *12*, 2488. [CrossRef]
18. Corona-Rivera, J.R.; Bobadilla-Morales, L.; Corona-Rivera, A.; Peña-Padilla, C.; Olvera-Molina, S.; Orozco-Martín, M.A.; García-Cruz, D.; Ríos-Flores, I.M.; Gómez-Rodríguez, B.G.; Rivas-Soto, G.; et al. Prevalence of orofacial clefts and risks for non-syndromic cleft lip with or without cleft palate in newborns at a university hospital from West Mexico. *Congenit. Anom.* **2018**, *58*, 117–123. [CrossRef] [PubMed]
19. Ceceña-Mateos, O.A.; Robles-Cervantes, J.A.; Ledezma-Rodríguez, J.C.; González-Gutiérrez, H.O.; Gómez-Díaz, A.E.; Ledezma-Gómez, V. Relación de variables demográficas y presencia de labio y paladar hendido en pacientes atendidos en el Instituto Jalisciense de Cirugía Reconstructiva Dr. José Guerrero Santos. *Cir. Plástica* **2021**, *31*, 56–61. [CrossRef]
20. Pons-Bonals, A.; Pons-Bonals, L.; Hidalgo-Martínez, S.M.; Sosa-Ferreyra, C.F. Estudio clínico-epidemiológico en niños con labio paladar hendido en un hospital de segundo nivel. *Bol. Med. Hosp. Infant. Mex.* **2017**, *74*, 107–121. [CrossRef] [PubMed]
21. Ibarra-Lopez, J.J.; Duarte, P.; Antonio-Vejar, V.; Calderon-Aranda, E.S.; Huerta-Beristain, G.; Flores-Alfaro, E.; Moreno-Godinez, M.E. Maternal C677T MTHFR polymorphism and environmental factors are associated with cleft lip and palate in a Mexican population. *J. Investig. Med.* **2013**, *61*, 1030–1035. [CrossRef]
22. Acuña-González, G.; Medina-Solís, C.E.; Maupomé, G.; Escoffie-Ramírez, M.; Hernández-Romano, J.; Márquez-Corona Mde, L.; Islas-Márquez, A.J.; Villalobos-Rodelo, J.J. Family history and socioeconomic risk factors for non-syndromic cleft lip and palate: A matched case-control study in a less developed country. *Biomedica* **2011**, *31*, 381–391. [CrossRef]
23. Vargas-Zacatenco, G.; Hernández-Trejo, N.G.; Cabrera-Serrano, M.S.; Gutierrez-Brito, M. Prevalencia de factores de riesgo asociados a la presencia de fisuras labiales y palatinas en pacientes que acudieron al Hospital para el Niño Poblano, en el periodo de enero de 2018 a diciembre de 2019. *Oral* **2022**, *23*, 2050–2056.
24. González, B.S.; López, M.L.; Rico, M.A.; Garduño, F. Oral clefts: A retrospective study of prevalence and predisposal factors in the State of Mexico. *J. Oral Sci.* **2008**, *50*, 123–129. [CrossRef] [PubMed]
25. Mejía, A.C.; Suárez, D.E. Factores de riesgo materno predominantes asociados con labio leporino y paladar hendido en los recién nacidos. *Arch. Investig. Matern. Infant.* **2012**, *4*, 55–62.
26. Mejía, G.G.; Hidalgo, H.O.M.; Arizmendi, L.J.D.; Cruz, E.C. Estudio epidemiológico de pacientes con labio y paladar fisurado en dos centros especializados. *Rev. Odont. Mex.* **2020**, *24*, 268–275.
27. Acosta, M.R.; Montes, D.P.; Flores Mesa, B.; Mónica, D.; Rangel, A. Frecuencia y factores de riesgo en labio y paladar hendidos del Centro Médico Nacional «La Raza». *Rev. Mex. Cir. Bucal Maxilofac.* **2013**, *9*, 109–112.
28. Estandia-Ortega, B.; Velázquez-Aragón, J.A.; Alcántara-Ortigoza, M.A.; Reyna-Fabian, M.E.; Villagómez-Martínez, S.; González-del Angel, A. 5,10Methylenetetrahydrofolate reductase single nucleotide polymorphisms and gene-environment interaction analysis in non-syndromic cleft lip/palate. *Eur. J. Oral Sci.* **2014**, *122*, 109–113. [CrossRef] [PubMed]
29. Pérez-González, A.; Lavielle-Sotomayor, P.; Clark, P.; Tusie-Luna, M.T.; Palafox, D. Factores de riesgo en pacientes con fisura de labio y paladar en México. Estudio en 209 pacientes. *Cir. Plást. Iberolatinoam.* **2021**, *47*, 389–394.
30. Pérez-González, A.; Lavielle-Sotomayor, P.; López-Rodríguez, L.; Pérez-Días, M.E.; Vega-Hernández, D.; Domínguez, J.N.; Clark, P. Characterization of 554 Mexican Patients With Nonsyndromic Cleft Lip and Palate: Descriptive Study. *J. Craniofac. Surg.* **2023**, *34*, 1776–1779. [CrossRef] [PubMed]
31. González-Osorio, C.A.; Medina-Solís, C.E.; Pontigo-Loyola, A.P.; Casanova-Rosado, J.F.; Escoffié-Ramírez, M.; Corona-Tabares, M.G.; Maupomé, G. Estudio ecológico en México (2003–2009) sobre labio y/o paladar hendido y factores sociodemográficos, socioeconómicos y de contaminacion asociados. *An. Pediatría* **2011**, *74*, 377–387. [CrossRef]
32. Cerón-Zamora, F.; Scougall Vichis, R.J.; Contreras-Bulnes, R.; González-López, B.S.; Vera-Hernández, M.A.; Lucas-Rincón, S.E.; Escoffié-Ramírez, M.; Medina-Solis, C. Trends in cleft lip and/or palate prevalence at birth in Mexico. A national (ecological) study between 2003 and 2019. *Cleft Palate Craniofac. J.* **2023**, *60*, 1353–1358. [CrossRef]
33. Donkin, I.; Barrès, R. Sperm epigenetics and influence of environmental factors. *Mol. Metab.* **2018**, *14*, 1–11. [CrossRef] [PubMed]
34. Nguyen, R.H.; Wilcox, A.J.; Moen, B.E.; McConnaughey, D.R.; Lie, R.T. Parent.s occupation and isolated orofacial clefts in Norway: A population-based case-control study. *Ann. Epidemiol.* **2007**, *17*, 763–771. [CrossRef] [PubMed]
35. Bille, C.; Skytthe, A.; Vach, W.; Knudsen, L.B.; Andersen, A.M.N.; Murray, J.C.; Christensen, K. Parent's age and the risk of oral clefts. *Epidemiology* **2005**, *16*, 311–316. [CrossRef] [PubMed]
36. James, O.; Erinoso, O.A.; Ogunlewe, A.O.; Adeyemo, W.L.; Ladeinde, A.L.; Ogunlewe, M.O. Parental Age and the Risk of Cleft Lip and Palate in a Nigerian Population—A Case-Control Study. *Ann. Maxillofac. Surg.* **2020**, *10*, 429–433. [CrossRef] [PubMed]
37. Jugessur, A.; Wilcox, A.J.; Lie, R.T.; Murray, J.C.; Taylor, J.A.; Ulvik, A.; Drevon, C.A.; Vindenes, H.A.; Abyholm, F.E. Exploring the effects of methylenetetrahydrofolate reductase gene variants C677T and A1298C on the risk of orofacial clefts in 261 Norwegian case-parent triads. *Am. J. Epidemiol.* **2003**, *157*, 1083–1091. [CrossRef]

38. Chevrier, C.; Perret, C.; Bahuau, M.; Zhu, H.; Nelva, A.; Herman, C.; Francannet, C.; Robert-Gnansia, E.; Finnell, R.H.; Cordier, S. Fetal and maternal MTHFR C677T genotype, maternal folate intake and the risk of nonsyndromic oral clefts. *Am. J. Med. Genet. A* **2007**, *143A*, 248–257. [CrossRef]
39. Garland, M.A.; Reynolds, K.; Zhou, C.J. Environmental mechanisms of orofacial clefts. *Birth Defects Res.* **2020**, *112*, 1660–1698. [CrossRef]

Disclaimer/Publisher's Note: The statements, opinions and data contained in all publications are solely those of the individual author(s) and contributor(s) and not of MDPI and/or the editor(s). MDPI and/or the editor(s) disclaim responsibility for any injury to people or property resulting from any ideas, methods, instructions or products referred to in the content.

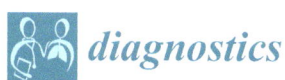

Systematic Review

Oral Health-Related Quality of Life in Temporomandibular Disorder Patients and Healthy Subjects—A Systematic Review and Meta-Analysis

Lujain AlSahman [1,*], Hamad AlBagieh [1] and Roba AlSahman [2]

[1] Oral Medicine and Diagnostic Sciences Department, College of Dentistry, King Saud University Riyadh, Riyadh 57448, Saudi Arabia
[2] Faculty of Dentistry, Royal College of Surgeons, D02 YN77 Dublin, Ireland
* Correspondence: 442203369@student.ksu.edu.sa

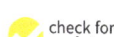

Citation: AlSahman, L.; AlBagieh, H.; AlSahman, R. Oral Health-Related Quality of Life in Temporomandibular Disorder Patients and Healthy Subjects—A Systematic Review and Meta-Analysis. *Diagnostics* 2024, *14*, 2183. https://doi.org/10.3390/diagnostics14192183

Academic Editor: Daniel Fried

Received: 28 July 2024
Revised: 10 September 2024
Accepted: 14 September 2024
Published: 30 September 2024

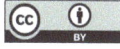

Copyright: © 2024 by the authors. Licensee MDPI, Basel, Switzerland. This article is an open access article distributed under the terms and conditions of the Creative Commons Attribution (CC BY) license (https://creativecommons.org/licenses/by/4.0/).

Abstract: (1) Background: Temporomandibular disorders (TMD) signs and symptoms affect the quality of life of patients because they impose an incapacity to participate in daily life activities, causing both physical and psychological discomfort. This review aims to provide the most accurate, comprehensive, and up-to-date description of all information available regarding OHRQoL in TMD. (2) Methods: A systematic search of articles from January 2013 till August 2023 was performed on five databases to identify articles, including TMD and oral health-related quality of life. Two calibrated reviewers performed the search following inclusion and exclusion criteria. A manual search of reference articles was also performed. The data were analyzed qualitatively by combining a meta-analysis and GRADE evidence. The Newcastle–Ottawa scale for cross-sectional and case-control studies was utilized to assess the quality of the included studies. (3) Results: The initial search consisted of 738 articles without the removal of duplicates. Fifteen articles were included in this systematic review, and ten were included in the meta-analysis. Almost all the included observational studies reported poor OHRQoL among patients with different types of TMD. The results of the meta-analysis with a standard mean difference (SMD) and that included seven studies suggest high heterogeneity with I^2 = 99%, SMD (95% CI) = 3.18 (1.90, 4.46), p-value < 0.01. The odds ratio analyzed for three included articles in the meta-analysis reported statistical significance (p-value < 0.01) with OR = 8.21 (2.39, 28.25) and a heterogeneity of 86%. The certainty of evidence by GRADE resulted in a downgraded level of evidence, indicating that the OHRQoL of TMD patients may differ slightly from the healthy controls. (4) Conclusions: The impact of OHRQoL on the TMD was deemed to be significant. Overall, the OHRQoL is low for any type and intensity of pain among TMD patients and controls.

Keywords: oral health-related quality of life; temporomandibular disorders; meta-analysis; GRADE analysis

1. Introduction

Temporomandibular disorders (TMD) is a group of musculoskeletal disorders that affect the masticatory muscles, the temporomandibular joint (TMJ), and the related structure according to the American academy of orofacial pain [1]. The common signs and symptoms of TMD include muscular and/or articular pain, joint stiffness, clicking, asymmetric joint movements, and limited mouth opening. Additionally, patients with sleep disorders are more predisposed to TMD signs and symptoms, increasing the psychological issues of the patients [2,3]. Due to physical and psychological discomfort, patients with TMDs show poor oral health-related quality of life [4]. The World Health Organization (WHO) defined oral health-related quality of life (OHRQoL) as an individual's perception of oral health and how it impacts their overall well-being, daily functioning, and quality of life [5]. Measuring OHRQoL is not limited to diagnosing oral diseases and considers the perspective of a person on their subjective experience, including their ability to eat, speak, and socialize without discomfort or embarrassment [6]. Previous models on oral health-related quality of life were directly associated with oral conditions and quality of life [7]. While the present models are designed to connect a person's mind and overall health as a single unit and concentrate on socioenvironmental factors along with oral diseases. OHRQoL questionnaires consider how oral health conditions can affect a person's physical, psychological, and social well-being [8]. This concept recognizes that oral health is an integral part of general health and that improving oral health can positively impact a person's overall quality of life. This approach ultimately helps policymakers and investors plan strategies in favor of oral health and improving the well-being of an individual. In an observational study by Almoznino et al., reduced OHRQoL was reported in patients with TMD compared to healthy adults [9]. Similarly, in a systematic review of clinical studies by Dahlstrom and Carlsson (2010), all included studies measured reduced general quality of life in patients with TMD than the controls [10]. The advancement of research that focuses on the relationship between oral health-related quality of life and various prevalent oral diseases is crucial for effectively allocating public and private financial companies to address urgent and impactful healthcare needs guided by the principle of equitable care [11]. Recent studies have explored the association between temporomandibular disorders (TMD) and quality of life, but these studies exhibit varying methodologies and reported diverse outcomes concerning both quality of life and a TMD diagnosis [10,12–14]. A systematic review indicated that TMD patients experience a lower quality of life than non-TMD individuals [15]. However, this review did not provide specific data for TMD diagnostic groups categorized under the Research Diagnostic Criteria for Temporomandibular Disorders (RDC/TMD) axis I, such as muscle disorders (group I), disc displacements (group II), and joint dysfunction (group III). Introduced in 1992, the RDC/TMD became a standard tool in TMD research until the development of the Diagnostic Criteria for Temporomandibular Disorders (DC/TMD), which, as an enhanced version, has since become the more reliable tool. The DC/TMD provides clinicians with evidence-based criteria for assessing patients and improving communication about consultations, referrals, and prognoses. The importance of these criteria relay on providing a comprehensive framework for assessing TMD, and both clinicians and researchers can identify and classify the type and severity of TMD accurately [16].

Moreover, none of these reviews also conduct a meta-analysis and GRADE evidence [15]. Moreover, all the reviews examined the overall quality of life and its association with TMD [10,15]. Therefore, this systematic review and meta-analysis with GRADE evidence focuses on the observational studies on TMD and oral health-related quality of life utilizing validated diagnostic tools. Hence, the aim of this prospective systematic review and meta-analysis is to compare the oral health-related quality of life between the patients with TMDs and healthy controls in observational settings that have utilized one of the diagnostic criteria (RDC/TMD and\or DC/TMD) and a valid questionnaire to measure OHRQoL. Moreover, the aim is to present the most up-to-date and comprehensive overview of all the data on TMD and oral health-related quality of life.

2. Materials and Methods

The present systematic review and meta-analysis followed the PRISMA guidelines (preferred systematic review and meta-analysis guideline) [17]. The research protocol was designed prior to the commencement of the study, and the protocol was registered in the PROSPERO database under registration number CRD42023417542.

2.1. Research Question

This review aimed to answer the research question: "Is there a difference in oral health-related quality of life in individuals with (Group 1 DC/TMD) compared to healthy adults?" The PECOT strategy followed was (P) 18–60-year-old patients with TMD; (E) diagnosis of TMD evaluated by RDC/TMD or DC/TMD; (C) individuals without any TMDs;

(O) outcome measured with OHRQoL; and (T) observational studies (cross-sectional and case-control).

2.2. Inclusion and Exclusion Criteria

Inclusion criteria were as follows: (a) the study had to be observational (cross-sectional and case-control studies) and involve subjects aged 18 to 60 years, (b) the diagnostic criteria for temporomandibular disorders had to be the RDC/TMD or the DC/TMD (both axis I and axis II), and (c) standard questionnaires measuring the quality of life (OHIP-14 or OHIP-49) had to be used. The studies must have been published in peer-reviewed journals since January 2013 and be in English.

The exclusion criteria were as follows: (a) studies that did not focus on TMD and myofascial pain as the primary disease or outcome (b) studies involving patients who had undergone previous TMD treatments (such as oral splints, medication, joint replacement, etc.), (c) studies involving patients with a history of facial trauma or rheumatic diseases, and (d) studies that did not use standard research diagnostic questionnaires for TMD and/or quality of life assessments. Review articles, letters to editors, and interventional studies like RCTs were excluded.

2.3. Search Strategy

A systematic search was conducted on five databases, PubMed/MEDLINE, Cochrane, Embase, Scopus, and Web of Science, from January 2013 to August 2023. The database searches commenced on 5 October 2023. The title and abstract searches used general search terms with Medical Subject Headings (MeSH) from PubMed and MEDLINE. These terms and descriptors are listed in Table 1 alongside the articles extracted from various databases. Boolean operators 'AND' and 'OR' were employed to refine and broaden the search scope.

Additionally, two investigators conducted reference chasing and manual searches of articles. The reference lists in the bibliographies of the identified articles were also reviewed. Two investigators independently screened the titles and abstracts of all the papers from the initial search. Any disagreements between these two authors were resolved through the consensus of a third reviewer.

2.4. Data Extraction and Study Selection

The articles from the databases were organized using EndNote 21 (Thomson Reuters®, New York, NY, USA), and duplicates were removed. The article screening and selection process consisted of two stages, each conducted by two independent investigators: (a) the first stage involved reading and evaluating the titles and abstracts, and (b) the second stage involved reading the full-text articles and reaching a consensus. A third investigator was consulted in any disagreement, and their decision was considered final. The articles that were excluded during the full-text reading stage and the reasons for exclusion are listed in Table S1. For articles without the full text or that were missing information, attempts were made to contact the authors. In cases where no reply was obtained from the authors, the articles were purchased.

For data extraction, a customized Excel (Microsoft Office 365, Redmond, WA, USA) worksheet was created based on the "Cochrane Handbook for Systematic Review and Meta-analysis" following STROBE guidelines for cross-sectional and case-control studies by two investigators [18,19].

Based on recommendations following the guidelines, the information extracted from the articles were as follows: (1) Authors/Country/Year; (2) study design; (3) age range of participants and gender; (4) the number of patients and controls; (5) diagnostic criteria for TMD; (6) instrument utilized for measuring oral health-related quality of life; (7) data collection method; and (8) outcome of the study (comparison with control and effect on OHRQoL).

Table 1. MesH terms utilized in various databases.

Databases Searched	MesH Terms	Articles Found
PubMed	"Temporomandibular disorders [MeSH Terms] OR Temporomandibular Joint Disorders OR TMD" [MesH Terms] OR "temporomandibular joint disorder" [All Fields] OR "temporomandibular joint disease" [All Fields] OR "temporomandibular joint diseases" [All Fields] OR "temporomandibular joint dysfunction syndrome" [MeSH Terms] OR "temporomandibular joint dysfunction syndrome" [All Fields] OR "temporomandibular joint syndromes" [All Fields] OR "tmj disease" [All Fields] OR "tmd" [All Fields] OR "tmj" [All Fields] OR "tmjd" [All Fields] OR "tmj disorders" [All Fields] OR "tmj disorder" [All Fields] OR "tmj diseases" [All Fields] AND "orofacial pain" [Mesh term] OR "craniofacial pain [MesH term]" AND "Oral health [MeSH Terms] OR Oral Health OR Oral Health-Related Quality of Life [All Fields] OR OHRQoL [All Fields] OR Oral Health-Related Quality of Life [Mesh Terms] OR OHRQoL [MesH terms]	Initial search 205 Abstract and Title 26
Scopus	TITLE-ABS-KEY (temporomandibular disorders OR temporomandibular joint disorders OR TMD) AND (oral health-related quality of life OR oral health OR OHRQoL) AND (orofacial pain OR craniofacial pain)	Initial search 145
Web of science	(TS = ("temporomandibular joint disorder" OR "temporomandibular joint disorders" OR "temporomandibular dysfunctions" OR "temporomandibular joint syndrome" OR "tmj disease" OR tmjd OR "tmj disorder" OR "tmj diseases" OR "temporomandibular joint dysfunction syndrome") AND TI = ("oral health related quality of life" OR "OHRQoL")) AND TI = ("orofacial pain" OR "craniofacial pain") AND DOCUMENT TYPES: (Article)	Initial search 189
EMBASE	#1 = ('temporomandibular joint disorders':ta,ab OR 'tmj disorder':ta,ab OR 'temporomandibular joint disease':ta,ab 'temporomandibular joint dysfunction syncrome':ta,ab) #2 = ('oral health related quality of life':ta,ab OR 'OHRQoL':ta,ab) #3 = ('orofacial Pain' OR craniafacial pain') AND #4 = ([article]/lim) #5 = #1 AND #2 AND #3 AND #4	Total articles: 160
Cochrane	(TS = ("temporomandibular joint disorder" OR "temporomandibular joint disorders" OR "temporomandibular dysfunctions" OR "temporomandibular joint syndrome" OR "tmj disease" OR tmjd OR "tmj disorder" OR "tmj diseases" OR "temporomandibular joint dysfunction syndrome") AND TI = ("oral health related quality of life" OR "OHRQoL")) AND TI = ("orofacial pain" OR "craniofacial pain") AND DOCUMENT TYPES: (Article)	Total articles: 39 Abstract and title: 2

2.5. Risk of Bias and Data Analysis

The quality of articles included in this review was measured by the New Castle Ottawa (NOS) scale. This scale is based on the star system used to classify observational studies. A single star is assigned to measure the quality of specific items, providing a maximum score of seven. The NOS system for case-control study has three main domains: (a) selection of cases and control; (b) compatibility between the group; and (c) exposure and outcome variables of the study [20]. For cross-sectional studies, the major domains are (a) case selection (representativeness of cases, sample size, and surveillance tools), (b) compatibility, and (c) outcome (assessment of the outcome and statistical tests) [21]. Concerning data analysis, results were combined in a meta-analysis by graphical presentation with the forest plot. Only studies presenting sufficient data (sample of cases and control; mean and standard deviations for TMD patients and controls) were included. Articles without a control group that was not divided by the group of TMD were excluded from the meta-analysis. Ten articles were included for meta-analysis and I^2 measured heterogeneity.

2.6. Certainty of Evidence (GRADE Analysis)

The evidence for comparison of included studies was evaluated with the grading of recommendation, assessment, development, and evaluation tool (GRADE tool, available online at gradepro.org). The GRADE evidence was assessed using each effect generated by comparison of all included studies. For all included studies, the certainty of the evidence was rated down if there was a problem due to the risk of bias, indirectness, inconsistency, imprecision, and publication bias. Also, evidence was rated if the study design was proper and the outcome measured was consistent [22].

3. Results

A total of 738 studies were initially retrieved from various databases and synchronized in Endnote 21 (Clarivate, NY, USA). Among these, 378 studies were removed due to duplication and 228 due to other reasons (irrelevant study, letter to editors, etc.). The remaining 132 records underwent screening based on title and abstract, resulting in the removal of 74 studies (Figure 1). Subsequently, 58 articles were selected for full-text retrieval, but 2 could not be retrieved. Finally, 56 articles were considered for full-text reading, and 41 were excluded for various reasons (Table S1). Ultimately, 15 articles were included in this systematic review, with 10 were eligible for the meta-analysis.

3.1. Characteristics of Included Studies

Table 2 illustrates the summary and characteristics of the included 15 studies. Of all studies, eight were case-control [9,23–29], and seven were cross-sectional studies [2,30–35] reporting the OHRQoL of TMD patients; the oldest study was from 2013 [26,34]. A total of 4821 participants (cases 3945; control 1943) were included in this systematic review. All the included studies evaluated patients with TMD in hospital settings, and none were population based. The RDC/TMD axis I was applied in 11 studies [2,23,25,26,29–35], while DC/TMD with axes I and II were applied in 4 studies [9,24,28,36]. Four case-control studies utilized RDC/TMD analysis for all the cases [23,25,26,29], while three studies utilized DC/TMD [24,28,36], and one study utilized both RDC/TMD and DC/TMD for a diagnosis of TMD in the cases and controls [9]. Regarding the questionnaire measuring oral health-related quality of life, 13 studies utilized the oral health impact profile (OHIP)-14, and one study utilized OHIP-49 and the World Health Organization Quality of Life (WHOQOL) [34].

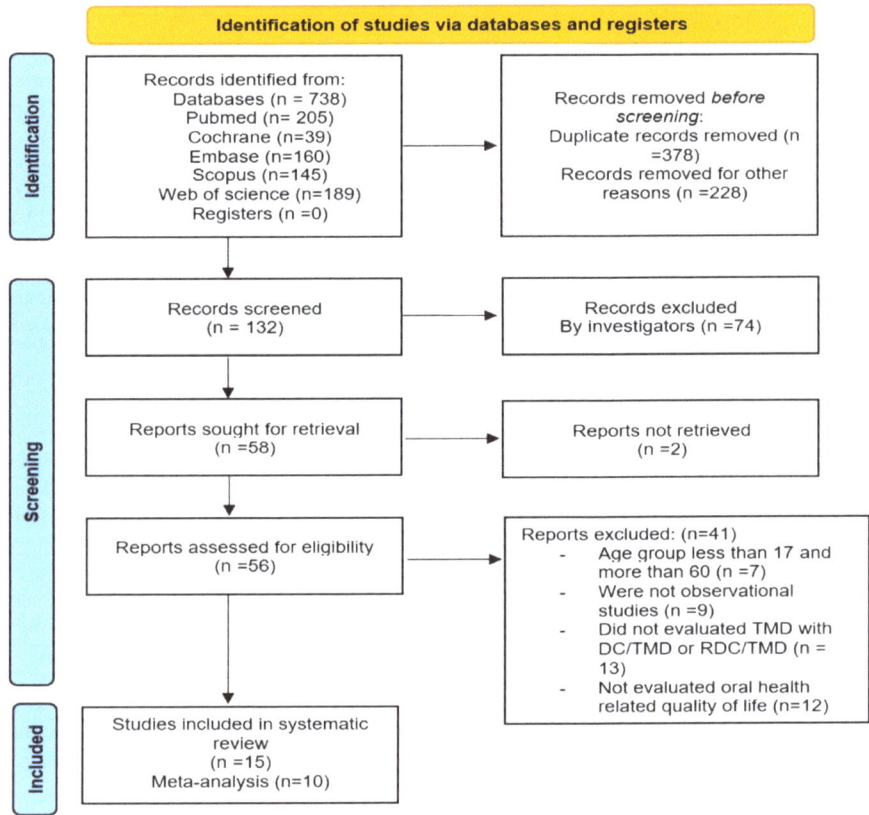

Figure 1. PRISMA flow chart for included studies.

Based on Table 2, the included participants were in the age group of 18–60 years, confirming that the data from all the included studies were from young and middle-aged individuals from both genders.

3.2. Oral Health-Related Quality of Life

All the included studies showed that TMD patients had worse oral health-related quality of life than healthy controls. Some studies have reported a direct relationship between the intensity of pain related to TMD and a worsened OHRQoL [28,34–36]. Coherently, two included articles on myofascial pain and TMD reported a worse OHRQoL of patients with severe pain compared to controls [34,35]. Additionally, two included cross-sectional studies have indicated that group I (with myofascial pain) and group III (with osteoarthritis) analyzed by RDC/TMD axis I had a worse OHRQoL compared to group II (with disc displacement) [33,34].

Table 2. Characteristics of included studies.

Study No.	Author/Year/ Country	Study Design	Number of Participants (Cases and Control)	Age (AR) and Gender	Case Selection Method	Control Selection Method	Diagnostic Criteria for TMD	Measurement of Oral Heath-Related Quality of Life	Method for Data Collection	Results/Conclusion
1	Celik et al., 2022 [24] Turkey	Case-Control Study	n = 200 (Case = 150; Control = 50)	AR = 18–60 years (F = 121; M = 79)	Patient seeking treatment for TMD	Not specified	DC/TMD for all cases	OHIP-14	Questionnaire	OHIP score was higher in patients with disc displacement and TMD-related pain compared to healthy controls
2	Pawar et al., 2022 [33] India	Cross-sectional comparitive study	n = 320 (Cases = 160; Control = 161)	AR = 18–60 years (F = 168; M = 152)	Patient seeking treatment for TMD (divided in three groups; G1 = myofacial pain, G2 = disc displacement, G3 = osteoarthritis	Patient seeking dental treatment for other reasons	RDC/TMD axis I and II for all the cases	OHIP-14	Questionnaire	Poor OHRQoL was reported in TMD patients compared to healthy controls
3	Ujin Yap et al., 2021 [28] China	Case-Control Study	n = 961 (Cases = 816; Control = 147)	AR = 18–40 years (F = 761; M = 200)	Not specified	Not specified	DC/TMD-SQ axis I for all cases	OHIP-14	Questionnaire	OHRQoL is affected by different types of TMD symptoms. Individuals having more and pain-related TMD symptoms with/without intra-articular features generally had greater OHRQoL impairments.
4	Ujin Yap et al., 2021 [36] China	Case-Control Study	n = 961 (Cases = 845; Control = 116;)	AR = 18–40 years (F = 761; M = 200)	Patient visted oral and maxillofacial clinics	Patients visited in prosthetic dental clinics	DC/TMD axis II for all the cases	OHIP-14	Questionnaire	Correlations between TMD severity OHRQoL were moderately strong to strong (rs = 0.42–0.72)
5	Filho et al., 2020 [25] Brazil	Case-Control Study	n = 765 (Cases = 153; Control = 612	AR = 18–25 years (F = 765)	Not specified	Not specified	RDC/TMD axis II for all the cases	OHIP-14	Questionnaire	Women with negative OHRQoL reports symptoms of TMD
6	Yildirim et al., 2020 [29] Turkey	Case-Control Study	n = 315 (Cases = 172; Controls = 143)	AR = 18–60 years (F = 192; M = 123)	Not specified	Not specified	RDC/TMD axis I and II for all the cases	OHIP-14 questionnaire	Questionnaire	Bruxers with TMD had poorer OHRQoL than those without TMD

Table 2. Cont.

Study No.	Author/Year/ Country	Study Design	Number of Participants (Cases and Control)	Age (AR) and Gender	Case Selection Method	Control Selection Method	Diagnostic Criteria for TMD	Measurement of Oral Heath-Related Quality of Life	Method for Data Collection	Results/Conclusion
7	Bayat et al., 2017 [23] Iran	Case-Control Study	n = 150 (Cases = 75; control = 75)	AR = 30–50 years (F = 119; M = 31)	Patient seeking treatment at clinic	Patients coming for follow-up of any dental treatment	RDC/TMD axis I and II for all the cases	OHIP-14	Interview	The TMD group had a worse quality of life than controls. The prevalence and severity of OHIP was 6 and 2 times higher, respectively, in the TMD group.
8	Balik et al., 2017 [30] Turkey	Cross-sectional study	n = 104 (Case and Control = not specified)	AR = 32–59 years (F = 64; M = 40)	Not specified	Not specified	RDC/TMD axis I and II for all the cases	OHIP-14	Questionnaire	OHIP score was higher in patients with disc displacement and TMD-related pain
9	Su et al., 2016 [35] China	Cross-sectional	n = 541 (Case and Control = not specified)	AR = 25–48 years (M = 134; F = 407)	Patient seeking treatment at clinic	Not specified	RDC/TMD axis I for all the cases	OHIP-14	Interview	OHIP score was worst in patients with muscular pain.
10	Almoznino et al. 2015, [9] Israel	Case-Control Study	n = 387 (Cases = 187 and Controls = 200	AR = 20–30 years (F = 111; M = 76)	Patient seeking treatment at clinic	Patient seeking treatment at clinic	DC/TMD and RDC/TMD axis I in cases	OHIP-14	Interview	TMD group showed statistical differences for the OHIP as compared to controls.
11	Lemos et al., 2015 [32] Brazil	Cross-sectional	n = 135 (Case and Control = not specified)	AR = 18–25 years (F = 77; M = 58)	Dental students	Not specified	RDC/TMD axes I	OHIP-14	Questionnaire	Severity of TMD impaired the oral health-related quality of life
12	Blanco-Aguilera et al. 2014, [2] Spain	Cross-sectional	n = 407 (Case and Control = not specified)	AR = 18–60 years (F = 365; M = 42)	Sample of the population of the Public Health System	Not specified	RDC/TMD (did not report axis)	OHIP-14	Interview	OHIP showed a significant and positive association in patients with painful TMD
13	Gui et al., 2014 [31] Brazil	Cross-sectional	n = 116 (Case = 76 and control = 40)	AR = 25–50 years (F = 116)	Sample from hospital records	Sample from hospital records	RDC/TMD for all the cases	OHIP-14	Questionnaire	Quality of life is significantly impaired by widespread TMD pain compared to healthy control

Table 2. *Cont.*

Study No.	Author/Year/ Country	Study Design	Number of Participants (Cases and Control)	Age (AR) and Gender	Case Selection Method	Control Selection Method	Diagnostic Criteria for TMD	Measurement of Oral Heath-Related Quality of Life	Method for Data Collection	Results/Conclusion
14	Rener-Sitar et al. 2014, [26] Slovenia	Case-Control Study	$n = 481$ (Cases = 81 and Control = 400)	AR = 18–60 years (F = 365; M = 115)	Patients seeking treatment at the dental clinic	Random patients without TMD taking treatment at hospital	RDC/TMD axis I in all the cases	OHIP-49	Interview	TMD patients are highly associated with a lower OHRQoL.
15	Resende et al. 2013, [34] Brazil	Cross-Sectional	$n = 43$ (Cases = 43 divided in 3 groups G1 = 30; G2 = 9; G3 = 4)	AR = 30–45 years (F = 32; M = 11)	Patients seeking treatment at the dental clinic	Patients seeking treatment at the dental clinic	RDC-TMD axis I for cases	WHOQOL-BREF	Interview	Impaired oral health-related quality of life is recorded in patient with myofacial pain associated with TMD.

N = number of subjects; DC/TMD = diagnostic criteria for temporomandibular disorder; RDC/TMD = research diagnostic criteria for temporomandibular disorder; OHIP-14 = oral health impact factor-14; OHIP-49 = oral health impact factor-49, WHOQOL-BREF = World Health Organization quality of life-BREF.

3.3. Result from Meta-Analysis

Ten studies of fifteen were included in the meta-analysis due to high variability among the studies (Figures 2 and 3). The included studies in the meta-analysis were the ones with an explicit inclusion of participants, standard deviation, and mean per group and compared OHRQoL between TMD and control groups. Studies included in this systematic review without proper comparison between TMD and controls were excluded from the meta-analysis. Two articles with the subgroups were not included as it was impossible to have accurate data for various groups.

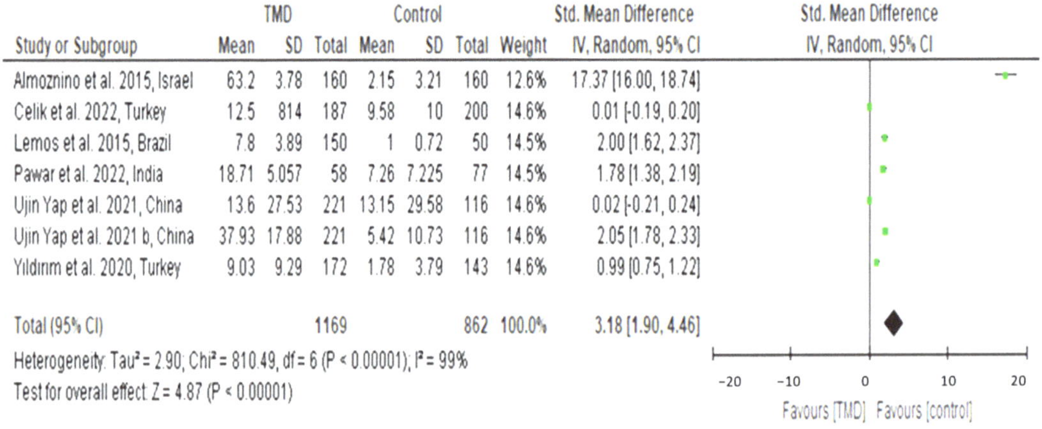

Study or Subgroup	TMD Mean	SD	Total	Control Mean	SD	Total	Weight	Std. Mean Difference IV, Random, 95% CI
Almoznino et al. 2015, Israel	63.2	3.78	160	2.15	3.21	160	12.6%	17.37 [16.00, 18.74]
Celik et al. 2022, Turkey	12.5	814	187	9.58	10	200	14.6%	0.01 [-0.19, 0.20]
Lemos et al. 2015, Brazil	7.8	3.89	150	1	0.72	50	14.5%	2.00 [1.62, 2.37]
Pawar et al. 2022, India	18.71	5.057	58	7.26	7.225	77	14.5%	1.78 [1.38, 2.19]
Ujin Yap et al. 2021, China	13.6	27.53	221	13.15	29.58	116	14.6%	0.02 [-0.21, 0.24]
Ujin Yap et al. 2021 b, China	37.93	17.88	221	5.42	10.73	116	14.6%	2.05 [1.78, 2.33]
Yıldırım et al. 2020, Turkey	9.03	9.29	172	1.78	3.79	143	14.6%	0.99 [0.75, 1.22]
Total (95% CI)			1169			862	100.0%	3.18 [1.90, 4.46]

Heterogeneity: Tau^2 = 2.90; Chi^2 = 810.49, df = 6 (P < 0.00001); I^2 = 99%
Test for overall effect: Z = 4.87 (P < 0.00001)

Favours [TMD] Favours [control]

Figure 2. Forest plot for calculating standarized mean for OHRQoL among TMD patients and controls [9,24,27,29,32,33,37]. *The green dots represent the **standardized mean differences (SMD)** for each study, with horizontal lines indicating the **95% confidence intervals (CI)**. Values left of the vertical line favor the TMD group, while those to the right favor the control group.*

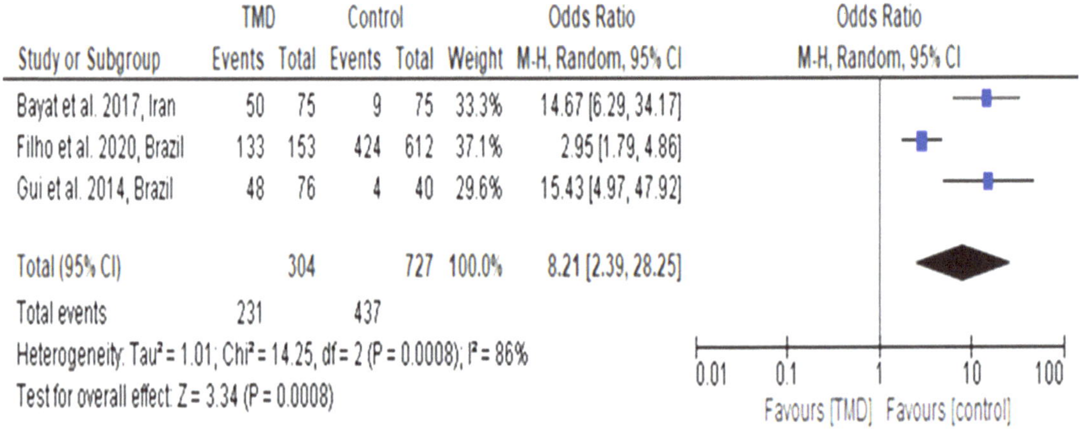

Study or Subgroup	TMD Events	Total	Control Events	Total	Weight	Odds Ratio M-H, Random, 95% CI
Bayat et al. 2017, Iran	50	75	9	75	33.3%	14.67 [6.29, 34.17]
Filho et al. 2020, Brazil	133	153	424	612	37.1%	2.95 [1.79, 4.86]
Gui et al. 2014, Brazil	48	76	4	40	29.6%	15.43 [4.97, 47.92]
Total (95% CI)		304		727	100.0%	8.21 [2.39, 28.25]
Total events	231		437			

Heterogeneity: Tau^2 = 1.01; Chi^2 = 14.25, df = 2 (P = 0.0008); I^2 = 86%
Test for overall effect: Z = 3.34 (P = 0.0008)

Favours [TMD] Favours [control]

Figure 3. Forest plot for calculating odds ratio for OHRQoL among TMD patients and controls [23,25,31]. The blue dot represents the pooled standardized mean difference (SMD) with its 95% confidence interval (CI) for the overall meta-analysis.

Figure 2 included seven articles that reported oral health-related quality of life in global TMD patients and controls. All the included studies utilized RDC/TMD (with axis I or II) for diagnosis and OHIP-14 for evaluating OHRQoL.

The meta-analysis result reported high significance among the OHRQoL of TMD patients compared to the controls. The results are as follows: total participants: 2031 subjects; the standard mean difference (95% CI): 3.18 (1.90, 4.46); heterogeneity I^2 99% and Z test: 4.87, with the $p < 0.01$.

In Figure 3, the results of three studies have been pooled to calculate the odds ratio for measuring the difference in the OHRQoL of TMD patients and controls. The results indicated $I^2 = 86\%$ and odds ratio = 8.21 (2.39, 28.25), which was found to be statistically significant ($p < 0.05$ and Z test = 3.34, respectively). Therefore, the findings of the meta-analysis indicate that patients with intense TMD pain had a worse OHRQoL compared to healthy adults.

3.4. Quality of Included Studies

Of the eight included case-control studies, four were of good quality, three were of moderate quality, and one was of poor quality on the NOS scale (Table 3). The studies lacked a proper diagnosis of TMD by utilizing RDC/TMD for controls, which caused hindrances in accurate diagnosis. Of the seven included in the cross-sectional study (Table 4), three were of good quality, two were of moderate and two poor quality on the NOS scale. The poor and moderate quality of the cross-sectional study was due to a comparison between the TMD group and control (most studies did not have controls) and an improper assessment of the findings.

3.5. GRADE Certainty of Evidence

The certainty of evidence among the included studies was low and downgraded, indicating imprecision, indirectness, inconsistency, and a high risk of bias (Table 5). The low level of the certainty of the evidence in this review indicates that the confidence in the effect estimate is limited, and the true effect may be substantially different from the estimate of the effect.

Table 3. Risk of bias using NOS tool for case-control studies [20].

Studies		Celik et al., 2022 [24] Turkey	Ujin Yap et al., 2021 [28] China	Ujin Yap et al., 2021 [36] China	Filho et al., 2020 [25] Brazil	Yıldırım et al., 2020 [29] Turkey	Bayat et al., 2017 [23] Iran	Almoznino et al., 2015 [9] Israel	Rener-Sitar et al., 2014 [26] Slovenia
Selection	Case definition adequate	*	*	*	*	*	*	*	*
	Representativeness of cases	*	*	*	*	*	*	*	*
	Selection of controls	*	*	*	*	*	*	*	*
	Definition of controls	*	–	*	–	*	*	–	*
Comparability		**	**	**	*	**	**	**	**
Exposure	Ascertainment of exposure	–	*	*	–	*	–	–	*
	Same method of ascertainment for case and control	–	–	–	–	–	–	–	–
	Nonresponse rate	–	*	*	*	–	–	*	–
Quality		Moderate	Good	Good	Poor	Good	Moderate	Moderate	Good

NOS tool for cross sectional study is represented by * where; 1. **Representativeness of the sample**: a. Truly representative of the average in the target population. * 2. **Sample size**: a. Justified and satisfactory (≥100 patients included). * 3. **Non-respondents**: a. The response rate is satisfactory (≥90% of patients have anti-Ro levels available). * 4. **Ascertainment of the exposure (risk factor)**: a. Validated measurement tool used and anti-Ro52 has been distinctly measured. ** b. Validated measurement tool used but no distinction is made between anti-SSA/Ro and anti-Ro52. * **comparability**: (Maximum 1 stars) (a) The study investigates potential confounders. * **Outcome**: (Maximum 3 stars) (1) **Assessment of the outcome**: (a) Independent blind assessment. ** (b) Record linkage. ** (c) Self report. * (2) **Statistical test**: (a) The statistical test used to analyze the data is clearly described and appropriate *.

Table 4. Risk of bias using NOS tool for cross-sectional study [21].

Studies		Pawar et al., 2022 [33] India	Balik et al., 2017 [30] Turkey	Su et al., 2016 [35] China	Lemos et al., 2015 [32] Brazil	Blanco-Aguilera et al., 2014 [2] Spain	Gui et al., 2014 [31] Brazil	Resende et al., 2013 [34] Brazil
Selection	Representativeness of sample	*	*	*	*	*	*	*
	Sample size	*	*	*	*	*	*	*
	Nonrespondent	—	—	*	*	*	*	*
	Uncertainty of exposure	—	—	—	—	—	*	*
Comparability		**	—	*	—	—	**	**
Outcome	Assessment of outcome	*	*	*	*	*	*	*
	Statistical tests	*	*	*	*	*	*	*
Quality		Moderate	Poor	Good	Moderate	Poor	Good	Good

The NOS tool is represented by stars (*) as follows: **Representativeness of the Sample:** (*): Truly representative of the target population (all subjects or random sampling). (*): Somewhat representative of the target group (non-random sampling). (0 stars): Selected group of users/convenience sample. (0 stars): No description of the derivation of included subjects. **Sample Size:** (*): Justified and satisfactory (≥100 patients included). (0 stars): Not justified (<100 patients included). **Non-respondents:** (*): Response rate is satisfactory ≥90% of patients have anti-Ro levels available). (0 stars): Response rate is unsatisfactory (<90% of patients have anti-Ro levels available). **Ascertainment of the Exposure (Risk Factor):** (**): Validated measurement tool used and anti-Ro52 distinctly measured. (*): Validated measurement tool used but no distinction made between anti-SSA/Rc and anti-Ro52. (0 stars): Measurement methods not described. **Comparability:** (Maximum 2 stars) (*): The study investigates potential confounders through subgroup analysis or multivariable analysis. (0 stars): The study does not investigate potential confounders. **Outcome:** (Maximum 3 stars) **Assessment of the Outcome:** (**): Independent blind assessment. (**): Record linkage. (*): Self-report. (0 stars): No description. **Statistical Test:** (*): The statistical test used is clearly described and appropriate. (0 stars): The statistical test is not appropriate, not described, or incomplete.

Table 5. Certainty of evidence (GRADE) (https://gdt.gradepro.org/app/#project) (accessed on 5 October 2023).

Outcomes	№ of Participants (Studies) Follow-Up	Certainty of the Evidence (GRADE)	Relative Effect (95% CI)	Anticipated Absolute Effects	
				Risk with Healthy Control	Risk Difference with Temporomandibular Disorder Patients
TMD and Myofascial pain and oral health-related quality of life (TMD) assessed with: Relative risk timing of exposure: mean 6 months	3945 cases 1943 controls (7 observational studies)	Low [a,b]	RR 3.18 (1.90 to 4.46)	Low	
				520 per 1000	1134 more per 1000 (468 more to 1799 more)
				Study population	
				307 per 1000	477 more per 1000 (358 more to 619 more)
TMD and Myofascial pain and oral health-related quality of life assessed with odds ratio follow-up: mean 6 months	304 cases 727 controls/exposed 304/991 unexposed (3 observational studies)	Low	OR 8.21 (2.39 to 28.25)	Low	
				307 per 1000	477 more per 1000 (358 more to 619 more)

The risk in the intervention group (and its 95% confidence interval) is based on the assumed risk in the comparison group and the **relative effect** of the intervention (and its 95% CI). **CI:** confidence interval; **OR:** odds ratio; **RR:** risk ratio. Moderate certainty: moderately confident in the effect estimate: the true effect is likely to be close to the estimate of the effect, but there is a possibility that it is substantially different. Low certainty: confidence in the effect estimate is limited: the true effect may be substantially different from the estimate of the effect. Very low certainty: very little confidence in the effect estimates: the true effect is likely to be substantially different from the estimate of effect. [a]: inconsistency in findings due to high heterogeneity related to study designs and recruitment of participants. [b]: impression in findings was high due to high effect size and lower confidence interval.

4. Discussion

This systematic review and meta-analysis aimed to compare the perception of oral health-related quality of life in patients with and without TMD. The included studies used RCD/TMD and/or DC/TMD and validated questionnaires for diagnosing the condition. Based on the analysis of this systematic review and meta-analysis with GRADE evidence, it was observed that oral health-related quality of life is worse for the patients suffering from TMD compared to the control group. Moreover, the patients diagnosed on RDC/TMD axis I with myofascial pain and osteoarthritis had a worse oral health-related quality of life than patients with disc displacement. Additionally, there was a direct relationship between the intensity of pain and a worse oral health-related quality of life.

Most articles included in this systematic review utilized RDC/TMD axis I for diagnosing TMD. However, RDC/TMD axis II has not been applied in several studies [24,27,36]. This is paramount when the study evaluates the OHRQoL, as axis II is used to diagnose the psychological factors associated with TMD (stress, anxiety, depression, and somatization). In the literature, it is mentioned that TMD pain not only worsens OHRQoL but also affects the psychological well-being of an individual [38]. Published systematic reviews and meta-analyses measured high depressive symptoms in patients with chronic TMD pain [10,39]. Oral health-related quality of life variables were evaluated by OHIP 14 and 49. These questionnaires are reliable and identify major aspects associated with OHRQoL [2,3,40]. One study has used the World Health Organization Quality of Life questionnaire, which mainly involves the general quality of life; however, one section of this questionnaire is mainly for evaluating OHRQoL [34]. Additionally, the WHOQOL also has a section involving the environment and the individual [34]. All the studies included in this analysis evaluated patients' OHRQoL subscales, revealing that individuals with temporomandibular disorder (TMD) experience a compromised quality of life across all the subscales. Notably, pain emerged as the predominant factor affecting the quality of life in all subsets. Furthermore, the origin and etiology of TMD-related pain vary among individuals. Particularly, myofascial pain, associated with TMD, exhibits an intense pain of muscular origin [41]. Psychological complaints like depression and anxiety are common among patients suffering from TMD with muscular pain [14]. This is supported by the findings of an interventional study where patients receiving injections for TMD pain had a better quality of life compared to the placebo [42]. Additionally, the subscale of oral pain in patients with intervention was improved. Nowadays, researchers use a four-dimensional approach to evaluate the OHIP scale [43]. This approach includes oral pain, appearance, function, and psychological factors combined. Moreover, this approach provides a comprehensive result on oral health and its association with the intensity of pain [43]. Therefore, studies should report all seven subscales in OHIP to maintain the compatibility of the data provided.

In relation to meta-analyses, only ten studies were included due to high heterogeneity related to the methodological analysis, a lack of exposure, and the absence of the necessary data required for an analysis. However, it was observed that TMD negatively affects individual's OHRQoL when compared to the non-TMD subjects. Additionally, OHRQoL was worsen in TMD patients in group I (myofascial pain) and group III (arthritis) compared to group II (disc displacement), with a statistically significant difference. These factors can be explained mainly by the worst pain levels in group I and III patients compared to group II, as reported in a systematic review on TMD pain and chronic pain analysis. Additionally, the presence of anxiety, depression, and somatization was reported worse in group I TMD patients compared to group II and III, also negatively impacting OHRQoL [44]. A systematic review on the therapeutic intervention of TMD reported improvement in pain intensity if the psychological factors along with pain medication are controlled in the patients with severe pain [45]. Most of the included studies measured that females with chronic TMD have two times worse OHRQoL than males. This difference could be attributed to the role of gender, considering that females are more likely to develop TMD-related pain and seek treatment faster compared to males. However, the literature suggests contradictory results when comparing the severity of pain and quality of life among genders, and only one study found functional limitations in females suffering from TMD-related pain [37]. Due to the heterogeneity among the included studies, a random effect model was used, and the study reported that the observed effect is an estimate of the real effect and follows the general distribution of the studies with smaller sample sizes gaining the weight compared to larger sample sizes. To improve future systematic reviews with a meta-analysis and to reduce the heterogeneity, it is suggested that the future systematic reviews should either apply the RDC/TMD or DC/TMD with axis I and II and comparing the overall quality of life measures in observational studies with larger sample size. Additionally, studies should clearly report the sample size, the mean, median, and standard deviation for the RDC/TMD diagnosis with axis I, II, and III groups. The use of RDC/TMD axis II is important, as it demonstrates the psychological aspects of the patients suffering from TMD-related pain. These findings are important when considering a person's OHRQoL. Finally, studies should also report the sample source, method of randomization, qualification of examiner, and inclusion and exclusion criteria for both cases, and controls should be provided to avoid the bias related to the selection of participants.

Based on this systematic review and meta-analysis, several recommendations could be made for future studies. Firstly, studies should include both axis I and II for TMD patients, as this could not only focus on the intensity of pain but also the psychological variables associated with the severity of pain. Future studies should also focus more on the general quality of life because of the various etiological factors associated with TMD. It is paramount that future studies be more focused on investigating cases and controls with either RDC/TMD or DC/TMD to avoid bias related to case selection. In addition, the role of gender should also be assessed to evaluate the difference in OHRQoL among the genders. Finally, more clinical studies are required that focus on the data collection process of TMD and quality of life among various subgroups of TMD.

In summary, this systematic review with a meta-analysis and GRADE evidence shows that the OHRQoL is directly related to chronic TMD. The disability associated with TMD pain is also mentioned in this review. Therefore, TMD with (disc displacement) have an acceptable OHRQoL compared to myofascial pain and arthritis patients.

Strengths and Limitations

Three qualified researchers conducted the evaluation, and the present systematic review adhered to PRISMA guidelines. Despite adhering to PRISMA guidelines and conducting a thorough quality appraisal of all included studies to comprehensively assess the oral health-related quality of life (OHRQoL) in patients with temporomandibular disorders (TMD), there are certain limitations that need consideration.

First, many included studies lacked important information, and some studies only provided details on TMD patients without a specific comparison to healthy subjects.

This systematic review and meta-analysis may be influenced by selection and measurement biases. All the included studies were of an observational nature, which limits the ability to establish causal relationships between TMD and OHRQoL. The inclusion criteria that required studies to be published in English since January 2013 and to use particular diagnostic criteria and questionnaires might have led to the exclusion of relevant research, such as studies in other languages or those using different diagnostic approaches. Additionally, the variability in diagnostic criteria (RDC/TMD or DC/TMD) and OHRQoL measurement tools (e.g., OHIP-14, OHIP-49) across studies could affect the comparability of results and the consistency of findings.

Second, all the included studies were of an observational nature, which limits their ability to establish causal relationships between TMD and OHRQoL. Additionally, the heterogeneity in study designs and measurement tools used to assess OHRQoL may introduce variability in the results. Most of the studies did not present the results in the function of RDC or DC subgroups. Therefore, in future research, standardizing diagnostic criteria using DC/TMD would ensure consistency in the definition and classification of TMD across studies. Uniform study designs to minimize variability in research methodologies will allow for straightforward comparisons between studies and contribute to a more coherent body of evidence, thereby enhancing the generalizability of findings.

5. Conclusions

Based on the results of this systematic review and meta-analysis with GRADE evidence, it can be concluded that patients with temporomandibular disorders (TMD) experience a lower oral health-related quality of life (OHRQoL) compared to healthy adults. This decline in OHRQoL is directly associated with the intensity of pain and disability as reported in individuals diagnosed with RDC/TMD and DC/TMD with axis I and II. Furthermore, the analysis revealed that pain intensity was higher among groups with arthritis and myofascial pain in comparison to those with disc displacement and healthy individuals. To gain a more comprehensive understanding of the impact of TMD on patients' quality of life, further investigations are required. These should include the assessments of general quality of life, OHRQoL questionnaires, population-based data, and the diagnosis of TMD patients and controls using validated recent methods, such as DC/TMD, for a more accurate analysis of the effects on the quality of life of TMD patients.

Supplementary Materials: The following supporting information can be downloaded at https://www.mdpi.com/article/10.3390/diagnostics14192183/s1, Table S1: Excluded studies for TMD-OHRQoL.

Author Contributions: Conceptualization, L.A. and H.A.; methodology, L.A.; software, R.A.; validation, L.A., H.A. and R.A.; formal analysis, L.A.; investigation, L.A.; resources, L.A. and R.A.; data curation, L.A. and R.A.; writing—original draft preparation, L.A. and R.A.; writing—review and editing, L.A. and R.A.; supervision, H.A.; project administration, L.A.;All authors have read and agreed to the published version of the manuscript.

Funding: This study received no external funding.

Institutional Review Board Statement: Not applicable.

Informed Consent Statement: Not applicable.

Data Availability Statement: The data that support the findings of this study are available on request from the corresponding author.

Conflicts of Interest: The authors declare no conflicts of interest.

References

1. De Leeuw, R.; Klasser, G. Orofacial pain: Guidelines for assessment, diagnosis, and management. *Am. J. Orthod. Dentofac. Orthop.* **2008**, *134*, 171. [CrossRef]
2. Blanco-Aguilera, A.; Blanco-Hungría, A.; Biedma-Velázquez, L.; Serrano-Del-Rosal, R.; González-López, L.; Blanco-Aguilera, E.; Segura-Saint-Gerons, R. Application of an oral health-related quality of life questionnaire in primary care patients with orofacial pain and temporomandibular disorders. *Med. Oral Patol. Oral Cir. Bucal* **2014**, *19*, e127–e135. [CrossRef] [PubMed]
3. Cao, Y.; Yap, A.U.; Lei, J.; Zhang, M.J.; Fu, K.Y. Oral health-related quality of life of patients with acute and chronic temporomandibular disorder diagnostic subtypes. *J. Am. Dent. Assoc.* **2022**, *153*, 50–58. [CrossRef] [PubMed]
4. Hanna, K.; Nair, R.; Amarasena, N.; Armfield, J.M.; Brennan, D.S. Temporomandibular dysfunction experience is associated with oral health-related quality of life: An Australian national study. *BMC Oral Health* **2021**, *21*, 432. [CrossRef]
5. World Health Organization. The World Health Organization Quality of Life assessment (WHOQOL): Position paper from the World Health Organization. *Soc. Sci. Med.* **1995**, *41*, 1403–1409. [CrossRef] [PubMed]
6. Shearer, D.M.; MacLeod, R.J.; Thomson, W.M. Oral-health-related quality of life: An overview for the general dental practitioner. *N. Z. Dent. J.* **2007**, *103*, 82–87. [PubMed]
7. McGrath, C.; Bedi, R. An evaluation of a new measure of oral health related quality of life--OHQoL-UK(W). *Community Dent. Health* **2001**, *18*, 138–143. [PubMed]
8. Namvar, M.A.; Moslemkhani, C.; Mansoori, K.; Dadashi, M. The Relationship between Depression and Anxiety with Temporomandibular Disorder Symptoms in Dental Students. *Maedica J. Clin. Med.* **2021**, *16*, 590. [CrossRef]
9. Almoznino, G.; Zini, A.; Zakuto, A.; Sharav, Y.; Haviv, Y.; Avraham, J.; Chweidan, H.; Noam, Y.; Benoliel, R. Oral Health-Related Quality of Life in Patients with Temporomandibular Disorders. *J. Oral Facial Pain. Headache* **2015**, *29*, 231–241. [CrossRef]

10. Dahlström, L.; Carlsson, G.E. Temporomandibular disorders and oral health-related quality of life. A systematic review. *Acta Odontol. Scand.* **2010**, *68*, 80–85. [CrossRef]
11. Karaman, A.; Sapan, Z. Evaluation of temporomandibular disorders, quality of life, and oral habits among dentistry students. *Cranio* **2023**, *41*, 316–322. [CrossRef]
12. Oberoi, S.S.; Hiremath, S.S.; Yashoda, R.; Marya, C.; Rekhi, A. Prevalence of Various Orofacial Pain Symptoms and Their Overall Impact on Quality of Life in a Tertiary Care Hospital in India. *J. Maxillofac. Oral Surg.* **2014**, *13*, 533–538. [CrossRef]
13. Potewiratnanond, P.; Limpuangthip, N.; Karunanon, V.; Buritep, A.; Thawai, A. Factors associated with the oral health-related quality of life of patients with temporomandibular disorder at the final follow-up visit: A cross-sectional study. *BDJ Open* **2022**, *8*, 30. [CrossRef]
14. Turcio, K.H.; Neto, C.M.; Pirovani, B.O.; Dos Santos, D.M.; Guiotti, A.M.; Bertoz, A.M.; Brandini, D.A. Relationship of bruxism with oral health-related quality of life and facial muscle pain in dentate individuals. *J. Clin. Exp. Dent.* **2022**, *14*, e385–e389. [CrossRef]
15. Qamar, Z.; Alghamdi, A.M.S.; Haydarah, N.K.B.; Balateef, A.A.; Alamoudi, A.A.; Abumismar, M.A.; Shivakumar, S.; Cicciu, M.; Minervini, G. Impact of temporomandibular disorders on oral health-related quality of life: A systematic review and meta-analysis. *J. Oral Rehabil.* **2023**, *50*, 706–714. [CrossRef]
16. Schiffman, E.; Ohrbach, R.; Truelove, E.; Look, J.; Anderson, G.; Goulet, J.P.; List, T.; Svensson, P.; Gonzalez, Y.; Lobbezoo, F.; et al. Diagnostic Criteria for Temporomandibular Disorders (DC/TMD) for Clinical and Research Applications: Recommendations of the International RDC/TMD Consortium Network* and Orofacial Pain Special Interest Groupdagger. *J. Oral Facial Pain. Headache* **2014**, *28*, 6–27. [CrossRef] [PubMed]
17. Moher, D.; Liberati, A.; Tetzlaff, J.; Altman, D.G. Preferred Reporting Items for Systematic Reviews and Meta-Analyses: The PRISMA Statement. *PLoS Med.* **2009**, *6*, e1000097. [CrossRef]
18. Cumpston, M.; Li, T.; Page, M.J.; Chandler, J.; Welch, V.A.; Higgins, J.P.; Thomas, J. Updated guidance for trusted systematic reviews: A new edition of the Cochrane Handbook for Systematic Reviews of Interventions. *Cochrane Database Syst. Rev.* **2019**, *2019*, ED000142. [CrossRef] [PubMed]
19. Von Elm, E.; Altman, D.G.; Egger, M.; Pocock, S.J.; Gøtzsche, P.C.; Vandenbroucke, J.P. The Strengthening the Reporting of Observational Studies in Epidemiology (STROBE) statement: Guidelines for reporting observational studies. *Lancet* **2007**, *370*, 1453–1457. [CrossRef]
20. Margulis, A.V.; Pladevall, M.; Riera-Guardia, N.; Varas-Lorenzo, C.; Hazell, L.; Berkman, N.D.; Viswanathan, M.; Perez-Gutthann, S. Quality assessment of observational studies in a drug-safety systematic review, comparison of two tools: The Newcastle–Ottawa scale and the RTI item bank. *Clin. Epidemiol.* **2014**, *6*, 359–368. [CrossRef]
21. Cook, D.A.; Reed, D.A. Appraising the quality of medical education research methods: The medical education research study quality instrument and the Newcastle–Ottawa scale-education. *Acad. Med.* **2015**, *90*, 1067–1076. [CrossRef] [PubMed]
22. Huguet, A.; Hayden, J.A.; Stinson, J.; McGrath, P.J.; Chambers, C.T.; Tougas, M.E.; Wozney, L. Judging the quality of evidence in reviews of prognostic factor research: Adapting the GRADE framework. *Syst. Rev.* **2013**, *2*, 71. [CrossRef]
23. Bayat, M.; Abbasi, A.J.; Noorbala, A.A.; Mohebbi, S.Z.; Moharrami, M.; Yekaninejad, M.S. Oral health-related quality of life in patients with temporomandibular disorders: A case-control study considering psychological aspects. *Int. J. Dent. Hyg.* **2018**, *16*, 165–170. [CrossRef]
24. Celik, O.; Secgin, C.K.; Gulashi, A.; Yuzugullu, B. Oral Health-Related Quality of Life in Patients with Temporomandibular Disorders and Effect of Anxiety: A Retrospective Case-Control Study. *Int. J. Prosthodont.* **2023**, *36*, 148–154. [CrossRef]
25. Filho, J.C.; Vedovello, S.A.S.; Venezian, G.C.; Vedovello Filho, M.; Degan, V.V. Women's oral health-related quality of life as a risk factor for TMD symptoms. A case-control study. *Cranio* **2023**, *41*, 139–143. [CrossRef]
26. Rener-Sitar, K.; Celebic, A.; Mehulic, K.; Petricevic, N. Factors Related to Oral Health Related Quality of Life in TMD Patients. *Coll. Antropol.* **2013**, *37*, 407–413.
27. Yap, A.U.; Cao, Y.; Zhang, M.J.; Lei, J.; Fu, K.Y. Comparison of emotional disturbance, sleep, and life quality in adult patients with painful temporomandibular disorders of different origins. *Clin. Oral Investig.* **2021**, *25*, 4097–4105. [CrossRef]
28. Yap, A.U.; Tan, S.H.X.; Marpaung, C. Temporomandibular disorder symptoms in young adults: Three-dimensional impact on oral health-related quality of life. *J. Oral Rehabil.* **2022**, *49*, 769–777. [CrossRef]
29. Yildirim, G.; Erol, F.; Guven, M.C.; Sakar, O. Evaluation of the effects of bruxism on oral health-related quality of life in adults. *Cranio* **2023**, *41*, 230–237. [CrossRef] [PubMed]
30. Balik, A.; Peker, K.; Ozdemir-Karatas, M. Comparisons of measures that evaluate oral and general health quality of life in patients with temporomandibular disorder and chronic pain. *Cranio* **2021**, *39*, 310–320. [CrossRef]
31. Gui, M.S.; Pimentel, M.J.; Gama, M.C.d.S.; Ambrosano, G.M.B.; Barbosa, C.M.R. Quality of life in temporomandibular disorder patients with localized and widespread pain. *Braz. J. Oral Sci.* **2014**, *13*, 193–197. [CrossRef]
32. Lemos, G.A.; Paulino, M.R.; Forte, F.D.S.; Beltrão, R.T.S.; Batista, A.U.D. Influence of temporomandibular disorder presence and severity on oral health-related quality of life. *Rev. D'or* **2015**, *16*, 10–14. [CrossRef]
33. Pawar, P.; Puranik, M.; Shanbhag, N. Relationship between Oral Health Status and Oral Health-Related Quality of Life among Patients with Temporomandibular Disorders in Bengaluru City: A Cross-Sectional Comparative Study. *J. Indian Assoc. Public Health Dent.* **2022**, *20*, 287–292. [CrossRef]

34. Resende CMBMd Alves, A.C.d.M.; Coelho, L.T.; Alchieri, J.C.; Roncalli, Â.G.; Barbosa, G.A.S. Quality of life and general health in patients with temporomandibular disorders. *Braz. Oral Res.* **2013**, *27*, 116–121. [CrossRef] [PubMed]
35. Su, N.; Liu, Y.; Yang, X.; Shen, J.; Wang, H. Correlation between oral health-related quality of life and clinical dysfunction index in patients with temporomandibular joint osteoarthritis. *J. Oral Sci.* **2016**, *58*, 483–490. [CrossRef] [PubMed]
36. Yap, A.U.; Cao, Y.; Zhang, M.J.; Lei, J.; Fu, K.Y. Number and type of temporomandibular disorder symptoms: Their associations with psychological distress and oral health-related quality of life. *Oral Surg. Oral Med. Oral Pathol. Oral Radiol.* **2021**, *132*, 288–296. [CrossRef]
37. Yap, A.U.; Cao, Y.; Zhang, M.J.; Lei, J.; Fu, K.Y. Age-related differences in diagnostic categories, psychological states and oral health-related quality of life of adult temporomandibular disorder patients. *J. Oral Rehabil.* **2021**, *48*, 361–368.
38. Kroese, J.M.; Volgenant, C.M.C.; van Schaardenburg, D.; van Boheemen, L.; van Selms, M.K.A.; Visscher, C.M.; Crielaard, W.; Loos, B.G.; Lobbezoo, F. Oral health-related quality of life in patients with early rheumatoid arthritis is associated with periodontal inflammation and painful temporomandibular disorders: A cross-sectional study. *Clin. Oral Investig.* **2022**, *26*, 555–563. [CrossRef]
39. Aranha, R.L.d.B.; Martins, R.d.C.; de Aguilar, D.R.; Moreno-Drada, J.A.; Sohn, W.; Martins, C.d.C.; de Abreu, M.H.N.G. Association between Stress at Work and Temporomandibular Disorders: A Systematic Review. *BioMed Res. Int.* **2021**, *2021*, 2055513. [CrossRef] [PubMed]
40. Bieganska-Banas, J.M.; Gierowski, J.K.; Pihut, M.; Ferendiuk, E. Oral health-related quality of life and cognitive functioning in myofascial temporomandibular disorders pain. *Arch. Psychiatry Psychother.* **2019**, *21*, 45–58. [CrossRef]
41. Rahimi, H.; Twilt, M.; Herlin, T.; Spiegel, L.; Pedersen, T.K.; Küseler, A.; Stoustrup, P. Orofacial symptoms and oral health-related quality of life in juvenile idiopathic arthritis: A two-year prospective observational study. *Pediatr. Rheumatol. Online J.* **2018**, *16*, 47. [CrossRef] [PubMed]
42. Su, N.; Wang, H.; van Wijk, A.J.; Visscher, C.M.; Lobbezoo, F.; Shi, Z.; van der Heijden, G. Prediction Models for Oral Health-Related Quality of Life in Patients with Temporomandibular Joint Osteoarthritis 1 and 6 Months After Arthrocentesis with Hyaluronic Acid Injections. *J. Oral Facial Pain. Headache* **2019**, *33*, 54–66. [CrossRef] [PubMed]
43. Oghli, I.; List, T.; Su, N.; Häggman-Henrikson, B. The impact of oro-facial pain conditions on oral health-related quality of life: A systematic review. *J. Oral Rehabil.* **2020**, *47*, 1052–1064. [CrossRef]
44. Tanner, J.; Teerijoki-Oksa, T.; Kautiainen, H.; Vartiainen, P.; Kalso, E.; Forssell, H. Health-related quality of life in patients with chronic orofacial pain compared with other chronic pain patients. *Clin. Exp. Dent. Res.* **2022**, *8*, 742–749. [CrossRef] [PubMed]
45. Song, Y.L.; Yap, A.U. Outcomes of therapeutic TMD interventions on oral health related quality of life: A qualitative systematic review. *Quintessence Int.* **2018**, *49*, 487–496.

Disclaimer/Publisher's Note: The statements, opinions and data contained in all publications are solely those of the individual author(s) and contributor(s) and not of MDPI and/or the editor(s). MDPI and/or the editor(s) disclaim responsibility for any injury to people or property resulting from any ideas, methods, instructions or products referred to in the content.

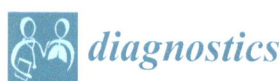

Systematic Review

Is There a Relationship between Salivary Cortisol and Temporomandibular Disorder: A Systematic Review

Lujain AlSahman [1,*], Hamad AlBagieh [1] and Roba AlSahman [2]

1. Oral Medicine and Diagnostic Sciences Department, College of Dentistry, King Saud University Riyadh, Riyadh 57448, Saudi Arabia; hamadnb@hotmail.com
2. Faculty of Dentistry, Royal College of Surgeons, D02YN77 Dublin, Ireland; robaalsahman@gmail.com
* Correspondence: alsahmanlujain@gmail.com

Abstract: Background: This systematic review examines and evaluates the relationship between salivary cortisol levels and temporomandibular disorder (TMD) in young adult patients. Method: Six databases—PubMed, Scopus, Web of Science, Google Scholar, ProQuest, and Cochrane Library—were utilized to screen eligible studies. A systematic search was performed based on PECO questions and eligibility criteria. The research question for this review was "Do salivary cortisol levels correlate with TMD in individuals aged 18–40?" The risk of bias for quality assessment was determined by the Cochrane tool. PRISMA guidelines were followed while performing this review. Result: A total of fourteen studies were included in this review. Of these, eleven were observational studies (four cross-sectional and seven case–control), and three were randomized control trials. Eleven of the included studies presented a low to moderate risk in the qualitative synthesis. The total sample size of the included studies was 751 participants. The included studies suggest higher salivary cortisol levels in TMD patients than in healthy individuals. Conclusions: The findings of this review indicate higher salivary cortisol levels in adult patients with TMD than in healthy controls. Thus, supportive psychological treatment and clinical modalities should be provided to patients with TMD. Moreover, higher-quality studies with low heterogeneity are required to support this finding.

Keywords: salivary cortisol; temporomandibular disorders (TMD); diagnostic tool; biomarkers

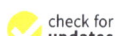

Citation: AlSahman, L.; AlBagieh, H.; AlSahman, R. Is There a Relationship between Salivary Cortisol and Temporomandibular Disorder: A Systematic Review. *Diagnostics* **2024**, *14*, 1435. https://doi.org/10.3390/diagnostics14131435

Academic Editor: Luis Eduardo Almeida

Received: 28 May 2024
Revised: 29 June 2024
Accepted: 30 June 2024
Published: 5 July 2024

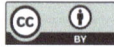

Copyright: © 2024 by the authors. Licensee MDPI, Basel, Switzerland. This article is an open access article distributed under the terms and conditions of the Creative Commons Attribution (CC BY) license (https://creativecommons.org/licenses/by/4.0/).

1. Introduction

The temporomandibular joint (TMJ) and its associated structures are pivotal in guiding mandibular movement and distributing stresses produced by everyday tasks like speaking, chewing, and swallowing [1]. Temporomandibular disorders (TMDs) are pathologic conditions affecting the TMJ, masticatory muscles, and surrounding tissues [2]. TMDs include abnormalities of the intra-articular disc's position and/or structure and dysfunction of the associated musculature [3]. The symptoms of TMDs include a reduced range of movement of the mandible, painful joint sounds, masticatory muscle pain, TMJ pain, and restriction/deviation in mouth opening [4]. TMD is the most common cause of chronic orofacial pain due to non-dental origin [5], with the prevalence of TMDs being about 31% in adults and about 11% in children and adolescents [6]. The aetiology of TMD is considered to be multifactorial, including biomechanical (occlusal overload and parafunction), neuromuscular, biological (e.g., elevated levels of oestrogen hormones), and psychosocial (e.g., stress, anxiety, depression) factors [7]. Psychological factors, especially stress, are considered one of the main areas of TMD aetiology, but their role in the occurrence of TMD is inconclusive [8]. Stress is a normal physiological response in humans. However, it leads to pathological conditions when it exceeds the body's adaptive capacity. It has also been found to strongly contribute to the formation and persistence of pain [9]. Additionally, pain and stress lead to parafunctional habits [9], like bruxism linked with signs and symptoms of TMD [8]. Mental stress is believed to stimulate the hypothalamic–pituitary–adrenal (HPA) axis, which triggers a series of reactions leading to increased cortisol secretion from the adrenal cortex [10]. As a product of the HPA axis, cortisol participates in anti-inflammatory and anti-stress activities and is considered a marker of stress and anxiety. Several studies have shown a correlation between HPA axis dysregulation and TMD [11,12]. Consequently, cortisol levels can be utilised to assess HPA axis activity [13] and evaluate TMD. Furthermore, cortisol level assessment can be developed as a diagnostic tool for TMD and to meet the specific treatment needs of TMD patients.

Cortisol levels can be measured using plasma, serum, urine, hair, and saliva specimens [14]. Considering its non-invasive mode of collection, saliva has become a good candidate for cortisol assessment. Moreover, salivary cortisol measurement indicates unbound active cortisol levels in contrast to bound plasma cortisol levels [15]. Previous studies have assessed salivary cortisol levels in TMD patients, with contradictory reports [16–18]. According to Kobayashi et al., no difference in salivary biomarkers was observed between children with and without TMD, although anxiety symptom scores were higher in children with TMD [18]. Contrary reports were provided by D'Avilla et al., who found significantly higher salivary cortisol values in their adult TMD group [17]. A recent study by Suprajith et al. concluded a significant impact of psychosocial stress on the etiopathogenesis of TMD [19]. Collaborating on these findings, Fritzen et al. stressed that the relationship between salivary cortisol and bruxism in adults and children could not be neglected [20]. Despite some existing studies, there is no conclusive evidence regarding the association of salivary cortisol levels in adult patients with TMD. Moreover, a significant increase in stress levels has been found in young adults compared to children and the elderly population. A literature search shows a systematic review by Lu et al. [21], but this review includes only case–control studies and a limited search period, from 2008 to 2020. Moreover, none of the existing studies focus on adult patients' salivary cortisol concentrations. So, we aimed to search all the available data regarding salivary cortisol levels in adult TMD patients between 18–40 years old. Hence, this systematic review was conducted in order to determine whether a correlation exists between salivary cortisol levels and TMD in adult patients.

2. Materials and Methods

This systematic review evaluates the relationship between salivary cortisol levels and temporomandibular disorders (TMDs) in individuals aged 18–40.

2.1. Protocol and Registration

A preliminary literature search was run to identify the research problem, focus question, and eligibility criteria in January 2023. Following this, a protocol was prepared and registered with PROSPERO before the systematic review began (CRD42022378756).

2.2. Eligibility Criteria

The focus question was formulated using the PECO (population, exposure, comparison, and outcome) framework. Population (P) was young adults aged 18–40 with TMD and without any other oral pathology or disorder; exposure (E) was salivary cortisol levels measured in observational and randomized control trials; comparison (C) was healthy participants without TMD; and outcome (O) was changes in salivary cortisol levels in patients diagnosed with TMD. Consequently, the focus question was, "Do salivary cortisol levels correlate with temporomandibular disorders (TMDs) in individuals aged 18–40?"

The inclusion criteria for the studies were as follows: (1) studies including patients between 18–40 years of age, (2) studies including patients diagnosed with TMDs according to RDC/TMD or DC/TMD, (3) clinical studies (mainly case–control studies, randomized control trials, and observational studies), and (4) studies evaluating salivary cortisol/biomarkers for stress.

Studies were excluded using the following criteria: (1) case report/series, (2) conference papers, (3) in vitro studies, (4) editorials, (5) commentaries, (6) literature reviews, (7) animal studies, and (8) studies not in the English language.

2.3. Information Sources and Search Strategies

The PRISMA 2020 statement [22] was followed to report this systematic review. Two researchers performed the literature search on all major databases, such as PubMed, Scopus, Web of Science, Google Scholar, ProQuest, and Cochrane Library, to include all relevant studies related to TMDs and salivary cortisol levels. An experienced librarian was always available to assist with the literature search.

After developing the protocol, the initial search began in March 2023. The PECO criteria were utilized to run the search using keywords and MeSH terms related to temporomandibular disorders ("temporomandibular joint disorders" OR "temporomandibular joint dysfunction" OR "craniomandibular disorders" OR "TMJ osteoarthritis") and salivary cortisol levels (Table 1), until December 2023 A manual search was also performed in the reference sections of already identified articles.

Table 1. Search string for various databases.

PubMed	(hydrocortisone) "[MeSH Terms] OR "hydrocortisone"[All Fields] OR "cortisol"[All Fields]) AND ("Temporomandibular disorder"[MeSH Terms] OR "TMD"[All Fields]) OR ("temporomandibular disfunction"[MeSH Terms] OR ("Facial muscle pain"[All Fields] AND young Adults [All Fields].
Scopus	(TITLE-ABS-KEY ("craniomandibular disorder*" OR "temporomandibular joint disorder*" OR "temporomandibular disorder*" OR tmjd OR tmd OR "tmj disorder*" OR ((facial OR jaw OR orofacial OR craniofacial OR trigem*) AND pain))) AND (TITLE-ABS-KEY (pcs OR "Salivary cortisol" OR Hydrocortisone* OR cortisol AND (Young adults))))
Web of science	cortisol* OR hydrocortisone* AND Temporomandibular disorder* OR TMD* AND Young adults.
Google scholar	(cortisol OR Salivary cortisol AND Temporomandibular disorder OR TMD AND Young Adults).

2.4. Study Selection

After identifying the articles from various databases, the titles and abstracts were screened independently by two reviewers to include all studies that satisfied the inclusion and exclusion criteria for this systematic review. This step removed duplicates using citation or reference manager (Endnote 21). Finally, two researchers retrieved and scrutinized full texts, and any disagreements were resolved by discussion.

2.5. Data Extraction and Data Items

Two reviewers extracted the following data from the full-text articles: author, year, country, study population, study design, sample size, test/control group size, age range, salivary cortisol levels in tests and controls, saliva collection techniques, the statistical significance of the results, and conclusion. The data retrieved were tabulated in Excel sheets. Both the reviewers confirmed the data obtained, and any disagreements were resolved by a third reviewer. The inter-examiner kappa coefficient between the examiners was measured and was above 0.9 for all the questions during data extraction.

2.6. Data Synthesis (Meta-Analysis)

The studies included in this systematic review are heterogenous in nature. Hence, no meta-analysis was planned. Overall, analysis of the studies included in this review was done by narrative summary of the included studies. The quality of the included studies was evaluated by deducing the risk of bias for randomized control trials, cross sectional studies, and case–control studies. Due to high heterogeneity among the included studies, the authors performed GRADE analysis to evaluate the certainty of the evidence of the studies included in this systematic review. The Grading of Recommendations Assessment, Development and Evaluation (GRADE) methodology for grading the certainty of evidence was utilized for the observational studies and RCTs [23].

2.7. Risk of Bias in Individual Studies

A panel comprising two researchers assessed the risk of bias among the included studies. The Cochrane Risk of Bias Tool II [24] was utilised for the risk of bias assessment of randomized control trials, and the Newcastle–Ottawa quality assessment scale was used for case–control studies [25]. The Newcastle–Ottawa quality assessment scale (adapted for cross-sectional studies) was applied for the risk of bias assessment of cross-sectional studies [26]. Scoring for the Newcastle–Ottawa scale (for cross-sectional and case–control studies) ranges from 0 to 10, with 0 meaning a high risk, 4 to 6 a medium risk, and 7 and above a low risk of bias. Scores for the Cochrane Risk of Bias Tool are measured as "low", "high", and "some concern".

3. Results

The survey identified 18,070 studies on different databases, out of which 666 studies were duplicates. A total of 17,404 studies were directed to the reading of the title and abstract, out of which 17,375 were removed. A final 29 studies were selected for full-text reading, and 15 were removed for various reasons; the study selection process is explained in Figure 1.

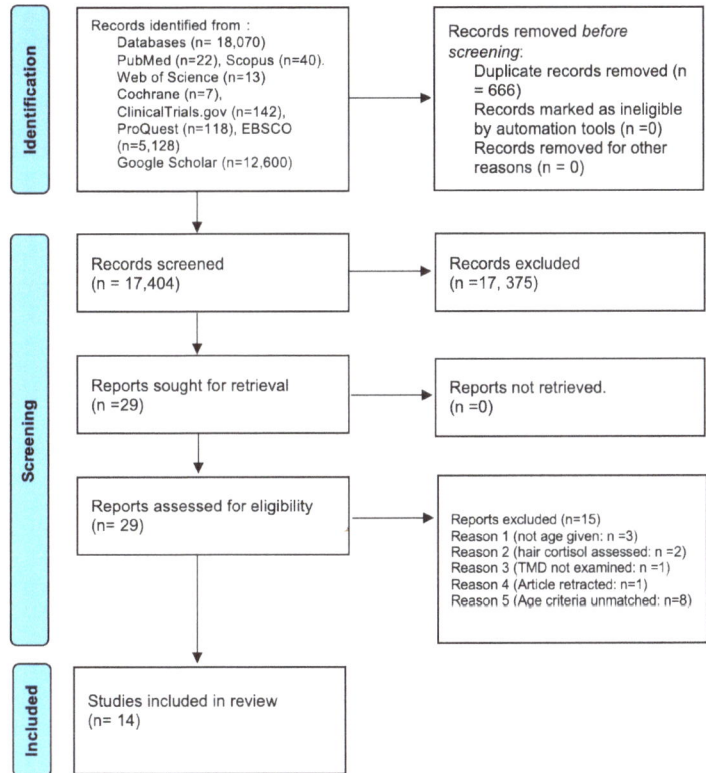

Figure 1. PRISMA flowchart.

Fourteen primary studies involving 751 participants (tests = 424 and controls = 327) met the criteria included in Table 2. The studies included in this review were published between 1997 and 2022.

3.1. Characteristics of Included Studies (Table 2)

Among the fourteen studies selected for data extraction were three randomized control trials [27–29], four cross-sectional studies [17,30–32], and seven case–control studies [16,33–38]. The included studies were from Brazil, Bosnia and Herzegovina, Thailand, Sweden, India, Canada, Iran, the USA, and China.

The study population in the test group consisted of young adult patients with TMD. All included studies—except one by Tosato et al.—had male and female participants, mostly university students. In the included studies, mainly female participants were affected by TMD, with higher stress and anxiety levels and elevated salivary cortisol [31]. As well as salivary cortisol levels, two studies by Rosar et al. studied bruxism and TMD [27,30]. Moreover, all three RCTs evaluated the effect of the treatment of TMD on salivary cortisol levels, and all of them reported a significant decrease in salivary cortisol levels after the treatment. The results of almost all included studies show that increasing salivary cortisol levels are seen in TMD patients with higher stress and anxiety levels. Goyal et al. [28] further verified that a significantly higher value of salivary cortisol was detected in TMD patients with depression than in TMD patients without depression, and treatment of TMD resulted in decreasing salivary cortisol levels. The Research Diagnostic Criteria for Temporomandibular Disorders (RDC/TMD) and clinical diagnosis were used to diagnose TMDs in almost all studies. The comparator group was mainly healthy controls without TMD. However, one study evaluated the salivary cortisol levels of TMD patients with normal occlusion and those with malocclusion [17]. A study by Magri et al. measured salivary cortisol levels with low-level laser therapy [29]. Goyal et al. measured salivary cortisol levels in cohorts of depressed and non-depressed TMD patients, as well as in a group of healthy controls [28]. Although the included studies were heterogenous, eleven of the included studies reported a higher salivary cortisol level in TMD patients than in controls.

3.2. Salivary Parameters of the Participants of the Included Studies (Table 3)

Seven primary studies used unstimulated saliva to assess cortisol ($n = 381$) [16,28,29,31,34,35,37], and the remaining five studies used stimulated saliva ($n = 267$) [17,27,30,36,38]. In seven studies, salivary samples were collected in the morning [27,29–32,34,37], while one study performed sampling both in the morning and evening [28]. However, in three studies, the timings of saliva sampling were not mentioned [17,33,36]. Six studies [16,28,33,34,36,37] collected saliva without extra stimulation, while five studies [17,27,29,30,35] collected saliva that was stimulated by chewing the swab and cotton roll. All the studies evaluated elevated cortisol levels with an ELISA kit, except for one study.

All the included studies utilized different measures for saliva collection. Quartana and colleagues collected salivary samples before and after 20 min of treatment [38]. While a stress test was performed by Jones et al., salivary samples were collected at three different intervals—at baseline, peak secretion (30 min), and 20 min after the rest [35].

Nine studies assessed salivary cortisol levels in adults with TMD compared to healthy controls. Seven of these were case–control study designs [16,33–38], and two were cross-sectional [31,32]. However, four of the included studies (three randomized control trials, and one cross-sectional study) evaluated salivary cortisol levels before and after treatment of TMD and controls. Ten of the included studies noted statistically significant differences between the salivary cortisol levels of both the groups. The statistical analyses reported in the included studies were in favour of the control group [17,27–34,37], showing higher cortisol levels in TMD patients. In contrast, four studies showed no statistical correlation between cortisol levels and TMD [16,35,36,38].

3.3. Risk of Bias Assessment (Tables 4–6)

The risk of bias assessment for the randomized controlled trials was performed by utilising the Cochrane Risk of Bias Tool-II [24]. One study was found to have a high risk [27], and two had a low risk of bias [28,29]. The high risk was due to inconsistency in measuring the exposure and differences in the sample allocation.

The Newcastle–Ottawa quality assessment scales for cross-sectional [26] and case–control studies [25] measured the risk of bias for corresponding studies. Among the seven case–control studies in the review, two had low risk [33,38], four had medium [16,34–36], and one had a high risk of bias [37]. The high- and medium-risk studies had higher heterogeneity in sample representativeness and exposure. Outcome measures were inconsistently reported among those studies.

Out of the four cross-sectional studies included, three had a low risk of bias [17,27,31], while one study had a medium risk of bias [32]. The observational studies, especially the case–control and cross-sectional studies, had a higher risk of publication bias due to a lack of proper registration procedures. Hence, the overall bias measured in these study designs is higher compared to clinical trials.

3.4. Certainty of Evidence (GRADE Analysis) (Table 7)

The certainty of the evidence from randomized control trials for the effect of salivary cortisol on the development of TMD was low (Table 7). The certainty was downgraded because of indirectness and imprecision, as according to the RCTs included, the level of salivary cortisol has minimal or no effect on the development of TMD. Evidence of the effect of salivary cortisol on the development of TMD in the observational studies was also downgraded due to indirectness, impression, and risk of bias. Moreover, for the observational studies all the four criteria for certainty of evidence were downgraded.

Because the certainty of their evidence for the effect of salivary cortisol on TMD development was high quality, randomized control trails and observational studies were included. Therefore, the certainty of evidence for all the included studies was low and IMPORTANT. This result is of IMPORTANCE because salivary cortisol levels are considered as a critical outcome measure in the development of TMDs.

Table 2. Characteristics of included studies

Author, Year, Region	Study Design	Age Range/Average (yrs)	Sample Size (Test/Control)	Study Population	Key Findings	Conclusion
Rosar et al., 2021, Brazil [30]	Cross-sectional	19–30	43 (28/15)	TMD group Healthy group	Similar salivary cortisol levels found between groups on awakening and after 30 min	Cortisol levels were not associated with the number or duration of bruxism (TMD) episodes
Venkatesh et al., 2021, India [32]	Cross-sectional	18–23	44 (22/22)	Test with TMD Controls without TMD	Salivary cortisol levels showed statistically significant difference between the TMD and control groups	Salivary cortisol can be used as a biological marker of stress in TMD
Goyal et al., 2020, India [28]	RCT	24.05 ± 2.3	60 (20/20/20)	TMDs and positive depression levels TMDs and no depression Healthy control	Statistically significant higher value of salivary cortisol in TMD with depression, as compared to TMD without depression and control	Salivary cortisol could be a promising tool in identifying underlying psychological factors associated with TMDs
D'Avilla, 2019, Brazil [17]	Cross sectional	25.3 ± 5.1	60 (45/15)	Group I: No TMD and clinically normal occlusion Group II: With TMD and malocclusion Group III: TMD and clinically normal occlusion Group IV: No TMD and with malocclusion	Salivary cortisol level was significantly higher in individuals with TMD (G2 and G3), independent of the presence/absence of malocclusion	Quality of life, pain, and emotional stress are associated with and impaired by the TMD condition, regardless of malocclusion presence
Bozovic et al., 2018, Bosnia and Herzegovina [33]	Case-control	19.35	60 (30/30)	TMD group Healthy controls	Levels of salivary cortisol were found to be significantly higher in the study group compared to the control group	Salivary cortisol plays a vital role in TMD development
Chinthakanan et al., 2018, Thailand [34]	Case-control	24	44 (21/23)	TMD group Control group	The salivary cortisol level of the TMD group was significantly greater than that of the control group	Patients with TMD demonstrated autonomic nervous system (ANS) imbalance and increased stress levels
Magri et al., 2018, Brazil [29]	RCT	18–40	64 (41/23)	Laser group (TMD) Placebo group Without treatment group	Women with lower cortisol levels (below 10 ng/mL) were more responsive to active and placebo laser treatment than women with higher cortisol levels (above 10 ng/mL)	Most responsive cluster to active and placebo LLLT was women with low levels of anxiety, salivary levels below 10 ng/mL

Table 2. Cont.

Author, Year, Region	Study Design	Age Range/Average (yrs)	Sample Size (Test/Control)	Study Population	Key Findings	Conclusion
Rosar et al., 2017, Brazil [27]	RCT	19–30	43 (28/15)	Sleep bruxism group (Gsb) Control group (Gc)	Salivary cortisol showed a significant decrease between baseline and T1 in test, which was not observed in control	Short-term treatment with interocclusal splints had positive affect on salivary cortisol levels in subjects with sleep bruxism
Poorian et al., 2016, Iran [37]	Case–control	19–40	41 (15/26)	TMD patients Healthy people	Salivary cortisol levels in TMD patients are significantly higher than in healthy people	Increase in salivary cortisol levels increases the probability of suffering from TMD
Tosato et al., 2015, Brazil [31]	Cross-sectional	18–40	49 (26/25)	Women with TMD Healthy women	Moderate to strong correlations were found between salivary cortisol and EMG activities of the women with severe TMD	Increase in cortisol levels corresponded with greater muscle activity and TMD severity
Almeida et al., 2014, Brazil [16]	Case–control	19–32	48 (25/23)	With TMD Without TMD	Results show no difference between groups	No relationship between saliva cortisol, TMD, and depression
Nilsson and Dahlstrom, 2010, Sweden [36]	Case–control	18–24	60 (30/30)	RDC/TMD criteria I RDC/TMD criteria II Control group with no TMD	No statistically significant differences were found between any of the groups	Waking cortisol levels were not associated with symptoms of TMD and were not differentiated between the groups
Quartana et al., 2010, USA [38]	Case–control	29.85	61 (39/22)	TMD patients Healthy controls	Pain index was not associated with cortisol levels	There was no association between markers of pain sensitivity and adrenocortical responses
Jones et al., 1997, Canada [35]	Case–control	27.07	75 (36/39)	TMD group Control group	No significant differences found between TMD and control cortisol levels at baseline, but values were significantly higher in the TMD group at both 30 and 50 min	No relationship was found between psychological factors and hypersecretion of cortisol in TMD group

Temporomandibular joint (TMJ), temporomandibular disorder (TMD), randomized controlled trial (RCT), low-level laser therapy (LLLT), research diagnostic criteria (RDC).

Table 3. Salivary parameters of the included studies.

Study (Author, Year)	Saliva Collection	Salivary Cortisol Levels in Tests/Morning/Night	Salivary Cortisol Levels in Controls	Statistical Significance
Rosar et al., 2021 [30]	Stimulated saliva Collection time: immediately after waking up and 30 min after waking up	Upon waking: 0.19 ± 0.21, After 30 min: 0.24 ± 0.28 μg/dL	Upon waking: 0.16 ± 0.13, After 30 min: 0.16 ± 0.09 μg/dL	No $p > 0.05$
Venkatesh et al., 2021 [32]	Stimulated saliva Collection time: 9:30 a.m. to 10:00 a.m.	1.107 ± 0.17	0.696 ± 0.16	Yes $p < 0.001$
Goyal et al., 2020 [28]	Unstimulated saliva Collection time: twice between 7.00 and 8.00 h, and again between 20.00 and 22.00 h	Morning: TMD with depression: 52.45 ± 18.62 TMD without depression: 20.35 ± 10.59 Evening: TMD with depression: 28.13 ± 10.88 TMD without depression: 12.33 ± 6.15	Morning: 12.85 ± 4.28 Evening: 8.51 ± 4.32	Yes $p = 0.0001$
D'Avilla, 2019 [17]	Stimulated whole saliva was collected	G2: 7.45 ± 4.93, G3: 7.87 ± 3.52, G4: 4.35 ± 2.59 μg/dL	3.83 ± 2.72 μg/dL	Yes $p < 0.05$
Bozovic et al., 2018 [33]	Stimulated saliva	2.8 μg/dL	0.6 μg/dL	Yes $p < 0.001$
Chinthakanan et al., 2018 [34]	Unstimulated saliva Collection time: morning, over five minutes	29.78 ± 2.67 ng/ml	22.88 ± 1.38 ng/mL	Yes $p < 0.05$
Magri et al., 2018 [29]	Unstimulated saliva Collection time: between 7 and 10 a.m.	Under 10 ng/mL: 5/7 Above 10 ng/mL: 15/14	Under 10 ng/mL: 6 Above 10 ng/mL: 17	Yes $p < 0.05$
Rosar et al., 2017 [27]	Stimulated saliva Collection time: morning	Baseline: 5.9, T1: 2.6, T2: 2.5	Baseline: 4.9, T1: 4.4, T2: 4.3	Yes $p < 0.05$
Poorian et al., 2016 [37]	Unstimulated saliva Collection time: between 9–11 a.m.	29.0240 ± 5.27835 ng/ml	8.8950 ± 9.58974 ng/mL	Yes $p = 0.000$

Table 3. *Cont.*

Study (Author, Year)	Saliva Collection	Salivary Cortisol Levels in Tests/Morning/Night	Salivary Cortisol Levels in Controls	Statistical Significance
Tosato et al., 2015 [31]	Unstimulated saliva Collection time: between 8 and 9 a.m.	Mild: 25.39, moderate: 116.7, severe: 250.1 μg/dL		Yes $p < 0.05$ for moderate and severe
Almeida et al., 2014 [16]	Unstimulated saliva Collection time: between 9:00 and 9:25 a.m.	0.272 μg/dL	0.395 μg/dL	No $p = 0.121$
Nilsson and Dahlstrom, 2010 [36]	Stimulated saliva	$10.53 \pm 5.05/12.61 \pm 8.17$ nmol/L	13.68 ± 9.96 nmol/L	No $p > 0.05$
Quartana et al., 2010 [38]	Stimulated saliva Collection time: immediately prior to the start of pain testing, immediately following the pain testing procedures, and 20 min after the pain testing procedures	High PCS: BL: 0.8 Post-pain: 0.85 20 min after pain: 0.9 μg/dL	Low PCS: BL: 0.92 Post-pain: 0.75 20 min after pain: 0.7 μg/ml	No $p > 0.05$
Jones et al., 1997 [35]	Unstimulated saliva Collection time: baseline (time, 0 min), peak secretion (time, 30 min), and after 20 min of rest (time, 50 min)	0 min: 6.41, 30 min: 11.96, 50 min: 10.28	0 min: 5.89, 30 min: 7.63, 50 min: 6.39	Yes $p < 0.01$

Temporomandibular disorder (TMD), randomized controlled trial (RCT), pain catastrophising scale (PCS).

Table 4. Risk of bias of randomized controlled trials using Cochrane Risk of Bias Tool II.

Authors/Year	Randomization Process	Deviation from Intended Intervention	Missing Outcome Data	Measurement of the Outcome	Selection of the Reported Results	Overall Bias
Goyal, 2020 [28]	Low	Low	Low	Some concern	Low	Low
Magri, 2017 [29]	Low	Low	Low	Low	Low	Low
Rosar, 2017 [27]	High	High	Low	High	High	High

Table 5. Risk of bias of case–control studies using the Newcastle–Ottawa quality assessment scale.

Author, Year	Selection				Comparability	Exposure			Risk of Bias
	Is the Case Definition Adequate?	Representativeness of the Cases	Selection of Controls	Definition of Controls	Comparability of Cases and Controls Based on the Design or Analysis	Ascertainment of Exposure	Same Method of Ascertainment for Cases and Controls	Non-Response Rate	
Almeida et al., 2014 [16]	1	0	1	1	1	0	1	1	Medium (6)
Bozovic et al., 2018	1	1	1	1	1	1	1	1	Low (8)
Chinthakanan et al., 2018 [34]	1	1	1	1	0	0	1	1	Medium (6)
Jones et al., 1997 [35]	1	1	0	1	1	0	1	1	Medium (6)
Nilsson and Dahlstrom, 2010 [36]	1	1	0	1	1	0	1	0	Medium (5)
Poorian et al., 2016 [37]	1	0	0	0	0	0	1	1	High (3)
Quartana et al., 2010 [38]	1	1	1	1	1	1	1	1	Low (8)

Table 6. Risk of bias of cross-sectional studies using the Newcastle–Ottawa quality assessment scale.

	Representativeness of the Sample	Sample Size	Non-Respondents	Ascertainment of the Exposure (Risk Factor)	The Subjects in Different Outcome Groups are Comparable, Based on the Study Design or Analysis; Confounding Factors are Controlled	Assessment of the Outcome	Statistical Test	Risk of Bias
D'Avilla, 2019 [17]	1	1	1	2	1	1	1	Low (8)
Rosar et al., 2021 [30]	1	1	1	2	1	1	1	Low (8)
Tosato et al., 2015 [31]	1	1	1	1	1	2	1	Low (8)
Venkatesh et al., 2021 [32]	1	1	0	1	0	1	1	Medium (5)

Table 7. GRADE analysis for certainty of evidence.

No. of Studies	Study Design	Certainty assessment					Effect			Certainty	Importance
		Risk of Bias	Inconsistency	Indirectness	Imprecision	Other Considerations	No. of Events	No. of Individuals	Rate (95% CI)		
3	Randomized trials	not serious	serious [a]	serious [b]	very serious [c]	Strong association; all plausible residual confounding would reduce the demonstrated effect	We cannot provide examples extracted from our review since our review was not intentionally limited to a specific prognostic factor. Instead, our goal has been to explore salivary cortisol levels at different times of day that have been investigated to date as potential risks for the persistence of a variety of chronic pain conditions and their associated TMDs. However, this poor representation would happen, for instance, if we were interested in exploring the effects of various levels of salivary cortisol on types of TMD. The studies included were only investigating the prognostic effect of salivary cortisol on TMD at a specific age.			⊕⊕⊕○ Low	IMPORTANT

Table 7. Cont.

No. of Studies	Study Design	Certainty assessment					Effect		Rate (95% CI)	Certainty	Importance
		Risk of Bias	Inconsistency	Indirectness	Imprecision	Other Considerations	No. of Events	No. of Individuals			
4	Observational studies (cross-sectional)	serious [d]	serious [e]	not serious	serious [f]	All plausible residual confounding would suggest spurious effect, while no effect was observed	151	196		⊕⊕⊕○ Low	IMPORTANT
7	Observational studies (case–control)	serious [g]	not serious	serious [h]	serious [i]	Publication bias strongly suspected; strong association; all plausible residual confounding would suggest spurious effect, while no effect was observed	When conducting comprehensive systematic reviews of the effects of cortisol levels on TMD incidence among young adults, authors reported that the evidence of increasing salivary cortisol as a prognostic factor for chronic TMD pain has serious limitations. This evidence comes from four studies, and all of them have a moderate risk of bias.			⊕⊕○○ Low	IMPORTANT

Explanations: [a] Variations in effect estimates across studies, with points of effect on either side of the line of no effect, and confidence intervals showing minimal overlap. [b] No precision in the estimation of the effect size within each primary study. [c] (1) Sample size justification is not provided and there are fewer than 100 cases reaching the endpoint (for continuous outcomes), and (2) no precision in the estimation of the effect size within each primary study. [d] Serious limitations, as most evidence is from studies with a moderate or unclear risk of bias for most bias domains. [e] Unexplained heterogeneity or variability in results across studies, with differences in results not clinically meaningful. [f] There are few studies and a small number of participants across the studies. [g] Serious limitations, as most evidence is from studies with a moderate or unclear risk of bias for most bias domains. [h] The study sample, the prognostic factor, and/or the outcome of the primary study do not accurately reflect the review question. [i] There are few studies and a small number of participants across the studies.

4. Discussion

This systematic review evaluated the relationship between salivary cortisol levels and temporomandibular disorder in young adult patients. The included studies suggest higher salivary cortisol levels in TMD patients than in healthy individuals. Cortisol is a hormone released by the adrenal glands in response to stress. Elevated cortisol levels over an extended period can have negative effects on the musculoskeletal system, including the muscles and joints around the temporomandibular joint (TMJ). Salivary cortisol levels can also serve as a diagnostic marker for evaluating the severity of stress experienced by an individual. Additionally, monitoring cortisol levels over time can provide valuable information about the effectiveness of stress management techniques in reducing TMD symptoms.

Higher cortisol levels were found in TMD patients compared to healthy participants in ten studies included in this systematic review (case–control and cross-sectional) [17,27–34,37]. In contrast, four studies demonstrated no significant association. Two randomized control trials showed reductions in salivary cortisol levels after treatment in patients with TMD compared to those treated with a placebo [28,29]. The possible correlation between TMD and higher salivary cortisol levels could be due to the etiological factors—mainly stress, anxiety, and depression. Recent studies have shown a positive association between stress, anxiety, and depression and the occurrence of TMD [6,39]. These psychological factors were eventually found to be associated with increased salivary cortisol levels.

4.1. Association of Cortisol and TMD

For decades, the measure of acute and chronic pain has been demonstrated by patients' responses to stress meters. Cortisol levels have a vital role in evaluating the level of stress. Cortisol is a glucocorticoid hormone secreted by the adrenal cortex. The activation of gluconeogenesis, the amplification of hepatic protein synthesis, and an increase in the utilization of fat for energy production are among the physiological effects of cortisol [40]. The hypothalamus increases the release of this hormone, known as the stress hormone, when a stressful condition occurs [6]. Stress is believed to not just function as an etiological factor, but also to exacerbate the symptoms of TMD, including pain in the TMJ area [39]. Stress affects the release of cortisol, an anti-inflammatory agent helping to mobilize glucose reserve and modulate inflammation. However, in prolonged or exacerbated stress responses, altered cortisol release leads to inflammation and pain [41]. Stress also activates the HPA axis, resulting in a cascade of responses leading to increased cortisol release from the adrenal cortex. Concerning TMD, patients frequently exhibit hyperactivity of the HPA axis [12]. The hyper-response of the HPA axis has been observed in anxiety disorders and depression. It is also important to note that the mediators for stress response also regulate pain modulation, which is why stress contributes to pain transmission and perception [12].

Various explanations for the association between painful TMD and depression or anxiety are given in the literature. Firstly, these symptoms may trigger muscle hyperactivity, followed by muscle abnormality and pain [42]. They may also induce a joint inflammatory process followed by biomechanical changes, leading to joint pain. Secondly, TMD may be associated with an abnormal trigeminal system process due to imbalances in neurotransmitters like serotonin and catecholamines [40].

4.2. Evidence from Randomized Controlled Trials

Three randomized control trials were included in this systematic review. All included studies have reported a positive association between higher cortisol levels and TMD [27–29]. Goyal et al. demonstrated a positive association between salivary cortisol levels and TMD in conjunction with depression compared to controls. The authors measured salivary cortisol levels in the morning and evening. In their findings, TMD patients with depression had higher cortisol levels than TMD patients without depression and healthy controls [28]. Student's t-test was performed to measure the difference in cortisol levels between males and females, and it was reported that females with TMD and depression had higher cortisol levels than their male counterparts. The study's design was a double-blinded control trial where the patients and investigators were unaware of the groups. Hence, the methodological quality of this study is high, and the results are conclusive.

Rosar and colleagues, in their parallel arm randomized trial, concluded that patients with sleep appliances had self-reported TMD with higher cortisol levels in the morning compared to the control. Researchers have also reported that females with TMD and occlusal appliances had higher cortisol levels than males. The authors of this study were unable to calculate awake bruxism. However, the findings of this study suggest higher cortisol levels in self-reported TMD patients compared to controls [27].

Magri et al., in their double-blinded randomized trial, assessed the effect of laser treatment on TMD patients and evaluated the salivary cortisol levels of affected females. The laser treatment was performed over two sittings across eight weeks, and the placebo patients received a light treatment at similar intervals. The salivary cortisol levels were reduced in females receiving laser treatment for TMD compared to controls. The salivary cortisol levels for controls were measured above 10 ng/mL compared to female receiving laser treatment. Findings of all the included RCTs in this review concluded that females with TMD had higher levels of salivary cortisol in the morning compared to controls [29].

4.3. Evidence from Case–Control Studies

The six case–control studies included in this review showed mixed results of salivary cortisol and TMD levels [33–38]. Four studies measured a positive association [33,34,37], while three studies indicated no significant correlation between the salivary marker and TMD [16,36,38]. Jasim et al. compared females with chronic and acute TMD and suggested no statistical significance in the levels of salivary cortisol among the group, even though perceived stress and depression were marked in both groups [43]. Similar findings were reported in the study by Almeida and colleagues, which compared individuals with and without TMD, with 64% of patients with TMD reporting having depression. Saliva cortisol levels were 0.272 g/dL in the group with TMD and 0.395 g/dL in the group without it, with no statistical significance [16]. In line with these results, studies by Nilsoson and Dahlstrom and Quartana reported no significant difference in salivary cortisol levels in patients with and without TMD. However, both studies showed a higher level of salivary cortisol in female TMD patients than their male counterparts [36,38].

On the other hand, Chinthakanan et al. reported a significant increase in cortisol levels in TMD patients compared to a control group; they concluded that TMD patients demonstrated an autonomic nervous system (ANS) imbalance and elevated stress levels [34]. Similarly, the study by Bozovic et al. on students with and without TMD reported a significantly higher level of salivary cortisol in TMD students with depression and stress [33]. The overall results of all the included studies report that females with TMD, depression, and stress have higher levels of salivary cortisol.

4.4. Evidence from Cross-Sectional Studies

Among the included cross-sectional studies (n = 43) [30] in this review, one half found no association between TMD and salivary cortisol, while the other showed a positive correlation [17,31,32]. The research by Tosato et al. correlated the cortisol concentration in saliva with the bioelectric activity of masticatory muscles [31]. They showed elevated levels of glucocorticosteroids with increased muscle tone and pronounced severity of TMD symptoms. Their work agrees with the hypothesis that increased muscle activity corresponds with hyperactivity of the HPA axis [7].

D'Avilla et al. indicated in their study that the concurrence of malocclusion and TMD has a significant negative influence on masticatory capacity, while salivary cortisol levels are higher in TMD patients regardless of the presence or absence of malocclusion. In contrast, the study by Rosar et al. reported no statistical significance of the level of salivary cortisol between the groups; moreover, the cortisol level was not increased in patients with psychological impairments. In conjunction with the findings of the case–

control studies and RCTs included in this review, the cross-sectional studies also reported higher salivary cortisol in young females with TMD, stress, and depression than their male counterparts [17].

4.5. Evidence from Systematic Reviews

Two systematic reviews on a similar topic were found in the literature. Lu et al. performed a meta-analysis of thirteen studies, including case–control studies, and stated the occurrence of increased cortisol levels in TMD patients. However, these results were inconclusive due to high heterogeneity among the included studies [21]. Their review included studies involving children and adult patients, while this review focused mainly on adults. Studies have suggested that adults aged 18–40 have higher stress levels than children and the elderly. Treatment of TMD and its associated psychological factors should be prioritized in this age group more than children and the elderly. Fritzen and colleagues performed the other systematic review; they checked salivary cortisol concentration in adults and children with bruxism and incorporated six studies into their data [20]. They concluded a positive correlation between bruxism and higher cortisol levels in saliva in patients with higher stress levels. Similar findings are reported in this review, but to strengthen our results, we incorporated all the clinical study designs and restricted the age group from 18–40 years.

To the best of our knowledge, this is the first review that focuses on the relationship between salivary cortisol levels and TMD in young adult patients, along with the patients' salivary cortisol concentrations. In this review, the authors have included every study's design to strengthen the findings. However, there are a few limitations to this systematic review. Firstly, heterogeneity was observed in the included studies; hence, a meta-analysis could not be performed. Secondly, gender dimorphism was not evaluated in the studies, as a few included only female patients [29], while in other studies, the female–male ratio was unequal [16]. Even though Quartana et al. stated in their results that there is a significant correlation between cortisol levels and TMD, the data they provided regarding salivary cortisol levels were unclear [38].

Furthermore, there were disparities in the timing of saliva collection among the studies; seven studies collected salivary samples in the morning [27,29–32,34,37,38,44], while one study collected it both in the morning and evening [28]. One study sampled saliva before and after the stress test [38]. Finally, due to the small sample size of the included studies, a conclusion cannot be drawn. Hence, more longitudinal studies with robust methodological approaches should be designed to support the findings of this review.

5. Conclusions

This systematic review demonstrates a relationship between salivary cortisol levels and TMD. The salivary cortisol levels were higher in TMD adults than healthy controls, which could be linked to probable exposure to stress, depression, and anxiety. Moreover, females suffering from TMD in conjunction with depression and stress had higher salivary cortisol levels. This is suggestive of the need for psychological and clinical treatment in patients with TMD. Considering the high heterogeneity and inconsistency of results in the included studies, higher-quality studies, with bigger sample sizes and follow-ups, are required.

Author Contributions: Conceptualization, L.A., H.A. and R.A.; methodology, L.A. and H.A.; validation, L.A., R.A. and H.A.; formal analysis, L.A.; investigation, L.A.; resources, L.A.; data curation, L.A. and R.A.; writing—original draft preparation, L.A. and R.A.; writing—review and editing, L.A.; visualization, H.A.; supervision, L.A. All authors have read and agreed to the published version of the manuscript.

Funding: This research received no external funding.

Institutional Review Board Statement: An international prospective register of systematic reviews was obtained before conducting the study.

Informed Consent Statement: Not applicable.

Data Availability Statement: The data that support the findings of this study are available on request from the corresponding author.

Conflicts of Interest: The authors declare no conflicts of interest.

References

1. Murphy, M.K.; MacBarb, R.F.; Wong, M.E. Temporomandibular Joint Disorders: A Review of Etiology, Clinical Management, and Tissue Engineering Strategies. *Int. J. Oral Maxillofac. Implants* **2013**, *28*, e393. [CrossRef] [PubMed]
2. Giannakopoulos, N.N.; Keller, L.; Rammelsberg, P.; Kronmüller, K.-T.; Schmitter, M. Anxiety and depression in patients with chronic temporomandibular pain and in controls. *J. Dent.* **2010**, *38*, 369–376. [CrossRef] [PubMed]
3. Tanaka, E.; Detamore, M.S.; Mercuri, L.G. Degenerative disorders of the temporomandibular joint: Etiology, diagnosis, and treatment. *J. Dent. Res.* **2008**, *87*, 296–307. [CrossRef] [PubMed]
4. Liu, F.; Steinkeler, A. Epidemiology, diagnosis, and treatment of temporomandibular disorders. *Dent. Clin. N. Am.* **2013**, *57*, 465–479. [CrossRef] [PubMed]
5. McNeill, C. Management of temporomandibular disorders: Concepts and controversies. *J. Prosthet. Dent.* **1997**, *77*, 510–522. [CrossRef] [PubMed]
6. Valesan, L.F.; Da-Cas, C.D.; Reus, J.C.; Denardin, A.C.S.; Garanhani, R.R.; Bonotto, D.; Januzzi, E.; de Souza, B.D.M. Prevalence of temporomandibular joint disorders: A systematic review and meta-analysis. *Clin. Oral Investig.* **2021**, *25*, 441–453. [CrossRef] [PubMed]
7. Chisnoiu, A.M.; Picos, A.M.; Popa, S.; Chisnoiu, P.D.; Lascu, L.; Picos, A.; Chisnoiu, R. Factors involved in the etiology of temporomandibular disorders—A literature review. *Med. Pharm. Rep.* **2015**, *88*, 473–478. [CrossRef] [PubMed]
8. Atsu, S.S.; Guner, S.; Palulu, N.; Bulut, A.C.; Kurkcuoglu, I. Oral parafunctions, personality traits, anxiety and their association with signs and symptoms of temporomandibular disorders in the adolescents. *Afr. Health Sci.* **2019**, *19*, 1801–1810. [CrossRef] [PubMed]
9. Ohrbach, R.; Michelotti, A. The Role of Stress in the Etiology of Oral Parafunction and Myofascial Pain. *Oral Maxillofac. Surg. Clin.* **2018**, *30*, 369–379. [CrossRef]
10. Smith, S.M.; Vale, W.W. The role of the hypothalamic-pituitary-adrenal axis in neuroendocrine responses to stress. *Dialogues Clin. Neurosci.* **2006**, *8*, 383–395. [CrossRef]
11. De Leeuw, R.; Bertoli, E.; Schmidt, J.E.; Carlson, C.R. Prevalence of traumatic stressors in patients with temporomandibular disorders. *J. Oral Maxillofac. Surg.* **2005**, *63*, 42–50. [CrossRef]
12. Gameiro, G.H.; da Silva Andrade, A.; Nouer, D.F.; Ferraz de Arruda Veiga, M.C. How may stressful experiences contribute to the development of temporomandibular disorders? *Clin. Oral Investig.* **2006**, *10*, 261–268. [CrossRef]
13. Cui, Q.; Liu, D.; Xiang, B.; Sun, Q.; Fan, L.; He, M.; Wang, Y.; Zhu, X.; Ye, H. Morning Serum Cortisol as a Predictor for the HPA Axis Recovery in Cushing's Disease. *Int. J. Endocrinol.* **2021**, *2021*, 4586229. [CrossRef]
14. El-Farhan, N.; Rees, D.A.; Evans, C. Measuring cortisol in serum, urine and saliva—Are our assays good enough? *Ann. Clin. Biochem.* **2017**, *54*, 308–322. [CrossRef]
15. Kirschbaum, C.; Hellhammer, D.H. Salivary cortisol in psychoneuroendocrine research: Recent developments and applications. *Psychoneuroendocrinology* **1994**, *19*, 313–333. [CrossRef]
16. Almeida, C.D.; Paludo, A.; Stechman-Eto, J.; Amenábar, J.M. Saliva cortisol levels and depression in individuals with temporomandibular disorder: Preliminary study. *Rev. Dor* **2014**, *15*, 169–172. [CrossRef]
17. D'Avilla, B.M.; Pimenta, M.C.; Furletti, V.F.; Vedovello Filho, M.; Venezian, G.C.; Custodio, W. Comorbidity of TMD and malocclusion: Impacts on quality of life, masticatory capacity and emotional features. *Braz. J. Oral Sci.* **2019**, *18*, e191679. [CrossRef]
18. Kobayashi, F.Y.; Gavião, M.B.D.; Marquezin, M.C.S.; Fonseca, F.L.A.; Montes, A.B.M.; Barbosa, T.S.; Castelo, P.M. Salivary stress biomarkers and anxiety symptoms in children with and without temporomandibular disorders. *Braz. Oral Res.* **2017**, *31*, e78. [CrossRef]
19. Suprajith, T.; Wali, A.; Jain, A.; Patil, K.; Mahale, P.; Niranjan, V. Effect of Temporomandibular Disorders on Cortisol Concentration in the Body and Treatment with Occlusal Equilibrium. *J. Pharm. Bioallied Sci.* **2022**, *14*, S483–S485. [CrossRef]
20. Fritzen, V.M.; Colonetti, T.; Cruz, M.V.; Ferraz, S.D.; Ceretta, L.; Tuon, L.; Da Rosa, M.I.; Ceretta, R.A. Levels of Salivary Cortisol in Adults and Children with Bruxism Diagnosis: A Systematic Review and Meta-Analysis. *J. Evid.-Based Dent. Pract.* **2022**, *22*, 101634. [CrossRef]
21. Lu, L.; Yang, B.; Li, M.; Bao, B. Salivary cortisol levels and temporomandibular disorders—A systematic review and meta-analysis of 13 case-control studies. *Trop. J. Pharm. Res.* **2022**, *21*, 1341–1349. [CrossRef]
22. Liberati, A.; Altman, D.G.; Tetzlaff, J.; Mulrow, C.; Gotzsche, P.C.; Ioannidis, J.P.; Clarke, M.; Devereaux, P.J.; Kleijnen, J.; Moher, D. The PRISMA statement for reporting systematic reviews and meta-analyses of studies that evaluate health care interventions: Explanation and elaboration. *PLoS Med.* **2009**, *6*, e1000100. [CrossRef]
23. Huguet, A.; Hayden, J.A.; Stinson, J.; McGrath, P.J.; Chambers, C.T.; Tougas, M.E.; Wozney, L. Judging the quality of evidence in reviews of prognostic factor research: Adapting the GRADE framework. *Syst. Rev.* **2013**, *2*, 71. [CrossRef]

24. Sterne, J.A.C.; Savovic, J.; Page, M.J.; Elbers, R.G.; Blencowe, N.S.; Boutron, I.; Cates, C.J.; Cheng, H.Y.; Corbett, M.S.; Eldridge, S.M.; et al. RoB 2: A revised tool for assessing risk of bias in randomised trials. *BMJ* **2019**, *366*, l4898. [CrossRef]
25. Stang, A. Critical evaluation of the Newcastle-Ottawa scale for the assessment of the quality of nonrandomized studies in meta-analyses. *Eur. J. Epidemiol.* **2010**, *25*, 603–605. [CrossRef]
26. Dubey, V.P.; Kievisiene, J.; Rauckiene-Michealsson, A.; Norkiene, S.; Razbadauskas, A.; Agostinis-Sobrinho, C. Bullying and Health Related Quality of Life among Adolescents-A Systematic Review. *Children* **2022**, *9*, 766. [CrossRef]
27. Rosar, J.V.; Barbosa, T.S.; Dias, I.O.V.; Kobayashi, F.Y.; Costa, Y.M.; Gaviao, M.B.D.; Bonjardim, L.R.; Castelo, P.M. Effect of interocclusal appliance on bite force, sleep quality, salivary cortisol levels and signs and symptoms of temporomandibular dysfunction in adults with sleep bruxism. *Arch. Oral Biol.* **2017**, *82*, 62–70. [CrossRef]
28. Goyal, G.; Gupta, D.; Pallagatti, S. Salivary Cortisol Could Be a Promising Tool in the Diagnosis of Temporomandibular Disorders Associated with Psychological Factors. *J. Indian Acad. Oral Med. Radiol.* **2021**, *32*, 354–359. [CrossRef]
29. Magri, L.V.; Carvalho, V.A.; Rodrigues, F.C.C.; Bataglion, C.; Leite-Panissi, C.R.A. Non-specific effects and clusters of women with painful TMD responders and non-responders to LLLT: Double-blind randomized clinical trial. *Lasers Med. Sci.* **2018**, *33*, 385–392. [CrossRef]
30. Rosar, J.V.; Marquezin, M.C.S.; Pizzolato, A.S.; Kobayashi, F.Y.; Bussadori, S.K.; Pereira, L.J.; Castelo, P.M. Identifying predictive factors for sleep bruxism severity using clinical and polysomnographic parameters: A principal component analysis. *J. Clin. Sleep Med.* **2021**, *17*, 949–956. [CrossRef]
31. de Paiva Tosato, J.; Caria, P.H.; de Paula Gomes, C.A.; Berzin, F.; Politti, F.; de Oliveira Gonzalez, T.; Biasotto-Gonzalez, D.A. Correlation of stress and muscle activity of patients with different degrees of temporomandibular disorder. *J. Phys. Ther. Sci.* **2015**, *27*, 1227–1231. [CrossRef]
32. Venkatesh, S.B.; Shetty, S.S.; Kamath, V. Prevalence of temporomandibular disorders and its correlation with stress and salivary cortisol levels among students. *Pesqui. Bras. Odontopediatria Clín. Integr.* **2021**, *21*, e0120. [CrossRef]
33. Božović, Đ.; Ivković, N.; Račić, M.; Ristić, S. Salivary cortisol responses to acute stress in students with myofascial pain. *Srpski Arhiv za Celokupno Lekarstvo* **2018**, *146*, 20–25. [CrossRef]
34. Chinthakanan, S.; Laosuwan, K.; Boonyawong, P.; Kumfu, S.; Chattipakorn, N.; Chattipakorn, S.C. Reduced heart rate variability and increased saliva cortisol in patients with TMD. *Arch. Oral Biol.* **2018**, *90*, 125–129. [CrossRef]
35. Jones, D.A.; Rollman, G.B.; Brooke, R.I. The cortisol response to psychological stress in temporomandibular dysfunction. *Pain* **1997**, *72*, 171–182. [CrossRef]
36. Nilsson, A.M.; Dahlstrom, L. Perceived symptoms of psychological distress and salivary cortisol levels in young women with muscular or disk-related temporomandibular disorders. *Acta Odontol. Scand.* **2010**, *68*, 284–288. [CrossRef]
37. Poorian, B.; Dehghani, N.; Bemanali, M. Comparison of Salivary Cortisol Level in Temporomandibular Disorders and Healthy People. *Int. J. Rev. Life Sci.* **2015**, *5*, 1105–1113.
38. Quartana, P.J.; Buenaver, L.F.; Edwards, R.R.; Klick, B.; Haythornthwaite, J.A.; Smith, M.T. Pain catastrophizing and salivary cortisol responses to laboratory pain testing in temporomandibular disorder and healthy participants. *J. Pain* **2010**, *11*, 186–194. [CrossRef]
39. Anna, S.; Joanna, K.; Teresa, S.; Maria, G.; Aneta, W. The influence of emotional state on the masticatory muscles function in the group of young healthy adults. *Biomed. Res. Int.* **2015**, *2015*, 174013. [CrossRef]
40. Apkarian, A.V.; Baliki, M.N.; Geha, P.Y. Towards a theory of chronic pain. *Prog. Neurobiol.* **2009**, *87*, 81–97. [CrossRef]
41. Hannibal, K.E.; Bishop, M.D. Chronic stress, cortisol dysfunction, and pain: A psychoneuroendocrine rationale for stress management in pain rehabilitation. *Phys. Ther.* **2014**, *94*, 1816–1825. [CrossRef] [PubMed]
42. Scrivani, S.J.; Keith, D.A.; Kaban, L.B. Temporomandibular disorders. *N. Engl. J. Med.* **2008**, *359*, 2693–2705. [CrossRef] [PubMed]
43. Jasim, H.; Louca, S.; Christidis, N.; Ernberg, M. Salivary cortisol and psychological factors in women with chronic and acute oro-facial pain. *J. Oral Rehabil.* **2014**, *41*, 122–132. [CrossRef]
44. Nadendla, L.K.; Meduri, V.; Paramkusam, G.; Pachava, K.R. Evaluation of salivary cortisol and anxiety levels in myofascial pain dysfunction syndrome. *Korean J. Pain* **2014**, *27*, 30–34. [CrossRef]

Disclaimer/Publisher's Note: The statements, opinions and data contained in all publications are solely those of the individual author(s) and contributor(s) and not of MDPI and/or the editor(s). MDPI and/or the editor(s) disclaim responsibility for any injury to people or property resulting from any ideas, methods, instructions or products referred to in the content.

MDPI AG
Grosspeteranlage 5
4052 Basel
Switzerland
Tel.: +41 61 683 77 34

Diagnostics Editorial Office
E-mail: diagnostics@mdpi.com
www.mdpi.com/journal/diagnostics

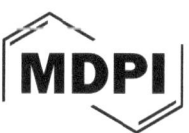

Disclaimer/Publisher's Note: The title and front matter of this reprint are at the discretion of the Guest Editor. The publisher is not responsible for their content or any associated concerns. The statements, opinions and data contained in all individual articles are solely those of the individual Editor and contributors and not of MDPI. MDPI disclaims responsibility for any injury to people or property resulting from any ideas, methods, instructions or products referred to in the content.

www.ingramcontent.com/pod-product-compliance
Lightning Source LLC
LaVergne TN
LVHW072321090526
838202LV00019B/2326